How to get through

NVQ2

for

Veterinary

Nurses

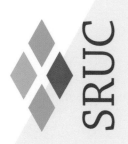
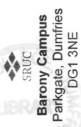

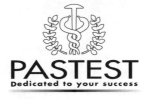

PASTEST
Dedicated to your success

About the authors

Alison Lomas qualified from the Royal Veterinary College in London. She is currently working in small animal practice at Hird & Partners in West Yorkshire.

Annaliese H. Magee qualified from Edinburgh's Telford College in 1997. She has worked in small animal and mixed practices. She gained the assessor examination in 2000 and the surgical diploma in 2003. She is now Head Nurse at Hird & Partners, Halifax, West Yorkshire.

Susan L. Roberts is a Glasgow graduate and was a clinician in small animal and mixed practice for 30 years. She now runs a peripatetic cardiology referral service in the north of England. Susan is also editor of *Veterinary Practice Nurse*.

Annaliese Magee would like to thank Jodie Foster VN of Hird & Partners, Halifax, for her help and advice on behaviour and training.

Level 2

How to get through

NVQ2

for

Veterinary

Nurses

Alison Lomas
B. Vet. Med. MRCVS

Annaliese H. Magee
VN, AVN Dip. (Surgical)

Edited by
Susan L. Roberts
BVMS, Cert VC, MRCVS

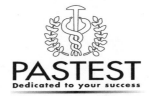

PASTEST
Dedicated to your success

First published 2003
Reprinted 2004

ISBN: 1 901198 78 2

A catalogue record for this book is available from the British Library.

PasTest Revision Books and Intensive Courses

PasTest has been established in the field of postgraduate medical education since
1972, providing revision books and intensive study courses for doctors preparing
for their professional examinations. Books and courses are available for the
following specialties:

**MRCGP, MRCP Part 1 and 2, MRCPCH Part 1 and 2, MRCPsych, MRCS,
MRCOG, DRCOG, DCH, FRCA, PLAB.**

For further details contact:

PasTest, Freepost, Knutsford, Cheshire WA16 7BR
Tel: 01565 752000 Fax: 01565 650264
www.pastest.co.uk   enquiries@pastest.co.uk

Cover design by Andrew Shoolbred
Text prepared by Vision Typesetting, Manchester
Printed and bound in Great Britain by MPG Books Ltd, Bodmin, Cornwall

Level 2

Contents

Unit 4: Principles of animal management and nursing   231

Foreword

One is naturally suspicious of books that promise in the title that they will 'get you through' a subject. The temptation then is to look at these books more critically, trying to find ways in which they fall short of this lavish claim. All I can say of this book is it really delivers all it promises to.

In my view, it is one of the clearest textbooks available for NVQ level 2 nurses. The bullet points outlining the core objectives of each section make it easy to follow the syllabus. The portfolio tips give very good guidance to assessor and student alike on how to best complete the case logs. In addition, the calculation exercises and the multiple-choice self-assessments at the end of each chapter allow the student to gauge their progression through the course.

It is difficult to define this type of book: although it lacks some details found in the larger textbooks, it is in many ways more complete. The facts are laid out in a logical, easy to read manner and in a way that follows the occupational standards for NVQ2 veterinary nursing almost verbatim.

As a profession, we are fortunate to have a role in training and developing the nursing component of our clinical staff. There is no doubt that the veterinary nurses of today are every bit as enthusiastic and hard working as those of days gone by: the increased demands put on today's nurses by the veterinary profession and by the public has meant that the core syllabus has spread and enlarged. Nurse training has become complex as a result of this; with college study, portfolio production and 'in-house' education being required to fulfil the criteria laid down in the occupational standards and also to produce nurses who can work well as part of a team and also on their own, say in dental or diet clinics.

If we are to continue to expand the responsibilities of veterinary nurses and to demand more from them clinically, then it is only right that we make sure that their training is as complete and wide-ranging as possible.

As an assessor and lecturer to veterinary nurses, I have already found this book invaluable for preparing module assessments and lecture notes. I am sure other assessors will find it equally useful.

Student veterinary nurses will find the format friendly and the content informative; qualified nurses will find it a very handy reference book.

In short, I can foresee this book becoming one of the standards to be found in every veterinary clinic, whether a training practice or not.

Julian Hoad
NVQ assessor

Level 2
Introduction

This book is written for veterinary nurses who are revising for their NVQ2 exam. Written by experts who have had to sit the NVQ exam themselves, it is the only book that reflects the structure of the syllabus so that you can follow each element by element. *How to get through NVQ2* is designed to be used for constant reference. You can either read the book from cover to cover or dip into the areas which you find particularly difficult.

How to get through NVQ2 explains the exam and gives you top tips on how to prepare for it. It also has useful *How much have you learnt?* sections, which test you after revising a section. If you haven't got all the questions right, this indicates that you need to go over certain elements again. The answers can be found within the chapter.

There are also multiple choice questions at the end of each unit and the answers are thorough so that you understand why A, B, C, D or E is the correct answer to question 1, etc.

Each element is broken down into *What you need to learn* sections to help you pass your exam. You can then tick off what you have learnt so far and plan the rest of your revision.

There are useful bullet points for you to remember rather than long-winded paragraphs and the text is also broken up by invaluable diagrams and photographs to help you visualise the points being made.

At the back of the book is a chapter to help you prepare for your portfolio at NVQ2 level and there is also a chapter on calculations, as calculators are not allowed to be taken into the exam.

There is also a comprehensive index to help you find more specific areas.

How to prepare for your NVQ2

The National Vocational Qualification (NVQ) 2 exam is held every July and December. The awarding body is the Royal College of Surgeons.

The NVQ (and SVQ, the Scottish equivalent) are vocational qualifications that are based on agreed national standards of competence. Veterinary nurses train in a veterinary practice so that their skills can be assessed both at work and in an exam.

The NVQ2 exam consists of two written multiple choice question papers of 90 minutes each. Veterinary nurses are also expected to start a portfolio (modules 1–5) at NVQ2. This is a collection of evidence to demonstate your practical competence and the standard you have reached in your training. It is completed at NVQ3 level. See page 369 for guidance on how to complete your portfolio.

Multiple choice questions (MCQs)

MCQs are the most consistent, reproducible and internally reliable method we have of testing how much a person can remember. They also test reasoning ability and an understanding of basic facts, principles and concepts that can be assessed.

The best way of passing your exam is to know the answers to all of the questions, but you need to be able to transfer this knowledge accurately onto the answer sheet. All too often, people suffer because they haven't given themselves enough time, they haven't read the instructions carefully or they have failed to read and understand the questions.

First of all, make sure you have time to answer all the questions. If you're stuck on one MCQ leave it and go on to the next one, making a note that you need to return to that question later. The exam lasts for 90 minutes. Try and save some time to go over your answers and complete any that you may have missed.

You must read the question carefully. You should be clear that you know what you are being asked to do. Once you are sure, mark your answer boldly, correctly and clearly.

The best way to get a good mark is to have as wide a knowledge as possible of the topics being tested in the exam, rather than focusing on particular areas, hoping they will come up. Use this book to help test yourself and your colleagues. Go back over the areas which seem weak. Use the index to help you.

Last but not least, get a good night's sleep before the exam – you'll be more mentally alert to get through your NVQ2.

How NVQ assessors should use this book

As the Introduction explains, this book is designed primarily for veterinary nurses who are revising for their NVQ2 exam. However, it serves equally well as a teaching guide for the assessors.

As the book follows the occupational standards in a very logical and sensible way, the assessor can easily use it as a framework for planned tutorials: sections may be 'ticked off' once completed to ensure that the full syllabus has been covered.

The multiple choice questions at the end of each unit may be used either as self-assessment for the individual student or as ready-made planned assessments for the assessor to gauge the student's progress. This may be done either in a formal way, under simulated exam conditions, or, again, as part of a tutorial.

The bullet points at the beginning of each section ('What you need to learn . . . ') may be used to provide a framework for assessment: by asking the student to expand on each bullet point the assessor can examine both the underpinning knowledge and the range of knowledge of that student – the bullet points themselves can therefore be used as planned assessments, or to check against performance criteria. Any misunderstanding or confusion relating to those subjects may then be very readily addressed by reference to the more detailed text.

This book is especially useful as a companion to the assessment of portfolios. The occupational standards and syllabus for NVQ2 must be adhered to for portfolio assessment: this book presents the syllabus requirements in a concise manner. The case logs can be assessed by reference to this book more easily than with a standard nursing text as the range and underpinning knowledge required for each case is presented within each section.

The 'Portfolio tips' section of this book, covering occupational standards, RCVS annexes and case log formats, should be read together with the student. This section is probably the most practically useful section of the book for assessors as it not only gives the student clear advice on completing the portfolio, but it also points out the assessor's responsibilities in a way that is easy to read and to refer to.

Finally, the NVQ assessor should use this book to revise from: after all, it is impossible to perform an adequate assessment unless the information is fresh in the mind of the assessor!

Julian Hoad
NVQ assessor

Level 2: Unit 1
Health and safety

2.1.01   Principles of health and safety

What you need to learn

* You need to be able to explain the implications of the Health and Safety at Work etc Act 1974 in veterinary practice. This includes:
    * the Health and Safety Executive, safety officers, employers' and employees' duties.
* Describe the provisions of the Control of Substances Hazardous to Health Regulations (COSHH) 1999:
    * clinical waste
    * clinical reagents
    * medicines
    * laboratory chemicals
    * film-processing solutions
    * cleaning materials
    * anaesthetic agents.
* Describe common hazards that may exist in a veterinary practice. These include:
    * facilities
    * fixtures
    * furniture
    * floor coverings
    * access
    * electrical items
    * equipment
    * hygiene
    * hazardous substances.
* Describe the principles of maintaining equipment and facilities:
    * safety monitoring checks
    * maintenance contracts.
* Describe how clinical examination rooms should be prepared and maintained.

Implications of the Health and Safety at Work etc Act 1974

The objective of the Act is to provide a safe working environment where no one, including the general public, is risking their health and safety. The Health and Safety Executive (HSE) is responsible for enforcing and advising on the Act. Safety officers are people who are appointed within the practice or who are responsible for specific duties, eg safety officer, fire officer.

The **employer's duties** are to provide:

• safety rules and induction training for new staff
• appropriate supervision for experienced staff
• a safe working environment including providing safe equipment and protective clothing
• a written health and safety report if there are more than four employees.

The **employee's duties** are:

• to take responsibility and care for the health and safety of themselves and others
• to co-operate with the employer so any necessary duties under the act are complied with
• not to interfere, recklessly or intentionally with anything in the interests of health and safety.

Implications of the Control of Substances Hazardous to Health Regulations (COSHH) 1999

This Act aims to provide a more comprehensive cover of certain areas of the Health and Safety Act. It also requires all practices to make an assessment of all the potential hazards that are in the workplace.

• Clinical waste is defined as animal tissue, body fluids, excretions, drugs, any product that may be hazardous to health. See 2.1.03 for disposal of waste.
• Clinical reagents and medicines are disposed of as clinical waste. Any bottles or vials contaminated with pharmaceutical products are disposed of in 'special waste' (special separate yellow plastic bins). Controlled drugs are the exception.
• Laboratory chemicals are disposed of in clinical waste or as special waste.
• Film-processing chemicals should be placed in original containers and are then collected by an authorised person.
• Cleaning materials should be disposed of in clinical waste.
• Use active or passive scavenging anaesthetic agents. Good ventilation should also be available.

Common hazards

- Facilities, eg staff room facilities, should be provided away from the working areas. The sink should provide drinking water.
- All fixtures should be kept in a good state of repair, especially gas and electric fixtures.
- Furniture should be in a good state of repair to avoid injury.
- Floor coverings should be complete, with no loose or unfinished areas.
- Sufficient access should be provided to all areas such as the X-ray room and warning lights and signs should be clear.
- Electrical items are governed by the Electricity at Work Regulations 1989. The use of circuit breakers, trip switches and residual current devices (RCD) are recommended.
- Equipment, eg X-ray machines, anaesthetic machines, needs to be serviced regularly. Keep all service records.
- Hygiene – be aware if protective clothing is needed, eg gloves and apron.
- Hazardous substances are all clearly labeled as either:

Figure 1.1   Hazard warning labels.

Further classification of hazardous substances

The maximum exposure limit (MEL) of hazardous substances is assessed in relation to a specific reference period approved by the Health and Safety Commission.

The occupational exposure standard (OES) is used on inhalational agents. Control is regarded as adequate even if the level is exceeded, as long as the employer identifies the reasons for this and takes appropriate action to remedy the problem.

Maintaining equipment and facilities

All employers are legally liable for the safety of electrical appliances, under the Electricity at Work Regulations 1989. Portable appliance testing (PAT) should be carried out on any electrical equipment and will be labelled to prove it has been tested.

All equipment should be serviced regularly according to manufacturers' instructions. Keep all service records and contracts.

Preparing and maintaining clinical examination rooms

- Be aware of children near sharps and drugs. If possible store drugs outside the room or keep out of children's reach. Dispose of sharps immediately and keep the sharps bin out of children's reach.
- The floors and skirting boards should be swept and mopped with disinfectant before and after each consulting session.
- Dispose of clinical waste appropriately.
- The table and table legs should be wiped with disinfectant after each patient.
- Provide disposable towels/tissues for drying hands and equipment.

2.1.02   Manual handling

What you need to learn

- You need to be able to describe the implications of the Manual Handling Regulations Act 1992 for the veterinary practice. This covers:
  - furnishings
  - equipment
  - stores
  - animals
  - work clothing.
- Explain the principles of safe moving and handling practice:
  - animals
  - equipment
  - materials.

Implications of the Manual Handling Regulations 1992

- Avoid hazardous manual handling operations as far as reasonably practicable.
- Assess carefully any hazardous manual handling operations that cannot be avoided.
- Reduce the risk of injury as far as reasonably practicable.

The following are included under these regulations:

- furnishings
- equipment
- stores

• animals
• work clothing.

Safe moving and handling

There is no specific maximum weight of an individual animal that one person is allowed to carry. Animals lack rigidity, so be aware of this to avoid damaging the animal. Also be prepared for animals making sudden, unpredictable movements.

There is no specific maximum weight of a piece of equipment that one person is allowed to move. Assessment is based on the:

• load
• task
• working environment
• individual's capability.

2.1.03   Disposal of waste

What you need to learn

❧ You need to be able to describe the principles of safe handling and disposal of waste in a veterinary practice. This includes:
  ❧ commercial waste
  ❧ clinical waste
  ❧ pathological waste
  ❧ sharps
  ❧ office waste.

The Environmental Protection Act 1992

The Environmental Protection Act 1992 covers all domestic and industrial (including clinical) waste.

• Commercial waste is non-hazardous waste from commercial businesses. It is collected by council refuse collectors.
• Clinical waste is further governed by the Collection and Disposal Waste Regulations 1992 and the Control of Pollution Act 1974. It is defined as animal tissue, body fluids, excretions, drugs, or any product that may be hazardous to health. It is placed in yellow clinical waste bags and collected by reputable companies who then incinerate the waste.
• Pathological waste consists of any pathological specimens, eg

blood, lumps, culture plates. It should all be sterilised before placing in clinical waste.
- Sharps are scalpel blades, needles and sharp surgical instruments. Discard them immediately after use in yellow plastic tubs labelled 'sharps'.
- Office waste, eg paper, is collected by council/local authority refuse collectors or it can be recycled where appropriate.

Safe disposal of cadavers (dead bodies)

By the practice

These are wholly animal tissue and should be disposed of as clinical waste. The practice must dispose of the animal if it had a hazardous condition while alive. This involves placing the animal in a freezer. The body is collected by authorised cremation companies who cremate it.

By the owner

Unless the animal presented a hazard to health while alive it is classed as commercial waste and therefore can be buried at home.

If health and safety procedures are not followed:

- safety is decreased and injury is more likely
- health problems are increased, eg effects from radiation
- risk to the environment is increased, eg water could become contaminated.

2.1.04   Incidents in the workplace

What you need to learn

- You need to be able to describe the implications for veterinary practices of the Reporting of Injuries, Diseases and Dangerous Occurrences Regulations (RIDDOR) 1995. This includes:
  - responsibility
  - recording
  - accidents
  - incidents
  - notifiable diseases.
- Outline the actions to be taken when an accident occurs in the workplace. This includes:
  - first aid
  - accident book
  - reporting
  - emergency services.

❧ Explain the principles of dealing with an untoward emergency incident within the practice premises. This covers:
  ❧ fire
  ❧ flood
  ❧ water leakage
  ❧ gas leakage
  ❧ electrical fault.

Implications of the Reporting of Injuries, Diseases and Dangerous Occurrences Regulations (RIDDOR) 1995

Certain events must be reported directly to the HSE:

• Major/fatal accidents – report by telephone and by written confirmation within seven days.
• 'Over-three-day' accidents – the HSE will request a written report.
• Dangerous occurrences and near misses – report to the HSE.

The practice is obliged to record all accidents and report them directly to the HSE if appropriate. The HSE may request a written report.

Each accident or incident needs to be recorded (in full) in an accident book approved by the HSE.

For notifiable diseases, eg rabies, isolate the patient immediately and contact the Department for the Environment, Food and Rural Affairs (DEFRA).

Actions to take when an accident or incident occurs

• Initiate appropriate first aid treatment.
• Call 999 if appropriate.
• Record the accident/incident in the accident book.
• Report to the HSE if the accident/incident falls under RIDDOR.

How to record an accident or incident in the accident book

• Enter the name, address and occupation of the person who had the accident.
• The person recording the accident must sign and date the entry and include their address and occupation if they are not the person who had the accident.
• Enter where and when the accident occurred.
• Record details of the cause and any injuries.
• State if the injury needs to be reported under RIDDOR.

Dealing with unexpected emergencies

Fire

- Raise the alarm, follow the veterinary practice fire procedure.
- Call 999.
- An appropriate fire officer should ensure the building is evacuated and not re-entered.
- Fire-fighting equipment can be used but only if safe to do so.
- Ensure all staff know where fire-fighting equipment and fire doors are. Hold regular fire drills.

Flood

- Call the appropriate services.
- Ensure safety of all staff and animals.
- Raise animals above floor level or evacuate them.

Water leakage

- Turn the water off at the mains.
- Call the appropriate services.

Gas leakage

- Do not flick any switches, lighters or matches.
- Turn the gas off at the mains.
- Call Transco.

Electrical fault

- Turn off the electricity at the mains.
- Call an electrician.

2.1.05   Security

What you need to learn

- You need to describe the principles of ensuring the security of the practice premises and property. This includes:
  - intruder prevention
  - alarms
  - secure internal storage
  - secure loading/unloading
  - money
  - medicines

* electronic and paper records.
* Describe how personal security may be maintained at work. This includes:
  * personal conduct
  * personal alarms
  * panic buttons
  * personal belongings.

Ensuring the security of the practice premises and property

Check the following:

• intruder prevention, eg window locks
• alarms
• secure internal storage, eg safe
• secure loading and unloading, eg for deliveries
• money – keep in a locked till, store in a safe overnight
• medicines – all controlled drugs must be kept in a locked, unbreakable cabinet
• electronic and manual records – for electronic records a password should be given to the user, keep manual records in a locked filing cabinet.

Maintaining personal security

• Maintain personal conduct – be professional at all times.
• Carry a personal alarm.
• Install and know where any panic buttons are, eg under the reception desk, or at the side of an entrance.
• Keep personal belongings in a locked cupboard or out of sight.

2.01.06 First aid in the workplace

What you need to learn

* You need to be able to explain the priorities of first-aid treatment:
  * safety
  * airway
  * circulation
  * burns
  * fractures.
* Describe the principles of cardio-pulmonary resuscitation:
  * airway management
  * cardiac compression.
* Outline the principles of basic first-aid management of major injuries:
  * shock

* burns
* fractures
* head injuries
* major wounds.
* Describe the first-aid management of minor injuries and illness:
  * minor wounds
  * bites
  * stings
  * sprains and strains
  * syncope (fainting).

Priorities of first-aid treatment

- Maintain your own safety.
- Establish an airway.
- Check circulation.
- Protect and begin first-aid treatment for burns and fractures.

Cardio-pulmonary resuscitation (CPR)

- Ring 999. Keep the head and neck in a straight position to maintain the airway.
- Place the casualty on their back.
- Begin cardiac compression – 5 compressions to 1 breath if there are two people present or 15 compressions to 2 breaths if there is only one person present.

Consult the practice's designated first aider for training on human CPR.

First-aid management of major injuries

Shock

- Lay the casualty down on a blanket.
- Raise and support the casualty's legs.
- Treat any bleeding.
- Loosen tight clothing.
- Dial 999.
- Monitor pulse and breathing.

Burns

- Wear gloves.
- Pour cold water on the burn for 10 minutes.
- Remove any constrictions, eg watches.
- Cover the burn with sterile/clean material.
- Take or send the casualty to hospital. If severe, ring 999.

If it is an electrical burn ensure the current is switched off first.

Fractures

Open

- Wear gloves.
- Cover the wound with a clean/sterile dressing.
- Apply pressure to control bleeding – do not press on the bone end.
- If the bone is protruding, build up pads of soft non-fluffy material around the bone until it can be bandaged.
- Secure the dressing and immobilise the injured part.
- Call 999.

Closed

- Steady and support the limb above and below injured part.
- For firmer support secure the injured limb to a sound part of the body.
- Raise the limb.
- Dial 999.
- Check circulation beyond bandages.

Head injuries

- Wear gloves.
- Do not remove any protective head wear such as a crash helmet.
- Control bleeding.
- Secure a dressing over the wound.
- Lay the casualty down.
- Take or send the casualty to hospital.

If the casualty loses consciousness place them in the recovery position.

Major wounds

- Wear gloves.
- Cover with a clean/sterile dressing.
- Do not attempt to remove any foreign bodies or embedded implements.
- Take to hospital or dial 999.

First-aid management of minor injuries and illness

Minor wounds

- Wear gloves.
- Clean with antiseptic.
- Cover with a clean/sterile dressing.

Bites

- Control any bleeding.
- Wash thoroughly with dilute antiseptic.
- Cover superficial bites.
- See a doctor as antibiotics may be needed.

Stings

- If the sting is still present, pull it out with tweezers.
- Apply a cold compress.
- Advise the casualty to see a doctor if pain and swelling persist.
- Dial 999 if the casualty shows signs of anaphylactic shock.

Sprains and strains

- Rest and support the injured part.
- Apply a cold compress to the area, eg ice pack surrounded by a layer of padding.
- Raise and support the limb.
- Take or send the casualty to hospital, or see a doctor if the injury is minor.

Syncope (fainting)

- Lay the casualty down, raise and support their legs.
- Ensure there is plenty of fresh air – open a window.
- Reassure the casualty when they recover.
- Look for and treat any injuries.
- If they do not regain consciousness, open their airway, check breathing, be ready to resuscitate and dial 999.

2.1.07   Cross infection and infestation

What you need to learn

- You need to outline the hazards in the workplace associated with infection and infestation. This includes:
  - routes of transmission
  - relative risk
  - zoonoses.
- Describe measures to prevent infection and/or infestation:
  - hand washing
  - personal hygiene
  - protective clothing.

Cross infection is the risk of disease spreading from one animal to another.

Routes of transmission

- Direct contact
- Indirect contact
- By fomites on inanimate objects
- By vectors – animate carriers
- By aerosols.

See 2.4.04 for prevention of the spread of infection.

Weigh up each situation to determine the relative risk.

Zoonosis is a disease that can be transmitted from animals to humans. Be aware of zoonotic diseases and the protocols for dealing with them, eg salmonella, sarcoptic mange, leptospirosis, rabies.

Measures to prevent infection/infestation

- Wash hands after any contact with an infected animal.
- Maintain personal hygiene, eg bathe daily and wear clean clothes.
- Wear disposable aprons and gloves when dealing with patients, cleaning urine, faeces or vomit.
- Dry hands on disposable tissue as opposed to hand towels.

2.1.08   Protective clothing

What you need to learn

- You need to be able to describe the situations in which protective clothing should be worn when dealing with animals and/or equipment. These include:
  - radiography
  - laboratory
  - operating theatre
  - gross exposure to biological contamination
  - exposure to infection/infestation
  - kennel cleaning/disinfection.
- Explain the principles of using protective clothing
  - aprons
  - gloves
  - masks
  - goggles
  - lead aprons
  - lead mittens.

When you should wear protective clothing

Wear protective clothing in the following instances:

• radiography – lead aprons/lead gloves/thyroid protectors
• laboratory – white coat
• operating theatre – surgical gowns or scrub suits
• gross exposure to biological contamination – all-in-one body suits
• exposure to infection/infestation – disposable aprons, gloves, masks
• kennel cleaning/disinfection – disposable aprons, gloves.

Protective clothing is worn to protect:

• from cross infection
• skin, eg from chemical burns
• clothes
• from ionising radiation (X-rays)
• eyes from flying objects, eg extracted teeth, drill burs.

The following are all used as protective clothing:

• aprons
• gloves
• masks
• goggles
• lead aprons
• lead mittens
• thyroid protectors (throat protectors).

Multiple choice questions

1. For disposal purposes, which of the following is not classed as clinical waste?
   ☐ A   Cleaning materials, including halogens
   ☐ B   Controlled drugs
   ☐ C   Clinical reagents
   ☐ D   Blood contaminated swabs

2. If a client slipped and fell in your practice waiting room, what would be your first action?
   ☐ A   Record the incident in the accident book
   ☐ B   Put out the yellow *wet floor* signs
   ☐ C   Report to the HSE under RIDDOR regulations
   ☐ D   Initiate appropriate first-aid treatment

3. Which of the following is the legislation which states that the employer must provide a safe working environment?

    ☐ A Control of Substances Hazardous to Health Regulations 1999
    ☐ B Electricity at Work Regulations 1989
    ☐ C Health and Safety at Work etc Act 1974
    ☐ D Manual Handling Regulations 1992

4. Which of the following incidents need not be reported directly to the HSE?
    ☐ A An 'over-three-day' accident to an employee
    ☐ B A severe dog-bite injury to the face of a nurse
    ☐ C A dog showing clinical signs of rabies
    ☐ D A suspected leak in the X-ray tube head

5. A thyroid protector (shield) may sometimes be worn in veterinary practice to protect the nurse against:
    ☐ A spread of a zoonotic agent
    ☐ B ionizing radiation
    ☐ C aerosols
    ☐ D chemical burns and disinfectant splashes

6. Inanimate objects capable of transmitting disease are known as:
    ☐ A vectors
    ☐ B fomites
    ☐ C aerosols
    ☐ D direct carriers

7. A work colleague is burnt by the electric cable of an autoclave in the practice. Your first action should be to:
    ☐ A contact the practice manager or head nurse
    ☐ B cover the burn with a sterile dressing
    ☐ C switch off the machine at the mains
    ☐ D wear gloves and pour cold water over the burn for 10 minutes

8. In human first-aid situations the priority should be to:
    ☐ A wear gloves
    ☐ B call for the designated first aider
    ☐ C maintain your own safety
    ☐ D establish an airway

9. A client faints during a consultation for their cat. You should:
    ☐ A lay the casualty down
    ☐ B press the panic alarm
    ☐ C open a window
    ☐ D telephone 999

10. In relation to the Manual Handling Regulations 1992, which of the following is the most accurate?
    ☐ A The regulations include equipment and work clothing

☐ B   There is a specific weight limit for each employee
☐ C   Assessments do not need to include an individual's strength
☐ D   Conscious animals should always be handled by two persons

Communication, record keeping and practice organisation

2.2.01   Communication

What you need to learn

❧ You need to be able to explain the ways in which interpersonal communication takes place:
  ❧ verbal
  ❧ written
  ❧ non-verbal.
❧ Describe ways in which clients may obtain information about veterinary care and services. These include:
  ❧ general media (press, television, Internet)
  ❧ practice-generated information (written, verbal)
  ❧ commercial information
  ❧ other personal contacts (friends, family, other clients).
❧ Describe factors that may influence perception:
  ❧ age
  ❧ culture
  ❧ education
  ❧ sensory loss (hearing, sight)
  ❧ socio-economic background.

Communication methods

Communication between nurses and other colleagues is paramount. This can be achieved by:

- Verbal communication:
    in person
    over the phone.
- Written communication:
    letters (personal or general information)
    memoranda
    electronic mail (e-mail)
    faxes.

• Non-verbal communication
   body language
   sign language
   braille.

Clients may obtain information on veterinary care and its services by:

• media, eg television or radio, websites, adverts in the yellow pages and newspapers
• commercial information, eg advertisements on veterinary products placed by pharmaceutical companies on hoardings, in public transport, in the media
• information generated by the practice, eg newsletters, mail shots (written), puppy parties (verbal)
• word of mouth, eg information passed on by friends, family, previous clients.

Factors that may influence perception

These include:

• age
• education
• culture
• sensory loss (deafness/blindness)
• upbringing, social standing and background (socio-economic background).

2.2.02 Talking to clients and colleagues

What you need to learn

❧ You need to be able to explain the factors necessary for effective communication:
   ❧ environment
   ❧ interpersonal skills
   ❧ knowledge
   ❧ time.
❧ Describe factors which act as barriers to communication. These include:
   ❧ culture
   ❧ environment
   ❧ language
   ❧ stress
   ❧ understanding.
❧ Describe the ways in which questions may be framed:
   ❧ open
   ❧ closed

🐾 leading.
🐾 Explain how different types of question may be used effectively.
🐾 Describe common methods of non-verbal communication:
  🐾 facial expression
  🐾 posture
  🐾 gestures
  🐾 apparel.
🐾 Outline effective methods of dealing with a distressed, assertive or angry client
  🐾 listening
  🐾 acknowledgement
  🐾 focussing on a salient issue
  🐾 safety of self and others
  🐾 engaging further help.

Factors necessary for effective communication

- Environment – choose a place that is quiet and not subject to interruption (away from barking dogs, general chatter and phones ringing). This will help concentration and therefore memory.
- Interpersonal skills – ensure the communication is not made complicated by irrelevant information and that it is spoken/written clearly. Be confident.
- Knowledge – the speaker or writer needs a sufficient level of knowledge on the subject being discussed, otherwise they will appear hesitant and unclear.
- Time – make sure enough time is spent on communicating an issue. A rushed attempt will only cause confusion, forgetfulness and mistakes.
- Patience – a good communicator should be patient and may need to repeat the matter several times. Make sure the listener or reader understands the issue.

Barriers to communication

Barriers contribute to a breakdown of communication. The results of this are seen as mistakes or forgetfulness, and colleagues and clients may become angry or upset.

- Culture – some clients may have different beliefs.
- Environment – avoid places that are subject to noise and interruptions.
- Language – some clients/colleagues may not speak English or understand English and may have sensory loss (eg deafness, blindness or illness).
- Stress – keep the situation as calm as possible, concentration levels are low when the situation is stressful.

- Understanding – listening and sympathy are very important. Communication increases dramatically if both parties listen to one another.
- Written confirmations – try and have written notes where applicable. This applies to the receiver and the speaker.

How questions may be framed

- Open – encourage clients/colleagues to talk. The answer to an open question is left entirely to the client or colleague, eg What's his drinking like?
- Closed – use for collecting facts. The response to a closed question is a yes or no, eg So his drinking is normal?
- Leading – these questions lead the client or colleague into making a certain response, eg So has he been drinking more?

Methods of non-verbal communication

Methods of non-verbal communication affect the way in which you are perceived, eg:

- Facial expression – keep facial expressions consistent with the issue and emotion, eg don't smile if you are angry or delivering bad news.
- Posture – keep posture relaxed and upright, don't cross arms and legs.
- Gestures – clients appreciate gestures such as stroking/talking to their pet, as it makes them feel at ease and cared for. Gestures can be distracting if overdone.
- Eye contact – eye contact should be direct (but don't stare), this encourages listening and concentration.

Dealing with clients

- The distressed client – be calm and, most importantly, listen and respond.
- The assertive client – remain calm and confident. Listen and remain focused on the issue in question. If needed, call for extra help (eg someone with more knowledge on the subject).
- The angry client – try to have an assistant with you to act as a witness and never put yourself in a dangerous or potentially dangerous situation (call for extra help if needed). Remain focussed on the issue in question, acknowledge their concern and always try to remain calm; becoming angry with the client makes the situation worse.

2.2.03   Working with clients and colleagues

What you need to learn

☙ You need to be able to explain the factors necessary to maintain an effective and happy practice team:
  ☙ communication
  ☙ environment
  ☙ organisation
  ☙ rewards.
☙ Describe the factors that influence human motivation, eg theories of motivation such as Maslow's hierarchy of needs.
☙ Describe human reactions to criticism and anger and explain effective measures for dealing with these reactions.

Factors for maintaining a happy and effective practice team

- Good communication
- Clean and tidy working environment
- Good practice organisation
- Rewards/bonuses for good work
- Praise
- Constructive criticism as opposed to negative criticism
- Be proactive as opposed to reactive.

Factors influencing human motivation

- Rewards/bonuses for good work
- Praise
- Promotion.

Maslow's famous Hierarchy of Needs represents man functioning on different levels. Maslow identified the following need levels:

- self-actualisation (direction and meaning)
- ego needs (self-help, finding healthy pride, direction, empowerment in business)
- social needs (social self-help, finding love, how to escape bad feelings and alienation, how to achieve a sense of belonging)
- security needs (safety planning, food supplies, shelter requirements, emergency supplies)
- body needs (medical, emergency, rescue, coping).

The following diagram shows this hierarchic theory in a pyramid format. Each level is dependent on the previous level.

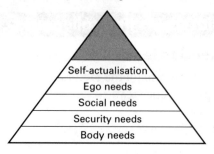

Maslow believed that once a person is self-actualised, they are content.

Reactions to criticism and anger

Psychological reactions may include:

- denial
- resenting criticism
- becoming upset
- becoming frightened or scared
- becoming angry.

How to deal with these reactions

- Always remain calm.
- Be consistent with the issue, don't back down.
- Listen to the other person and try to understand them. Each party should be given a fair hearing.
- Set review dates.
- Don't become angry yourself.
- Explain that the issue is work related and not personal.

Rationalisation: Put the problem into context. If an issue is not dealt with promptly or correctly, small issues may become very important, eg washing up, parking.

Offloading: Passing the responsibility to a third party (in effect, blaming the third party). Offloading is often used to avoid tackling an issue directly. All parties need to be involved in a discussion to solve the issue. Offloading is rarely a constructive way of dealing with the problem.

Displacement activity: Where a physical device is used for transferring anxiety during confrontation/discussion, eg biting nails, playing with hands or hair.

Supportive team ethos: In a supportive team the members tackle issues directly without appointing blame. In a good team the ethos is one of sharing problems and supporting colleagues.

Factors that lead to owner compliance

- Understanding – ensure the client understands the problem and the reason for the outcome. Use non-technical language.
- Skill – ensure the client can manage certain procedures, eg administering tablets.
- Conflicting beliefs – a client's own belief may conflict with the treatment (good communication would have prevented this problem).
- Perception – ensure everything is fully explained to the client, so the problem is perceived to be the same by both parties.
- Financial – the client should be made aware of **all** costs at the beginning of the treatment. Any issues related to or regarding the costs should be brought up at this stage.
- Interpersonal skills – ensure good communication is in place to avoid misunderstandings.

2.2.04　Grief and loss

What you need to learn

- You need to be able to explain the normal reactions which occur when a client faces loss:
  - denial
  - bargaining
  - anger
  - acceptance.
- Describe ways in which clients may be assisted through the process of grieving:
  - time
  - effective communication
  - emotional support
  - expert counselling.
- Explain effective and sensitive ways of breaking bad news:
  - time
  - environment
  - client-led discussion
  - giving and following cues.
- Consider euthanasia as a method of treatment.

Normal reactions to grief and loss

- Denial – the client can't believe it has happened, or believes it is not possible.
- Shock – the client feels the physical effect of bad news, eg feeling faint or sick, becoming pale, starting to sweat.

- Bargaining – clients argue about what you have said, eg you mean he's very ill, can't come home.
- Anger – the client shouts, postures, throws things, pushes.
- Acceptance – the client believes it has happened.
- Depression – the client feels dejected and dispirited.

These reactions may occur individually, at different stages, overlap one another or two or more reactions may occur at the same time.

How to assist in the grieving process

- Give the client as much time as they need as they may want to spend more time alone with their pet. Ask if they would like that option. Never try rushing a client out because there is a full surgery.
- Effective communication between all staff is essential, eg pre-warn all staff to prevent any embarrassing situations.
- Provide emotional support – listen and talk to the client. This may include telephoning them in a few days and sending them a condolence card.
- Expert (professional) counselling can be offered to the client if they seem to be stuck on one of the grieving processes and can't move forward. There are pet bereavement counsellors.

2.2.05   Developing self-awareness

What you need to learn

- You need to be able to explain the importance of self-awareness when working with other people. This covers:
  - self-perception
  - ability to recognise your strengths and weaknesses
  - self-development.
- Describe the process of reflection:
  - structured reflective process
  - learning from own performance.
- Describe the principles of effective self-organisation:
  - identifying priorities
  - setting goals
  - time management.

Importance of self-awareness

Self-awareness allows development of your skills both physically and mentally.

- Self-perception – think about how you react and interact with colleagues and clients. Can this be improved? Pay attention to how you communicate and your body language – this enables you to develop and produces confidence.

- Recognition of your own strengths and weaknesses makes you stronger and enables you to develop areas in which you feel weaker, while giving yourself confidence by recognising the areas in which you excel. Write them down, think about them and talk to another member of staff, eg head nurse or practice manager. This is good communication and they will be able to help develop your skills. Remember, they are not mind readers.
- Self-development – always keep this in mind and continue to develop it by the previous methods. Set goals for yourself – this instigates motivation and helps to develop your career.

The process of reflection

- The structured reflective process is a methodical process usually led by a senior colleague, eg appraisals.
- You also learn by your performance – look back at different mistakes and experiences and how they were handled. Could this be improved? Learn from successful experiences and share this success with other colleagues.

Self-organisation

Be organised to the best of your ability by:

- prioritising and identifying matters – what do I need to do first, what is most urgent?
- setting goals, eg finish a task by a certain time or date
- managing your time well, eg be realistic about how long tasks take, accept that you work better at certain times (morning people and evening people)
- identifying any problems and rectifying them.

2.2.06   Keeping records

What you need to learn

- ❧ You need to outline the methods of record keeping available in veterinary practice (manual and electronic).
- ❧ Describe the principles of effective record filing:
  - ❧ hierarchy
  - ❧ order
  - ❧ cross-referencing

☯ tracking extracted manual files.

☯ Explain the principles of recording written information in case records:

☯ accuracy

☯ legibility

☯ clarity

☯ objectivity.

☯ Explain what is meant by defamation and outline how this may be avoided in veterinary practice:

☯ libel

☯ slander

☯ objectivity

☯ discretion.

How to keep records

Records may be kept either:

• manually – cards with written information filed in a cabinet; or

• electronically – records are typed and stored on a computer system.

Principles of effective record filing

• Use a hierarchy (a graded, organised system).

• File items in order using an indexing system, eg alphabetical order, numerical order.

• Cross-reference items, eg animal species, related trends in laboratory results, radiographs.

• Track extracted manual files to prevent lost record cards. Use markers in removed file slots. File cards away immediately and keep a track on other people taking cards from the filing cabinet.

• When registering a new client always check they have not been before; this prevents duplicate record cards.

• A separate card should be used for each patient even if they belong to the same owner.

Principles of recording written information in case records

• Accuracy – correctness

• Legibility – readable handwriting

• Clarity – clear understandable language

• Objectivity – appropriate to the subject matter

• Identifiable – dated and initialled

• Permanent – written in indelible ink.

Defamation

Defamation damages the reputation or character of someone.

- Libel is written false or defamatory information.
- Slander is spoken false or defamatory information.

How to avoid defamation in the veterinary practice

- Objectivity – stick to speaking or recording only factual information and avoid making personal comments.
- Discretion – discuss client matters only within the practice. Be careful with whom you share information, don't talk about clients or professional matters in public, don't gossip.

2.2.07   Confidentiality

What you need to learn

- You need to outline the provisions of the Data Protection Acts and describe the implications for veterinary practice:
  - client access
  - mail shots.
- Describe circumstances in which client information may be disclosed:
  - criminal proceedings
  - public interest
  - insurance purposes.
- Discuss the ethical implications of information disclosure:
  - value judgements
  - professional/client relationship
  - public interest.
- Outline the RCVS guidance on record keeping and confidentiality (RCVS Guide to Professional Conduct).

Data Protection Acts

Case records, including radiographs and similar documents are the property of the veterinary surgeon, but remember – where a client has been charged specifically for radiographs or reports - they are entitled to them.

The provisions of the Data Protection Acts 1984 and 1998 give anyone the right to be informed about personal data relating to themselves on payment of a fee.

What does this imply?

A client can seek access to their pets' records. You can allow clients to see their records by making an appointment at the surgery at a mutually convenient time. Clients have to pay a fee to receive a copy of their pets' records according to the DPA.

Circumstances in which client information may be disclosed

- Criminal proceedings – court hearings may order disclosure of records or information.
- Public interest – in circumstances where the client has not given permission if the veterinary surgeon believes that animal welfare or public interest is compromised the RCVS must be contacted before divulging information.
- Insurance – an insurance company is entitled to receive all information relevant to the client's claim. This is called implied permission.
- Kennel club registered dogs – the veterinary surgeon can report acts that have altered the natural conformation of the dog to the kennel club.
- Express permission to disclose information – can be given by the client by word or in writing.

Ethical implications of information disclosure

- Value judgements – this is where you try to estimate the desirability or need for disclosure of information.
- Professional/client relationship – based on trust, veterinary surgeons and nurses are honour- and duty-bound to maintain confidentiality. Inappropriate disclosure of information may adversely affect this relationship with the client, you may lose the client and/or the practice's reputation may suffer.
- Public interest – giving information which involves the interests of the wider community.

Guidance on record keeping and confidentiality

The Royal College of Veterinary Surgeon's (RCVS) Guide to Professional Conduct states that information on the record card should include the following:

- Details of examination
- Any treatment to include medication
- Results of radiographs or diagnostic tests
- Advice given to the client
- Fees, estimates or quotes

- Consent – given or withheld
- Telephone conversations
- Contact details.

Storage of records

- Accident records – three years
- VAT records – six years
- PAYE records – at least three years
- There is no obligation to keep clients' record cards, any reports, consent forms or hospital records but the Veterinary Defence Society (VDS) recommends keeping them for two years. The RCVS recommends six years.
- If a case is referred to the Veterinary Defence Society it recommends to keep the records for six years and 364 days.

The RCVS Guide to Professional Conduct states that the veterinary surgeon/client relationship is founded upon trust. Information on the client, animal, clinical examination or post-mortem examination should not be disclosed to a third party. This confidentiality is to include all support staff employed by the practice.

2.2.08   Making appointments, receiving appointments, processing payments

What you need to learn

- You need to be able to explain the duties of a receptionist:
  - communicating with clients
  - retrieving information
  - filing and storing records
  - organising work areas
  - using materials and equipment
  - appreciating practice routines.
- Describe the principles of operating money control systems:
  - payments
  - credits
  - debits
  - cheques
  - credit cards
  - invoices
  - VAT.
- Describe systems available for making veterinary appointments:
  - manual
  - electronic.

☙ Describe the factors to be considered when prioritising veterinary appointments. Types of appointment include:
  ☙ routine or recall
  ☙ emergency
  ☙ urgent
  ☙ non-urgent
  ☙ re-examination.
☙ Describe the protocol required for second clinical opinions (as in the RCVS Guide to Professional Conduct).

The duties of the receptionist

- Communicating with clients – the receptionist is the first person a client will see or speak to, so good communication skills are essential.
- Retrieving information – you need to be able to know, memorise and recall information and clients' animals.
- Filing and storing records – you must be able to do this in an organised fashion.
- Organising work areas – the reception desk should be clean, tidy and uncluttered. The waiting room area should be free from dust, hair, urine, faeces and vomit. Keep it clean and ensure that there are well-stocked display stands. Make available posters and reading material to provide clients with information.
- Materials and equipment – you must be able to operate the telephone, fax, computer and till credit-card facilities correctly. You must be competent at receiving money and dealing with refunds or queries. Also ensure that equipment is regularly maintained.
- Appreciating practice routines – use the staff handbook to learn and understand all practice protocols, particularly for routine and common procedures, eg vaccination, neutering, worming and flea treatment, and second opinions. Use the appointment system or know the surgery times, know staff availability and know the procedure for advice calls.
- Personal appearance – wear a uniform or adopt a sensible, pleasant dress code. Wear a name badge, appropriate hair and jewellery, and also ensure good personal hygiene.

Operating money control systems

- Payments should be taken at the time of treatment.
- For credits, some practices may give long-standing clients credit. Unless instructed to do this, don't offer clients credit.
- Payment may be taken by debit card, cheque with guarantee card, credit card or cash.

• Always give the client an invoice or receipt which will state any transactions (including the VAT).

Appointments

Appointments can be made:

• manually – written in a diary
• electronically – on a computer system.

Prioritising appointments

Factors to be taken into account when booking appointments in order of priority are:

• Emergency – needs to be seen as soon as possible
• Urgent – needs to be seen that day
• Non-urgent – can wait until the following day
• Re-examination – when the veterinary surgeon has requested
• Routine/recall – can be seen any time.

Protocol for second clinical opinions

(Also see 2.4.01)

A second opinion is the opinion of a different veterinary surgeon for confirmation of a diagnosis. Clients have a right to request second opinions.

How to deal with a request for a second opinion from an existing client

• Accept that it is the client's right to make the request
• Refer to the veterinary surgeon involved
• Ensure details such as case history and radiographs are available.

How to deal with a request for a second opinion involving a client from a different practice

Before you make an appointment:

• ensure that the client has requested permission from their original practice
• get details of the original practice to allow your veterinary surgeon to make contact and request details of the case
• allow extra time for the appointment.

It is important not to speak or write disparagingly about the referring veterinary surgeon.

What you need to learn

* You need to be able to describe the factors to be assessed by the nurse when admitting an animal. These include:
    * general physical state
    * vital signs
    * feeding regime
    * routine management.
* Explain the factors which may render an animal a risk to other patients and practice staff. These include:
    * temperament
    * contagious disease
    * zoonotic disease.
* Explain the principles of obtaining valid consent to treatment:
    * written consent
    * informed consent
    * notification for insurance companies
    * design of consent forms
    * consent from a competent adult.
* Describe effective methods for identifying hospitalised animals and their belongings. These include:
    * identity tags
    * cage labels
    * admission and discharge procedures.
* Describe the factors/issues to be communicated to the clients when discharging an animal:
    * general physical state
    * nutrition and routine management
    * specific aftercare.

Admitting an animal

Admit patients in a separate room.

* General physical state – assess this by observation and by asking the owner if there has been any vomiting, diarrhoea, coughing, sneezing, exercise intolerance or any other changes since they were seen by the veterinary surgeon.
* Vital signs – take the patient's temperature, pulse and respiratory rate. Use a stethoscope to auscultate the thorax and listen to the heart. Assess mucous membrane colour, capillary refill time and hydration status.
* Feeding regime – ask the owner when the patient last ate and drank and if their pet has urinated and defaecated before admission.

- Routine management – make a note of the vaccination status and temperament and deal with the information accordingly. Weigh the patient and record its weight. Check the contact details, particularly a daytime telephone number. Make a note of any possessions, eg blanket, lead, toy. The owner must sign the consent form after confirming the animal's details. Give the owner a time to ring for a progress report or set a collection time.

Risk factors

There are a few factors that would make it inappropriate for the patient to be housed near other patients which include:

- treatment for aggressive or very timid patients
- contagious infections, eg parvo virus, cat flu
- zoonotic infections, eg salmonellosis.

Consent for treatment

- Written consent is required from the owner or agent for any procedure requiring a local or general anaesthetic.
- Informed consent – the client must be made fully aware of any procedures to be performed on their pet, including anaesthetic risk and post-operative care. Informed consent may be given over the telephone.
- Notification for insurance companies – the client is responsible for informing the insurance company of any procedure to be performed and obtaining their consent to pay for the procedure. It is helpful to note the insurance company and policy number on the consent form.
- An example of a consent form is given (see Figure 2.1).
- The person signing the form has to be 18 years old or above, ie a competent adult.

Identifying hospitalised animals

It is vital to ensure that correct procedures are carried out on animals. All patients and their belongings need to be correctly identified; this prevents items being lost or mislaid with other patients.

- Identity tags – these can be placed on animals at admission.
- Cage labels – once admitted a label can be tied on the kennel door identifying that patient. Cage labels can also be used for identifying belongings.
- Admission and discharge procedures – make a note on admission of any belongings and ensure these are collected by the owner at discharge.

Specimen Form of Consent for Anaesthesia and Surgical Procedures

SPECIMEN FORM OF CONSENT FOR ANAESTHESIA AND SURGICAL PROCEDURES

Species and Breed

Name

Colour

Age

Sex ☐ M ☐ F ☐ NM ☐ NF

Microchip/Tattoo/Brand

Owner s/Agent s* Name
*delete as applicable

Address

Telephone:
Home
Work
Mobile

Operation/Procedure

I hereby give permission for the administration of an anaesthetic to the above animal and to the surgical operation/procedure detailed on this form together with any other procedures which may prove necessary. The nature of these procedures and of other such procedures as might prove necessary has been explained to me and I understand that all anaesthetic techniques and surgical procedures involve some risk to the animal. I accept that the likely cost will be as detailed on the attached estimate, and that in the event of further treatment being required or of complications occurring which will give rise to additional costs, I shall be contacted as soon as practicable so that my consent to such additional costs may be obtained.

Signature:

Owner/Agent Name:
(Block capitals)

Notes and Instructions

The estimated cost of the procedures described above:

☐ will be £

☐ will be within the range:

£ to £

inclusive of:

☐ VAT ☐ Post-op Exam ☐ Post-op Treatment

Figure 2.1

Discharging patients

Discharge patients in a separate room. Speak to the owner alone first of all, (they are more likely to concentrate), then reunite them with their pet.

- General physical state – explain the procedure performed and relevant condition of the patient now.
- Nutrition and routine management – explain practice protocol on feeding and post-operative care.
- Specific aftercare – explain any specific requirements for the patient, eg medication, restricted exercise, darkened room, no noise.
- Return all belongings (check these against notes made on the consent form).
- Make a review appointment if needed and process the payment.

2.2.10 Nursing clinics

What you need to learn

- You need to be able to state types of common nursing clinics to promote client awareness with animal care. Types include:
  - puppy classes
  - dietary health
  - behaviour.

The following types of nursing clinics can be used to create client awareness and promote animal care. Full training in the relevant areas is needed before carrying out these clinics. Types of clinic include:

- puppy parties/classes – check on vaccination status, allow socialising at the optimal age, allow information exchange in relaxed conditions
- dietary health, eg weight-watcher clinics, specialised diets for illnesses, eg diabetic animals
- senior health clinics – dogs older than 8, cats older than 10
- behaviour clinics – normal and problem behaviour
- six-month-old puppy and kitten checks
- dental clinics – advice in dental hygiene and preventative care.

Multiple choice questions

1. When dealing with an angry client you should:
   - ☐ A make written notes throughout the conversation
   - ☐ B be assertive
   - ☐ C use non-verbal methods of communication
   - ☐ D remain calm and listen

2. Your reaction to an angry client should include:
   - ☐ A personal displacement activity
   - ☐ B non–rationalisation
   - ☐ C offloading
   - ☐ D supportive team ethos

3. Which of the following indicates the normal grieving process?
   - ☐ A anger, denial, acceptance
   - ☐ B denial, anger, depression
   - ☐ C bargaining, shock, depression
   - ☐ D depression, shock, acceptance

4. During training student VNs should gain a sense of self-awareness in order to develop both physical mental and nursing skills. They should:
   - ☐ A depend on their assessor to set personal goals
   - ☐ B prioritise problems but not rectify them immediately
   - ☐ C follow the practice's structured reflective process
   - ☐ D reflect on personal performance, both good and bad

5. The use of hierarchy in manual filing systems is:
   - ☐ A a system for cross referencing
   - ☐ B a graded organised system
   - ☐ C numerical order filing
   - ☐ D tracking of extracted files

6. Practice accident records should be kept for:
   - ☐ A 2 years
   - ☐ B minimum of 3 years
   - ☐ C 6 years
   - ☐ D 6 years and 364 days

7. To which of the following should client information not be disclosed:
   - ☐ A the client's insurance company
   - ☐ B the Kennel Club, if the dog is registered
   - ☐ C a neighbour
   - ☐ D a criminal court

8. In relation to *second opinions* which of the following is correct?
   - ☐ A the client need not contact the original practice
   - ☐ B clients have a right to request a second opinion
   - ☐ C the client should bring the case records from the original practice
   - ☐ D the second practice need not contact the original practice

9. If anyone in the practice expressed concern or spoke despairingly about another member of the veterinary profession, this would be known as:
   - ☐ A objectivity
   - ☐ B discretion
   - ☐ C slander
   - ☐ D libel

10. Which of the following piece of information is not confidential and may be disclosed to anyone who contacts the practice:
    - ☐ A an employee's home telephone number
    - ☐ B a fee paid by a client
    - ☐ C fees for veterinary services
    - ☐ D records of booster vaccinations

Level 2: Unit 3

Anatomy and physiology

2.3.01   Basic cell structure

What you need to learn

☙ You need to describe the structure of the components of a mammalian cell and different types of cells. Major cell types include epithelial, connective tissue, muscle, cartilage, bone, nerve and vascular cells.

☙ Describe the function of cell organelles and inclusions.

☙ Explain the basic methods of cell replication. This covers meiosis and mitosis (see pp. 46–50).

Cell structure

Nucleus

The nucleus contains DNA and within the nucleus is the nucleolus which contains RNA and ribosomes.

Cytoplasm

Cytosol:

- constitutes 50% of the cell volume
- is the site of protein synthesis
- is the site of most intermediate metabolism
- contains inclusions of stored products such as lipids, carbohydrates and proteins which are temporary structures within the cell, eg glycogen granules and pigment granules such as melanin
- centrioles involved in spindle termination during cell replication.

Organelles (membrane-bound components)

1 Endoplasmic reticulum (ER):
- Synthesis and storage of proteins. In places the ER is coated with small bodies called ribosomes. Protein synthesis occurs at the ribosomes. Where the ER is coated with ribosomes it is called rough ER, the rest of the ER is smooth ER.

• Lipid and steroid synthesis.
• Calcium store.

2 Golgi apparatus:
• Receives lipids and proteins from the ER then packages and dispatches them to a variety of destinations.

3 Mitochondria:
• Produce adenosine triphosphate (ATP) which generates energy to drive cellular reactions.

4 Lysosomes:
• Contain digestive enzymes for degrading materials such as ageing organelles or foreign particles from outside the cell.

Cell membrane

• This is also called the plasma membrane.
• It is a thin, flexible membrane separating the cell contents from the outside environment.
• It is selectively permeable, allowing transport of certain substances in and out of the cell.
• It consists of a double layer of phospholipid, proteins and some carbohydrates. Cholesterol is an important part of the cell membrane.

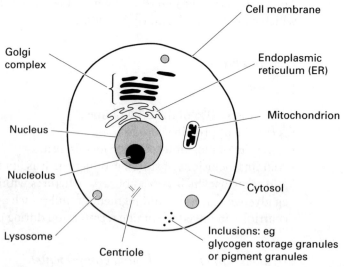

Figure 3.1 Basic cell structure.

2.3.02   Basic tissue types

What you need to learn

☙ You need to describe the structure and function of tissues.
☙ List the types of tissues that are found in the animal body. These are:
  ☙ epithelial
  ☙ glandular epithelial
  ☙ fibrous connective
  ☙ loose connective
  ☙ adipose
  ☙ muscle
  ☙ cartilage
  ☙ bone
  ☙ nerve
  ☙ vascular.
☙ You need to be able to describe the difference between the different types of tissue found in the body.

A **tissue** is defined as a group of cells of common origin with some specialised structure and a common function.

Examples of tissues are:

• epithelia (provide lining and protective layers)
• glandular epithelia (secrete hormones, enzymes and specialised fluids)
• fibrous connective tissue (provide strength and support in ligaments, tendons and fascia)
• adipose tissue (fatty tissue providing protection, insulation and energy storage)
• muscle
• cartilage
• bone
• neurones
• vessels (blood and lymph).

Cells become organised into tissues which can be further organised into organs.

Organs can be organised further to form systems. Examples of systems are:

• structural systems – the musculoskeletal system, the integumentary system and the cardiovascular system
• co-ordinating systems – the nervous system and the endocrine system
• visceral systems – the digestive system, the reproductive system, the respiratory system and the urinary system.

Types of tissue

1   Epithelial tissues

Table 3.1

Type of cell	Location
(a) Simple squamous epithelium	Capillary walls Alveoli Bowmann's capsule (kidney)
(b) Simple cuboidal epithelium	Thyroid gland Kidney tubules
(c) Simple columnar epithelium (i) Unciliated Basement membrane	Small intestine
(ii) Ciliated Basement membrane	Oviducts
(d) Simple pseudostratified epithelium Basement membrane *Often ciliated. Cells of different shapes and sizes, all contact the basement membrane.*	Trachea Bronchi Bronchioles
(e) Transitional epithelium *Several layers of cells of similar shapes and sizes capable of stretching to become 1-cell thick. There is no basement membrane.*	Lining of urinary bladder and ureters
(f) Stratified squamous epithelium Keratinised layer Germinal layer Basement membrane *Germinal layer divides providing new cells. Old cells are pushed to the surface and are sloughed off.*	Skin – keratinised Lining of: • mouth • pharynx • oesophagus • rectum • vagina are non-keratinised.

1(b)   *Glandular epithelial tissue*

Table 3.2

Type of cell	Location
Exocrine *Secretes material through a duct.* (see Figure 3.2(a))	Mucus gland Sweat gland Mammary gland Salivary gland Lacrimal (tear) gland *and many others*
Endocrine *Secretes hormones directly into body fluid – usually blood.* (See Figure 3.2(b))	Adrenal gland Thyroid gland Pituitary gland Ovary Testicle Parathyroid glands *and many others*

Note: The pancreas is a *mixed* gland because it has both endocrine (insulin, glucagon) *and* exocrine (digestive enzymes via the pancreatic duct) functions.

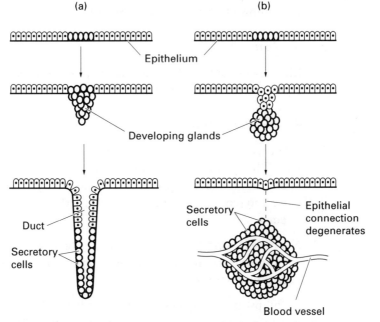

Figure 3.2   Exocrine gland (a) and endocrine gland (b).

2   *Connective tissue*

Connective tissue is a supporting structure consisting of various types of cells within an extracellular matrix (ECM). The ECM varies in consistency between liquid (eg blood) and solid (eg bone). The ECM can be amorphous (containing no fibres) or fibrous. The main types

Table 3.3

Cells	Extracellular matrix (ECM)
Fibroblasts: secrete ECM and various protein fibres.	Ground substance: consists of polysaccharides and proteins.
Adipocytes: fat cells which make up adipose tissue.	Fibres: (a) Collagen: loosely packed in areolar tissue; densely packed in tendons and ligaments (white fibrous tissue). Provide strength and support but have little elasticity.
Protective cells: such as *macrophages* and *mast cells* protect against infection and are involved in inflammatory response.	(b) Elastic: made of elastin fibres or sheets. Found in places where flexibility is needed such as blood vessels and lungs.
Chondrocytes: produce cartilage.	(c) Reticular fibres: delicate branching supportive network found in lymph nodes and endocrine glands.
Osteocytes : produce bone.	

Note: Cartilage, blood, bone and lymph are described elsewhere in greater detail.

of ECM are blood and lymph, haemopoietic tissue, loose connective tissue (adipose and areolar), dense connective tissue (white fibrous and yellow elastic), cartilage and bone.

3 Muscle tissue

Muscle is a contractile tissue made up of proteins. There are three types of muscle cell (see Table 3.4).

4 Nervous tissue

All nerve cells (neurones) possess:
• a cell body (contains the nucleus and a mass of cytoplasm)
• dendrites (receive impulses from other neurons)
• an axon (conveys impulses away from the cell body towards other neurons).

Nerve cells conduct electrical impulses (**action potentials**). They communicate with each other at **synapses,** or with muscles at a **neuromuscular junction.**

A synapse is the gap between the dendrites of two neurones. A **neurotransmitter** such as **acetylcholine** or **noradrenaline** is released from the first neurone and travels across the synapse, attaching to receptors on the second neurone. If the neurotransmitter creates another action potential in the second neurone it is an **excitatory** synapse. If not it is an **inhibitory** synapse. Neurotransmitters are then broken down and recycled.

Many axons are wrapped in a **myelin sheath** which increases the speed of conduction of the electrical impulse. The myelin sheath is

Table 3.4

Type of muscle	Function and location
(a) Skeletal muscle 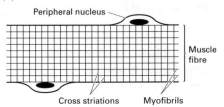	Responsible for virtually all voluntary movement. Can only contract or relax. Contractions are rapid and short lived eg biceps and triceps.

Each cell consists of many nuclei within a single cytoplasm – a syncitium. Skeletal muscle is striated and can only contract in one direction. The striations are myofibrils which are made up of filaments of protein which slide over one another during muscle contraction.

| (b) Cardiac muscle
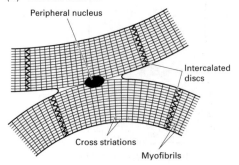 | Found only in the heart.
Movement is involuntary.
Contractions are generated from within the heart but are modified by the nervous system.
Contractions are rapid and short lived. |

Each cell consists of a single nucleus within a single cytoplasm. Cardiac muscle is also striated but the muscle fibres are branched, and divided into cells by intercalated discs which allow electrical conduction.

| (c) Smooth or visceral muscle
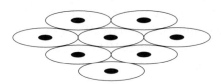 | Found in walls of the blood vessels, gut, respiratory tract and urogenital system.
Movement is involuntary.
Contractions are slow, rhythmic and sustained. |

Not striated. Contractile elements are criss-crossed to allow contraction in any direction.

created by **Schwann cells.** Gaps in the myelin sheath called the **nodes of Ranvier** allow the impulse to travel more quickly.

In the central nervous system there aren't any Schwann cells, instead the neural cells are supported and protected by a group of cells called **glial cells (neuroglia).**

An aggregation of neurones on a peripheral nerve is called a **ganglion.** Neurones can be multipolar (eg motor neurones), bipolar and unipolar (eg receptor sensory neurones) (see Figure 3.3).

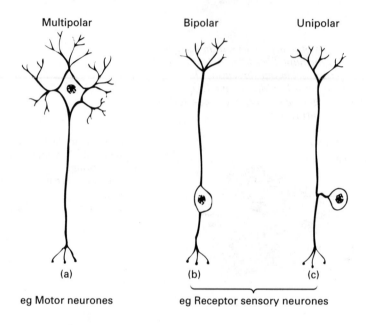

Multipolar   Bipolar   Unipolar

(a)   (b)   (c)

eg Motor neurones   eg Receptor sensory neurones

Figure 3.3 Examples of types of neurones.

Cell replication

During cell division the threads of DNA, along with histone proteins which help them to coil, are organised into **chromosomes.** Every species has a fixed number of chromosomes within the nucleus of each cell (known as the diploid number). Cats have 38 chromosomes whereas dogs have 78 chromosomes. A cat has 19 homologous pairs and a dog has 39 homologous pairs.

There are two ways in which cells divide.

Mitosis is the division of somatic (body) cells for addition to a multicellular organism during growth or to replace cells which are damaged. Most cells divide by mitosis. When a cell has divided by mitosis two identical daughter cells are produced, each containing the diploid number of chromosomes.

Meiosis is the division of cells to produce gametes. It occurs in organisms which reproduce sexually. When a cell divides by meiosis four daughter cells are produced, each containing the haploid number (half the diploid number) of chromosomes. Each gamete contains a different collection of genetic material.

Mitosis

Interphase

- This is the stage of the replication cycle before division begins. Although there is no visible activity a great deal of metabolic activity is occurring.
- DNA replication and synthesis of nuclear proteins occur.
- Production of ribosomes and cell organelles such as mitochondria occurs.
- The centrioles divide.

Prophase

- Chromosomes become visible in the nucleus and change from long threads to short, organised structures. During this time the nucleolus disappears.
- The centrioles migrate to opposite poles of the cell, laying down microtubules which form the **spindle**.

Metaphase

- The nuclear membrane disappears.
- Each chromosome can be seen as two **chromatids** attached by a **centromere**. The chromosomes become attached along the equator of the spindle by their centromeres.

Anaphase

- The centromeres split and the chromatids move to opposite poles of the cell.

Telophase

- A new nuclear membrane forms around each group of chromatids.
- The chromatids uncoil and the nucleoli reform.

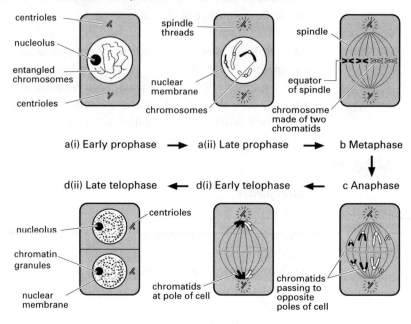

Figure 3.4 labels (top row):
Two cells, each with a diploid number of chromosomes

centrioles — spindle threads — spindle

nucleolus

entangled chromosomes — nuclear membrane — equator of spindle

centrioles — chromosomes — chromosome made of two chromatids

a(i) Early prophase → a(ii) Late prophase → b Metaphase

d(ii) Late telophase ← d(i) Early telophase ← c Anaphase

nucleolus — centrioles

chromatin granules

nuclear membrane — chromatids at pole of cell — chromatids passing to opposite poles of cell

Figure 3.4 Stages of mitosis (not all chromosomes are shown).

Shortly after nuclear division the cytoplasm divides into two approximately equal parts.

Meiosis

During meiosis there are two divisions of the nucleus producing four nuclei.

Interphase

• This is the same as that described for mitosis.

Prophase I

• The chromosomes become visible, first as entangled threads and then as the more organised shorter, thicker form.
• Homologous pairs of chromosomes come together to form **bivalents**. Crosslinks (called **chiasmata** between the chromosomes and their homologous partners develop. It is through the formation of chiasmata that genetic material is exchanged between chromosomes. For this reason meiosis is important in producing genetic variation.
• The nucleolus disappears and the spindle is laid down by centriole migration as happens during mitosis.

Metaphase I

- The nuclear membrane breaks down and the chromosomes become attached to the spindle by their centromeres.
- One chromosome from each bivalent is directed towards one pole of the cell while its homologous chromosome is directed towards the opposite pole.

Anaphase I

- The homologous chromosomes travel to opposite poles of the cell.

Telophase I

- A new nuclear membrane forms around each group of chromosomes.
- The chromosomes uncoil and the nucleoli reappear.
- Cleavage of the cytoplasm may occur.
- Note that each of the two new nuclei has the haploid number of chromosomes.

A short interphase may follow but no further DNA replication occurs.

Prophase II

- Chromosomes appear in the nuclei and a spindle is laid down by the centrioles.
- There is no pairing of chromosomes and no further crossing over occurs.

Metaphase II

- The nuclear membrane disappears.
- Each chromosome becomes visible as two chromatids.
- Chromosomes become attached to the spindle by their centromeres.

Anaphase II

- The centromeres split and the chromatids move to opposite poles of the cell.

Telophase II

- A new nuclear membrane forms around each group of chromatids.
- The chromatids uncoil and the nucleoli reform.

Shortly after nuclear division the cytoplasm divides into two approximately equal parts.

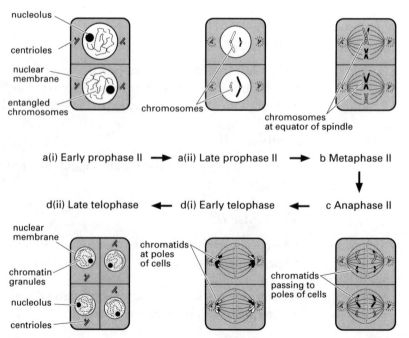

Compare metaphase I with metaphase of mitosis

centrioles

nucleolus

entangled
chromosomes

chiasma

a(i)
Early prophase I

a(ii)
Mid-prophase I

a(iii)
Late
prophase I

d(ii)
Late telophase I ← Early telophase I ← Anaphase I ← Metaphase I
d(i)   c   b

chromatin
granules

spindle

centrioles

nucleolus

nuclear
membrane

chromosomes
at poles of cell

homologous
chromosomes
passing to opposite
poles of cell

Four cells, each with a haploid number of chromosomes

nucleolus

centrioles

nuclear
membrane

entangled
chromosomes

chromosomes

chromosomes
at equator of spindle

a(i) Early prophase II → a(ii) Late prophase II → b Metaphase II

d(ii) Late telophase ← d(i) Early telophase ← c Anaphase II

nuclear
membrane

chromatids
at poles
of cells

chromatin
granules

chromatids
passing to
poles of cells

nucleolus

centrioles

Figure 3.5 Stages of meiosis.

The body cavities (see pp. 179-80)

The thorax

The thoracic cavity is enclosed by the thoracic vertebrae, sternum, ribs and caudally by the diaphragm. It contains the thoracic viscera (organs) which include the heart and lungs, along with the thoracic portions of the oesophagus and trachea. The pleural cavity is within the thoracic cavity.

The pleural cavity is a potential space between the pulmonary and parietal pleura and is filled with a small amount of pleural fluid. The pleural fluid is a lubricant and allows the organs to move smoothly over each other.

The **pleura** are serous membranes (thin layers of loose connective tissue) which cover the outer surfaces of the lungs (**pulmonary** or **visceral** pleura) and line the thoracic cavity (**parietal** pleura).

The parietal pleura consist of the following:

• **costal** pleura covering the inner surfaces of the chest wall
• **mediastinal** pleurae covering the partition between the pleural cavities
• **diaphragmatic** pleura covering the diaphragm.

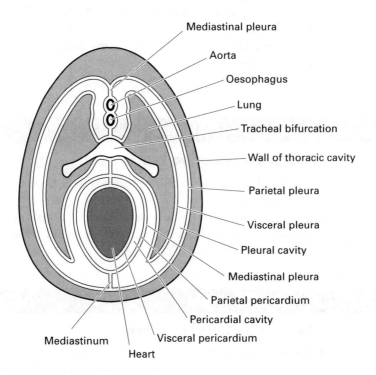

Figure 3.6 The pleural and thoracic cavities.

The **mediastinum** is the partition between the two pleural cavities. It includes the two mediastinal pleurae and the space between them. Within the mediastinal space are the thymus, heart, trachea, oesophagus and various nerves and vessels.

The abdomen

The abdominal cavity is formed by the abdominal wall, the diaphragm and the ribs. It contains the abdominal viscera (small and large intestines, liver, spleen, kidneys, bladder; and the uterus and ovaries in the female). It is lined by a serous membrane (the peritoneum) which encloses the peritoneal cavity. Peritoneal fluid is a lubricant and allows the viscera to move smoothly over each other.

The peritoneal cavity is a potential space. The **parietal** peritoneum lines the body wall whereas the **visceral** peritoneum covers and suspends the abdominal organs.

In places the peritoneum forms a double-layered sheet. Where this sheet suspends the gut from the body wall it is called **mesentery**. Where it bridges the gap between two organs it is called **omentum**.

The pelvic cavity

The pelvic cavity is contained within the bony pelvic girdle but is outside the peritoneum-lined part of the abdomen (retro-peritoneal). It contains the rectum, anal sacs, anus, bladder, urethra and reproductive organs.

2.3.03   Types of body fluids

What you need to learn

* You need to be able to describe the types of body fluid and their composition.
* You also need to describe how the different types of body fluid are formed. These fluids include cerebrospinal fluid (CSF), lymph, blood and synovial fluid (see Table 3.5).

2.3.04   Skeletal system

What you need to learn

* You need to be able to describe the components and functions of the axial, appendicular and splanchnic skeleton. This includes growth and development, epiphyseal closure and bone structure.

Table 3.5

Type of fluid	Composition	Function
Blood (discussed in detail on page 109)	Red blood cells White blood cells Platelets Serum Plasma proteins Electrolytes	Carriage of oxygen and nutrients throughout body via a network of blood vessels.
Cerebrospinal fluid	Ultrafiltrate of blood, similar to plasma but contains less glucose/protein and very few cells.	Cushions the brain and spinal cord. Compensates for changes in blood pressure in the central nervous system.
Lymph	Tissue fluid Antibodies Lymphocytes	Excess fluid in the tissues which is not reabsorbed into the blood enters the lymphatic system, preventing oedema. Lymph vessels are similar to veins but more delicate and with many valves. Passes through lymph nodes then returns to the blood through thoracic duct.
Synovial fluid (joint fluid)	Similar to plasma but contains hyaluronic acid which provides lubrication.	Lubricates joints. Nourishes articular cartilage.

- Identify obvious anatomical differences in skeletal structures between birds, rodents, lagamorphs, reptiles, amphibians and fish.
- You need to be able to describe the classification of bones according to their shape and give examples of bones in each group.
- Define intramembranous and endochondral ossification and state the sites in the body where each occurs.

Functions

- Provides support to body
- Protects soft tissues
- Locomotion.

The skeleton is made up of bone and cartilage which are connective tissues.

Axial skeleton: this part of the skeleton makes up a straight line from end to end and includes the skull, vertebral column and the ribcage.

Appendicular skeleton: this is the skeletal parts of the limbs.

Splanchnic skeleton: this includes bones which are found within organs. The os penis is a bone within the penis of the dog and cat. It protects the urethra and provides some rigidity to the penis.

The structure of bones

- Diaphysis (shaft)
- Epiphyses (ends of the bone)
- Periosteum (fibrous membrane covering the outer surface of the bone)
- Bone marrow (involved in blood cell production – haematopoiesis).

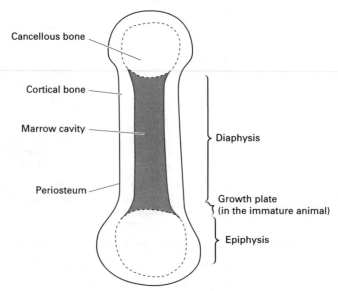

Figure 3.7 Schematic diagram of the structure of a bone.

Bone structure is described as being either spongy (cancellous) or compact (cortical).

Cortical bone

The matrix of bone consists of a collagen fibre mesh with concentric **lamellae** made of calcium salts (mainly phosphate). The bone cells, (**osteocytes**) which secrete the bone matrix, sit in cavities (**lacunae**) between the lamellae. The lacunae are linked by fine fibres (**canaliculi**). Running along the length of the bone are the **Haversian canals** which contain nerves and blood vessels, and connect with the periosteum and bone marrow.

Cancellous bone

The basic structure is the same but in cancellous bones there are fewer Haversian systems. The lamellae form a fine mesh of bone

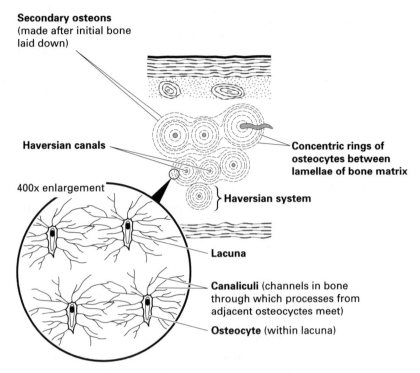

40x enlargement

Secondary osteons
(made after initial bone
laid down)

Haversian canals

400x enlargement

**Concentric rings of
osteocytes between
lamellae of bone matrix**

Haversian system

Lacuna

Canaliculi (channels in bone
through which processes from
adjacent osteocyctes meet)

Osteocyte (within lacuna)

Figure 3.8   Microscopic detail of the structure of bone.

known as trabeculae. The spaces within the network are filled with haemopoeitic and myeloid tissue.

Blood vessels pass through small holes in the cortex called **nutrient foramina**.

Bones can be classified according to their shape (see Table 3.6).

Development of bones

Endochondral ossification: the embryonic bone is made from cartilage. Calcium salts are deposited by cartilage cells (**chondroblasts**). Starting from the centre of ossification large cells called **osteoclasts** start to erode this calcified cartilage so that blood vessels can invade. **Osteoblast** cells then lay down a bony framework of trabeculae and ossification spreads outwards along the bone. Some osteoblasts become enclosed within the lacunae and become osteocytes.

Intramembranous ossification: cartilage is not involved in the development of certain bones such as the flat bones of the skull. Instead a membrane of connective tissue is formed which becomes

Table 3.6

Type of bone	Shape	Examples
Long bones	Generally cylindrical	Act as levers for locomotion. Main limb bones such as femur, humerus, tibia, etc.
Short bones	Length, width and breadth roughly the same	Allow complex movements. Carpal bones, tarsal bones.
Flat bones	Broad and flat	Large surface for muscle attachment, offer protection of soft tissues. Scapula, skull bones, wing of ilium (pelvis).
Irregular bones	Various shapes	Vertebrae, mandible.
Sesamoid bones	Various shapes	These alter the angle of pull of a tendon near a joint. Patella, fabellae.

calcified and is then remodelled by osteoclasts and organised by the osteocytes as for endochondral ossification.

Lengthening of the bones during growth occurs in the growth plates (**epiphyseal plates**). When growth has finished the growth plates are replaced with bone and are said to have closed. The age at which this occurs varies greatly between species and breeds.

Exotic species

Birds

There are many orders of bird. Those commonly encountered in veterinary medicine include:
• ducks, geese and swans (Anseriformes)
• birds of prey (Falconiformes)
• grouse, pheasants, domestic fowl (Galliformes)
• pigeons and doves (Columbiformes)
• parrots (Psittaciformes)
• perching birds such as finches and canaries (Passeriformes).

Bird skeletons are adapted for flight. Many of the features of the avian skeleton are designed to reduce the weight of the skeleton and to allow flight.

The bones have very thin cortices and some bones are hollow. Avian bones therefore shatter more easily than mammalian bones and are more difficult to repair. The forelimb of the bird is modified to form the wing. There is more variety in the number of vertebral bones in birds than in mammals. Some of the vertebral bones are fused. The

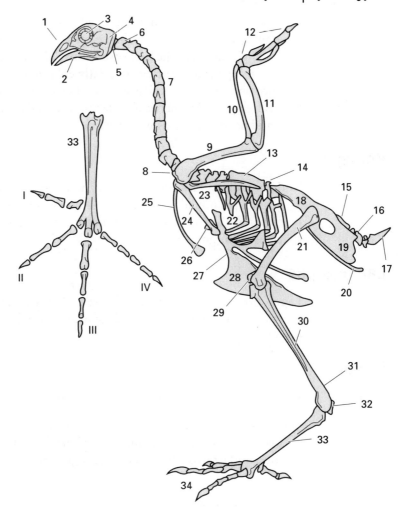

Figure 3.9 The skeleton of a bird.

KEY

1.	Facial part of skull	12.	Hand (manus)	23.	Scapula
2.	Mandible (hyoid bones protruding below)	13.	Nortarium	24.	Coracoid
3.	Orbit and sclerotic ring of eyeball	14.	Free thoracic vertebra	25.	Fused clavicles
4.	Cranium	15.	Synsacrum	26.	Manubrium sterni
5.	Atlas	16.	Caudal vertebrae	27.	Sternum
6.	Axis	17.	Pygostyle	28.	Keel
7.	Cervical vertebrae	18.	Ilium	29.	Patella
8.	Shoulder joint	19.	Ischium	30.	Fibula
9.	Humerus	20.	Pubis	31.	Tibiotarsus
10.	Radius	21.	Fermur	32.	Sesamoid bone (ossified tibial cartilage) in hock joint
11.	Ulna	22.	Ribs	33.	Tarsometatarsus
				34.	Digits: I–IV digits

ventral part of the sternum is modified to form the **keel**. It provides a large surface area for the attachment of the powerful pectoral (flight) muscles. The depth of the keel varies with the ability of that species to fly. The bony orbit of the eye is greatly enlarged, reflecting their reliance on vision. The pelvis is a fused box. The shape varies between species. The pelvis is wide in species which run or climb, but long and narrow in birds which swim.

Rodents

Rodents include rats, mice, gerbils, guinea-pigs and hamsters. The axial and appendicular skeletons resembles those of cats and dogs in many ways. Rodents have continuously erupting teeth which are specialised for gnawing.

Lagomorphs

Lagomorphs are the rabbits and hares. They are similar to rodents except that they have a third pair of incisors on the upper jaw – the **peg** teeth.

Reptiles

Reptiles are cold blooded and include four orders:

• **chelonians** (tortoises, turtles and terrapins)
• **crocodilians** (crocodiles, alligators, gharials, etc)
• **snakes and lizards** (this is the biggest group)

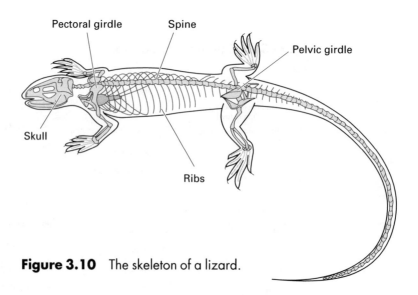

Figure 3.10 The skeleton of a lizard.

• **tuatara** (this order contains a single species similar to a lizard in New Zealand).

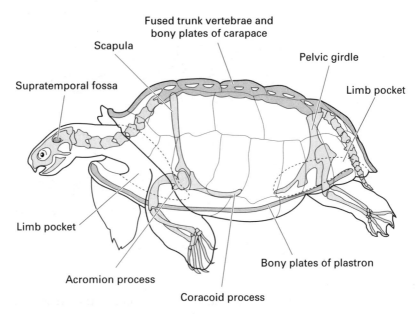

Figure 3.11 The skeleton of a tortoise.

Most reptiles possess four limbs. The exceptions are the snakes which are basically lizards without legs.

The chelonians possess a shell which consists of an upper bony plate (the carapace) and a lower plate (the **plastron**). The ribs are fused to the bony part of the shell. The horny scales which cover the bones of the shell are called **scutes**.

The structure of the limbs is basically similar to those of the mammals, although in the slow worm and snakes the limbs have become vestigial (remnants of the original structure). The vertebral column is very flexible and may contain several hundred vertebrae. Some species of lizard are able to discard part of the tail. The damaged tail is then able to regrow. In snakes the two halves of the mandible are not fused.

Amphibians

Amphibians are cold blooded and most live in a semi-aquatic environment. They include frogs and toads, newts, salamanders and axolotls. Amphibians have simpler skeletons with fewer bones than many of the other vertebrates. The spine is short with few vertebrae. The tail vertebra is called the urostyle. The ribs are poorly developed and sometimes absent. The skull is flat and broad with large orbits. In

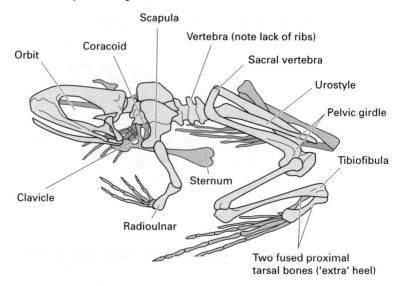

Figure 3.12 The skeleton of a frog.

some species (such as salamanders) the skeleton doesn't become completely ossified.

Fish

Fish are cold blooded. Nearly all fish are completely aquatic. Fish are divided into the bony fish, which have an ossified skeleton (such as cod, goldfish, trout); and the cartilaginous fish which have a cartilaginous skeleton (such as the sharks and rays). Fish have a number of appendices (fins) which vary between the species.

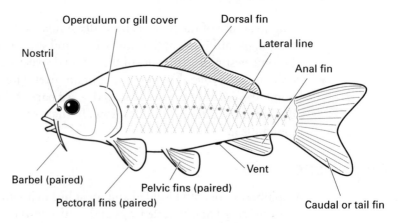

Figure 3.13 Diagram of the external anatomy of a fish.

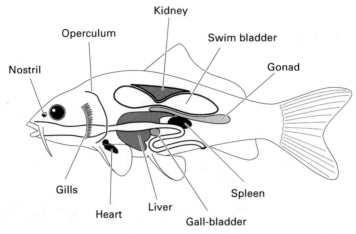

Figure 3.14 Diagram showing the digestive system of a fish.

2.3.05 Skull

What you need to learn

☙ You need to be able to name and locate the skull bones and structures. These are:
  ☙ maxilla
  ☙ mandible (see 2.3.06)
  ☙ foramen magnum
  ☙ incisive
  ☙ frontal
  ☙ temporal
  ☙ parietal
  ☙ orbit
  ☙ zygomatic arch
  ☙ sphenoid
  ☙ nasal
  ☙ tympanic bulla
  ☙ occipital.
☙ Define various skull types and state the difference between the types. These include:
  ☙ brachycephalic, mesocephalic and dolicocephalic types.
☙ Describe the location and function of the sinuses.

Lateral view of the skull

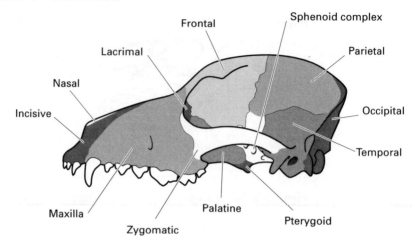

Figure 3.15 Lateral view of the bones of the skull.

The delicate scroll-shaped bones within the nasal cavity are called **turbinate** bones.

Ventral view of the skull

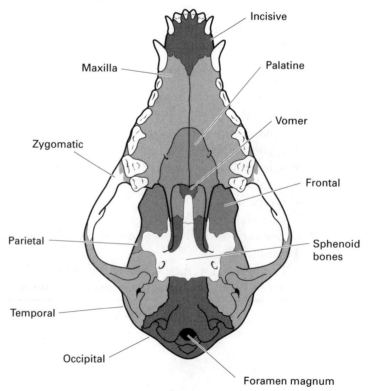

Figure 3.16 Ventral view of the bones of the skull.

2.3.06   Mandible

What you need to learn

🐾 You need to be able to describe the structure and functions of the mandible:
- 🐾 horizontal and vertical ramus
- 🐾 coronoid process
- 🐾 condylar process
- 🐾 the area of the mandibular symphysis and alveoli for various teeth.

- The mandible consists of two bones which are fused at the **mandibular symphysis.**
- The coronoid process forms a point of attachment of the powerful chewing (**masticatory**) muscles.
- The condylar process forms a synovial joint with the mandibular fossa of the temporal bone – the **temperomandibular joint.**

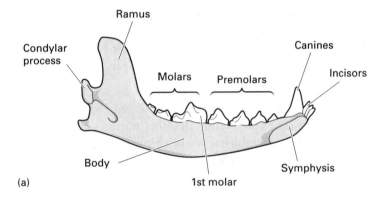

(a)

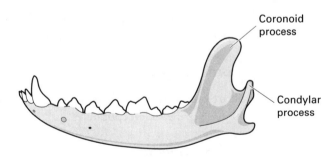

(b)

Figure 3.17   Medial view of the mandible (a) and lateral view of the mandible (b).

The sinuses

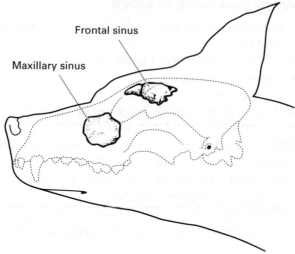

Figure 3.18 The sinuses.

The function of the sinuses is not fully understood but it has been suggested that they may do the following:

• provide insulation for the brain, eyes and nose
• allow development of a larger head without adding extra weight
• act as resonating chamber for the voice
• protect the brain from blows to the head
• mucous secretions in the sinuses may help keep the nasal mucosa moist.

Skull types

There is great variation in skull shapes between breeds (see Figure 3.19). The three basic shapes are as follows:

1 Brachycephalic

Short-faced breeds such as bulldogs, boxers, pugs and King Charles spaniels are brachycephalic.

2 Mesocephalic

Medium faced-breeds such as beagles, springer spaniels, red setters and German pointers are mesocephalic.

3 Dolicocephalic

Long-nosed breeds such as greyhounds, Afghan hounds, borzois and salukis are dolicocephalic.

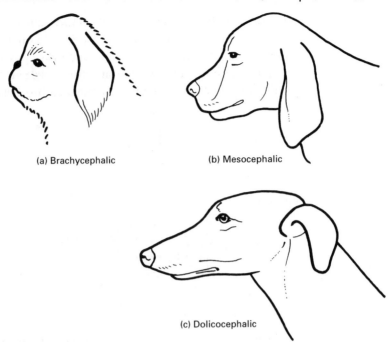

(a) Brachycephalic   (b) Mesocephalic

(c) Dolicocephalic

Figure 3.19 Diagram showing the three basic skull shapes seen in dogs.

2.3.07   Vertebral column

What you need to learn

❧ You need to be able to describe the basic structure of a vertebra and the vertebral column, and the sacrum.

❧ Itemise the regions of the vertebral column and state the number of vertebrae in each region. These include:

  ❧ atlas
  ❧ axis
  ❧ other cervical vertebrae
  ❧ thoracic vertebrae
  ❧ lumbar coccygeal vertebrae.

❧ Identify the differences between different types of vertebrae.

❧ Describe the structure and function of interverterbral discs.

The vertebral column or spine extends from the skull to the tip of the tail and consists of a number of separate bones – the vertebrae. The vertebral column protects the spinal cord and each vertebra provides points for attachment of muscles.

Each vertebra consists of:

• a **body** which is a cylindrical bone with a convex cranial end and concave caudal end

- an **arch** which encircles the **vertebral foramen,** each half of the arch is made from a lateral **pedicle** and a dorsal **lamina**
- **spinous and transverse processes** which vary in size along the vertebral column and provide sites for muscle attachment
- **articular processes** which form synovial joints between vertebrae.

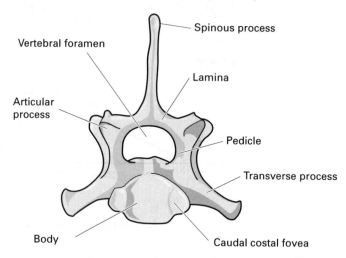

Figure 3.20 Diagram of the basic structure of a vertebra.

The vertebrae are divided into five groups:

1 **The cervical vertebrae:** (7 neck vertebrae) the first of these is the **atlas** which articulates with the skull and has flattened transverse processes – the **wings.** The second is the **axis** which has a process called the **dens** which projects cranially towards the atlas. These two bones form a pivot joint.

2 **The thoracic vertebrae:** (13 chest vertebrae) these have taller spinous processes and short bodies. On each side is an **articular facet** which articulates with a rib. T11 is the anticlinal vertebra. All spines of vertebra cranial to T11 are directed caudally. All spines of vertebra caudal to T11 are directed cranially.

3 **The lumbar vertebrae:** (7 lower back vertebrae) these have large bodies but small spinous processes. The transverse processes are long and are angled cranially.

4 **The sacral vertebrae:** 3 vertebrae are fused to form one bone – the **sacrum.** A cartilaginous joint, the **sacro-iliac joint,** attaches the pelvis to the spine.

5 **The caudal vertebrae:** there are on average 20 caudal vertebrae although there is great species variation. These bones support the tail.

The bodies of adjacent vertebrae are separated by fibrocartilage discs – the **intervertebral discs.** These act as shock absorbers and allow some movement between the vertebrae. They are composed of a semi-fluid centre, the **nucleus pulposus**, surrounded by a tough fibrous layer called the **annulus fibrosus**. With age the discs often become calcified making them less flexible and therefore more prone to damage.

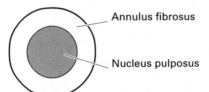

Figure 3.21   Schematic diagram of an intervertebral disc.

2.3.08   Ribs

What you need to learn

☙ You need to be able to describe the structure and functions of the ribs. This includes the number of ribs, costal arch, sternal rib, asternal rib, costal cartilage, floating rib and intercostal space.
☙ Describe the articulation of the ribs with the vertebral column and sternum.

The ribs and sternum complete the rib-cage which provides protection for the thoracic viscera, and allows expansion of the lungs during respiration.

There are 13 pairs of ribs or **costae**. Each rib consists of a bony dorsal part and a cartilaginous ventral part, the **costal cartilage**.

The bony part of each rib consists of the:

• tubercle which articulates with the articular process of the thoracic vertebrae.
• head
• neck of the rib which lies between the tubercle and the head
• body of the rib.

The costal cartilage articulates with the sternum. The costal cartilages of the ninth to twelfth rib overlap to form the **costal arch**.

The first nine pairs of ribs are **sternal** or **true** ribs because they articulate with the sternum. The caudal four pairs are called **false** or **asternal** ribs because they don't articulate directly with the sternum. While ribs 10, 11 and 12 articulate with the sternum only through their overlapping costal cartilages, the thirteenth ribs don't articulate with the sternum at all and are therefore called **floating ribs**.

The spaces between the ribs are called **intercostal spaces**. The ribs are joined to one another by **intercostal muscles**.

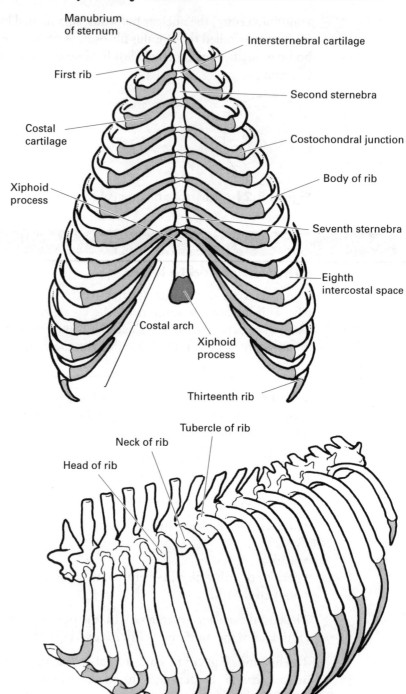

Figure 3.22 The ribs and sternum.

2.3.09   Sternum

What you need to learn

* You need to be able to describe the structure and functions of the sternum. These include:
  * manubrium
  * xiphisternum
  * xiphoid cartilage and intersternebral cartilage.

The sternum consists of eight bones, the **sternebrae** which articulate with each other through **intersternebral cartilages**. The first sternebra is called the **manubrium**. The last sternebra is called the **xiphoid process** (or **xiphisternum**) and is longer than the other sternebrae. A cartilage plate, the **xiphoid cartilage**, is attached to the xiphoid process. The xiphoid cartilage provides attachment for the muscles of the abdominal floor and provides attachment of the linea alba.

2.3.10   Appendicular skeleton

What you need to learn

* You need to be able to describe the bones of the fore and hindlimbs and state the differences in different species including exotics, birds, rodents and lagomorphs, reptiles, dogs and cats.
* Describe the structure and position of various bones:
  * scapula
  * humerus
  * radius
  * ulna
  * pelvis
  * femur
  * tibia
  * fibula
  * fibular tarsal and tibial tarsal bones
  * carpus
  * tarsus
  * metacarpus
  * metatarsus
  * phalanges
  * patella
  * fabella
  * clavicle.
* Recognise normal digital number in different species, including rodents, birds and lagomorphs.

The forelimb

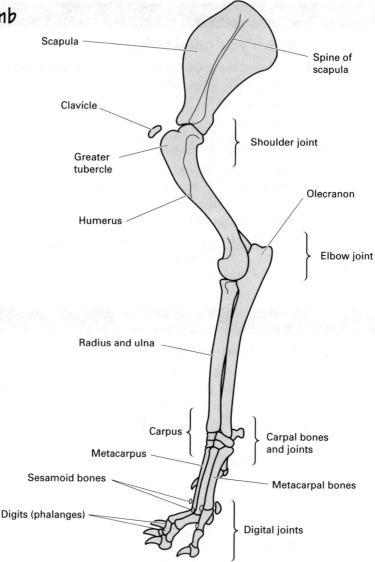

Figure 3.23 The bones of the forelimb.

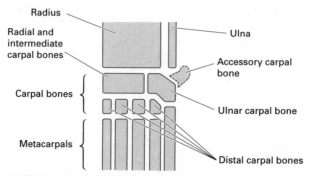

Figure 3.24 Schematic diagram of the carpal bones in cats and dogs.

The pelvis and hindlimb

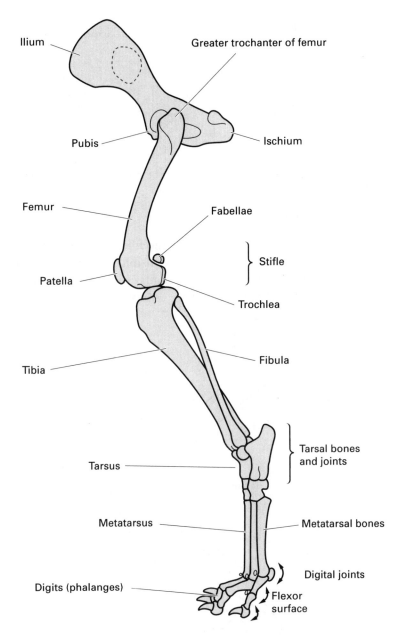

Ilium

Greater trochanter of femur

Pubis

Ischium

Femur

Fabellae

Stifle

Patella

Trochlea

Tibia

Fibula

Tarsal bones and joints

Tarsus

Metatarsus

Metatarsal bones

Digital joints

Digits (phalanges)

Flexor surface

Figure 3.25 Bones of the hindlimb.

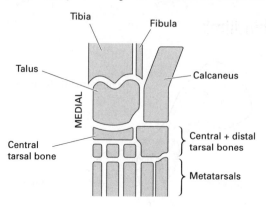

Figure 3.26 The bones of the tarsus in the dog and cat.

Exotics

Birds

In birds the forelimbs are modified to form wings. The humerus is hollow and contains an extension of the air sacs (**pneumatised bone**). The ulna and radius are similar to those in mammals. The distal bones of the forelimb are reduced and fused.

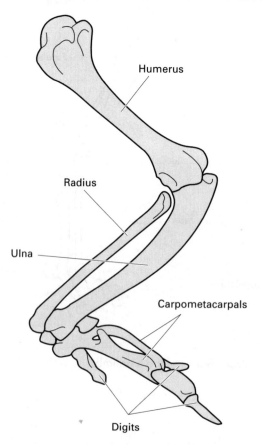

Figure 3.27 Diagram of the bones of the wing.

The hindlimbs are responsible for providing locomotion on the ground, they are also responsible for swimming, perching and landing. The femur is similar to that of the mammal. It is occasionally pneumatised. The more distal bones are fused and reduced. There are four digits. Some species perch with digits 2,3, and 4 pointing forwards (eg chicken) while other birds perch with only digits 2 and 3 pointing forwards (eg budgerigar).

Rodents and lagomorphs

The front limbs tend to be short. The hindlimbs tend to be long and powerful. The forelimb has five digits while the hindlimb has four digits.

Reptiles

In many species the limb bones are short and thick providing strength. The tarsal and carpal bones are often fused.

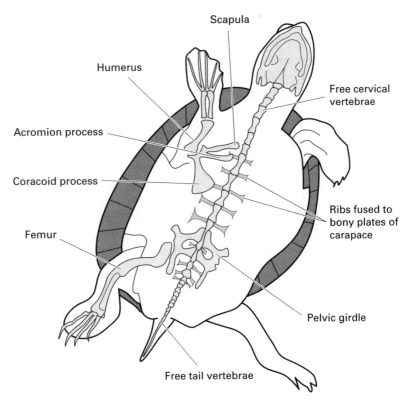

Figure 3.28   Ventral view of the skeleton of a chelonian.

The forelimb has five digits while the hindlimb has four or five depending on the species. Some primitive snakes such as the boas possess vestigial hindlimbs in the form of very small claws in the cloacal area.

2.3.11   Splanchnic skeleton

What you need to learn

☙ You need to be able to state the location of the os penis and describe its functions.

See 2.3.65, The Male Reproductive Tract, pp. 198–201, and 2.3.69 Mating, pp. 210–11. See also pp. 53–4.

2.3.12   Joints

What you need to learn

☙ You need to be able to describe the classification of joints according to their structure and the types of movement that can occur. These are:
  ☙ fibrous
  ☙ cartilaginous
  ☙ synovial
  ☙ extension
  ☙ flexion
  ☙ rotation
  ☙ over-extension
  ☙ adduction
  ☙ abduction
  ☙ gliding/sliding.
☙ Describe in detail the structure of a typical synovial joint.
☙ Describe the normal range of movement of these joints:
  ☙ shoulder
  ☙ hip
  ☙ elbow
  ☙ stifle joints carpus
  ☙ tarsus and digits.

Classification of joints

There are three types of joints:

1 Fibrous

• These are dense connective tissue joints between two adjacent bones.
• They allow very little movement.

- They occur mainly in the skull and are known as sutures. In the young animal they allow growth of the skull.
- They are also seen joining facing parts of two bones such as the joint between the radius and ulna. In these cases the joints are called syndesmoses.

2 Cartilaginous

- These are cartilaginous joints between two adjacent bones.
- They allow a small amount of movement and are sometimes called synchondroses.
- They include joints between symmetrical halves of the mandible and pelvis; the mandibular symphysis and pubic symphysis respectively.

3 Synovial

- A fluid-filled space, the **synovial cavity**, separates the articulating bones.
- They are freely movable joints.
- The synovial cavity is lined with a **synovial membrane** which produces the lubricating **synovial fluid**. The outside of the synovial membrane is protected by a tough fibrous joint capsule. Often parts of the joint capsule are strengthened by ligaments.
- The articular surfaces of the bones in a synovial joint are covered with articular cartilage (usually hyaline cartilage).
- A few synovial joints (eg the stifle) possess fibrocartilage discs or **menisci** which sit between the bones and aid the smooth movement of the joint.

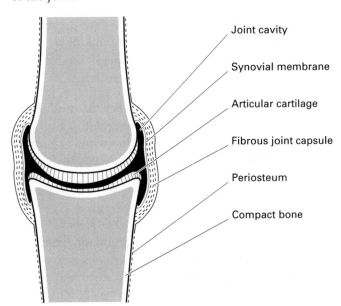

Joint cavity

Synovial membrane

Articular cartilage

Fibrous joint capsule

Periosteum

Compact bone

Figure 3.29 Schematic diagram of a synovial joint.

Movement of joints

Gliding: the articular surfaces glide smoothly over one another.

Angular:
* *Extension* – the angle of the joint is opened, eg straightening the knee. (**Overextension** is where a joint is extended past 180 degrees – this is possible in the carpus).
* *Flexion* – the angle of the joint is reduced, eg bending the knee.

Rotation: the bone rotates along its longitudinal axis.

Movement of complete limbs

Adduction: the moving part is brought medially towards the body.
Abduction: the moving part is moved away from the body.
Circumduction: the extremity of the limb moves in a circle. This movement involves flexion, extension, adduction and abduction.
Protraction: cranial movement of the limb.
Retraction: caudal movement of the limb.
Pronation: inward rotation of the paw.
Supination: outward rotation of the paw (think: thumbs up).

Specific examples

The shoulder: the humerus articulates with the glenoid cavity of the scapula in a ball and socket joint. Movement is mainly flexion and extension. Ligaments within the joint help prevent dislocation.

The elbow: the elbow is a hinge joint between the condyle of the humerus, the head of the radius and the trochlear notch of the ulna. Collateral ligaments prevent lateral movements so movement of this joint is mainly flexion and extension.

The hip: the articulation between the head of the femur and the acetabulum is a ball and socket joint. A ligament helps support this joint. Movement is mainly flexion and extension but abduction, adduction and circumduction are possible.

The stifle: this is a complex hinge joint connecting the femur, tibia, fibula and patella. There are two menisci between the femur and tibia. Four ligaments reinforce the joint. The **lateral** and **medial collateral ligaments** prevent lateral movement. The **anterior** and **caudal cruciate ligaments** are crossed ligaments which help prevent cranial and caudal movement of the tibia with respect to the stifle. The cruciate ligaments provide much of the stability of the joint and are commonly damaged when rotational forces are applied to the extended joint. Movement of the stifle is flexion and extension only.

2.3.13   Muscles, tendons and ligaments

What you need to learn

🐾 You need to be able to describe the structure, function and location of different types of muscle tissue. These include skeletal, smooth and cardiac muscle (also see Table 3.4, p. 45).

🐾 Define terms associated with skeletal muscle:
  🐾 bursa
  🐾 synovial sheath
  🐾 tendon
  🐾 origin
  🐾 insertion.

🐾 Describe how muscle contraction is controlled, including intrinsic, extrinsic and muscle tone.

🐾 Describe the location and function of the facial muscles.

🐾 Define the muscles of the trunk, including the paxial and hypaxial vertebral muscles and intercostal muscles.

🐾 Describe the muscular structure of the abdominal wall, including the:
  🐾 external abdominal oblique
  🐾 internal abdominal oblique
  🐾 transverse abdominis
  🐾 rectus abdominis
  🐾 linea alba and pre-pubic tendons.

🐾 Describe the basic structure and function of the cranial and caudal cruciate ligaments and medial and lateral collateral ligaments.

🐾 Describe the structure, functions and attachment of the diaphragm. These include:
  🐾 foramen vena cava
  🐾 aortic hiatus
  🐾 oesophageal hiatus.

🐾 State the position and function of the muscles and tendons of the forelimb. These include:
  🐾 trapezius
  🐾 brachiocephalicus
  🐾 latissimus dorsi
  🐾 supraspinatus
  🐾 infraspinatus
  🐾 triceps
  🐾 biceps brachii
  🐾 brachialis
  🐾 carpal and digital flexors and extensors.

🐾 State the position and function of the muscles and tendons of the hindlimb. These include:
  🐾 quadriceps femoris
  🐾 semimembranosus

❀ semitendinosus
❀ gastrocnemius
❀ biceps femoris
❀ pectineus
❀ cranial (anterior) tibialis
❀ digital flexors and extensors
❀ Achilles tendon.

Skeletal muscle

- The action of muscles on bones allows movement to occur.
- Muscles are attached to bones by **tendons**.
- The more proximal point from which the muscle arises (or the point which moves the least) is called the **origin**. The more distal point where the muscle attaches (or the point which moves the most) is called the **insertion**.
- Circular arrangements of muscle which allow the opening and closing of orifices are called **sphincters**.
- A flat sheet of tendon attaching a muscle to another muscle or bone is called an **aponeurosis**.
- Bones are connected to other bones by **ligaments**.
- Where tendons change direction they are at risk of damage from pressure and friction so at these points many tendons have areas of ossification called **sesamoid bones**.
- Another way the tendons are protected is with fluid-filled cushions or **bursae**. Occasionally the whole circumference of the tendon is wrapped in a protective fluid-filled sheath – the **tendon sheath** or **synovial sheath**.

Muscle contraction

- Most muscles are supplied by a single nerve which branches repeatedly until it reaches the neuro-muscular junction.
- An electrical impulse from a motor nerve stimulates a bundle of muscle cells (the muscle fibres stimulated by one nerve fibre is called a **motor unit**).
- The strength of the muscle contraction depends on how many motor units are stimulated.
- When the muscle is stimulated it tries to shorten. If the muscle is allowed to shorten the contraction is described as **isotonic**. If the muscle is prevented from shortening the contraction is described as **isometric** (common during standing).
- The degree of tension in a muscle is described as the **muscle tone**.

Head and face muscles

- Muscles which move the whole head are called **extrinsic** muscles.
- Muscles which move parts of the head are called **intrinsic** muscles.

Superficial facial muscles

- The superficial facial muscles are innervated by cranial nerve VII – the facial nerve.
- These are the muscles of facial expression.

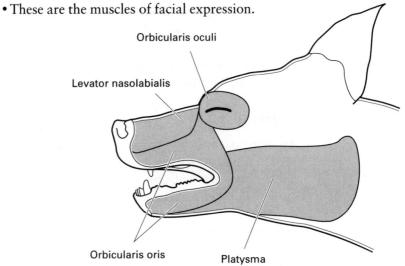

Orbicularis oculi

Levator nasolabialis

Orbicularis oris

Platysma

Figure 3.30 Diagram showing some of the superficial facial muscles of the dog.

Masticatory (chewing) muscles

- The masticatory chewing muscles are innervated by the mandibular branch of cranial nerve V – the trigeminal nerve.

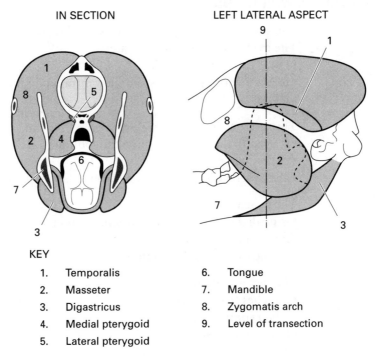

IN SECTION

LEFT LATERAL ASPECT

KEY

1.	Temporalis	6.	Tongue
2.	Masseter	7.	Mandible
3.	Digastricus	8.	Zygomatis arch
4.	Medial pterygoid	9.	Level of transection
5.	Lateral pterygoid		

Figure 3.31 The masticatory muscles of the dog.

Trunk muscles

Epaxial muscles

The epaxial muscles lie dorsal to the transverse processes of the vertebrae and are supplied by the dorsal branches of the spinal nerves. They are the muscles of the dorsal trunk, attaching to the vertebrae, ribs, and caudally to the pelvis. The major muscles are arranged in three parallel columns and are the extensors of the spine.

Hypaxial muscles

The hypaxial muscles lie ventral to the transverse processes of the vertebrae and are supplied by the ventral branches of the spinal nerves. They are the flexor muscles of the neck (and tail). This group also includes the muscles of the abdominal and thoracic walls.

Intercostal muscles

The intercostal muscles form part of the musculature of the thoracic wall.

- There are 12 external intercostal muscles on each side of the thorax. Their function is to draw the ribs together during respiration.
- The internal intercostal muscles are also involved in drawing the ribs together in respiration. Medial to these muscles are the pleurae.

Abdominal wall muscles

There are four abdominal muscles (see Figure 3.32).

The external abdominal oblique:
- fibres run caudoventrally
- forms a wide aponeurosis in the ventral abdominal wall which inserts on the linea alba.

The internal abdominal oblique:
- is deep to the external abdominal oblique
- fibres run cranioventrally
- also inserts on the linea alba through an aponeurosis.

The transversus abdominis:
- is medial to the internal abdominal oblique and rectus abdominis
- fibres run transversely
- aponeurosis attaches to the linea alba.

The rectus abdominis:
- attaches from the ribs to the pelvis, causing flexion of the spine when contracted
- fibres run craniocaudally

• forms part of **pre-pubic tendon** where the linea alba attaches to the pubis.

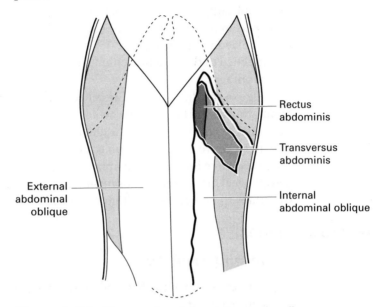

Figure 3.32 The muscles of the abdominal wall.

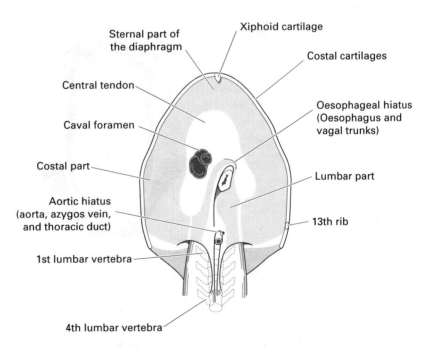

Figure 3.33 The diaphragm.

The diaphragm

- The diaphragm is a domed sheet of muscle which separates the thorax from the abdomen (see Figure 3.33).
- It is involved with respiration.
- It is attached to the vertebral column by paired muscles, the **crura** of the diaphragm.
- The edge of the diaphragm is attached to the ribs while the ventral point attaches to the xiphoid cartilage.
- The outer portion of the diaphragm is muscular.
- The inner, more cranial portion is a tendinous sheet.
- There are three holes in the diaphragm (the aortic hiatus, the oesophageal hiatus and the foramen vena cava) which allow certain structures to pass from the thorax to the abdomen.

The forelimb muscles

Pectoral girdle muscles

- These muscles attach the forelimb to the trunk as there is not a conventional joint.
- The **serratus ventralis** and the **pectoral** muscles form a sling while the dorsal muscles, the **trapezius** and **rhomboideus** elevate the limb and draw it forwards.

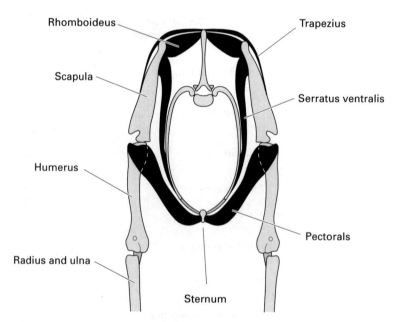

Figure 3.34 The pectoral girdle muscles.

Shoulder and neck muscles

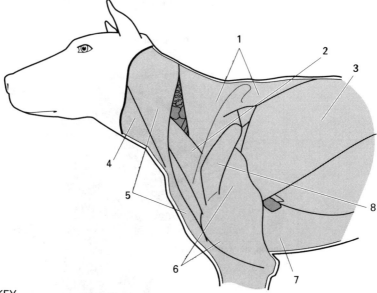

KEY

1. Cervical and thoracic parts of trapezius
2. Omotransversarius
3. Latissimus dorsi
4. Sternocephalicus
5. Brachiocephalicus
6. Triceps
7. Pectoral muscles
8. Deltoideus

Figure 3.35 The muscles of the neck and shoulder.

The muscles of the neck and shoulder are the:

• sternocephalicus (draws head and neck laterally, actions on the tongue and larynx)
• brachiocephalicus (advances the limb, extends shoulder, draws head and neck laterally)
• omotransversarius (advances the limb, draws neck laterally). Trapezius (elevates and abducts forelimb)
• deltoideus (flexes shoulder)
• latissimus dorsi (draws limb caudally and flexes shoulder)
• triceps (extends elbow and flexes shoulder)
• pectorals (adducts limb, extends shoulder).

Deep muscles of the upper forelimb

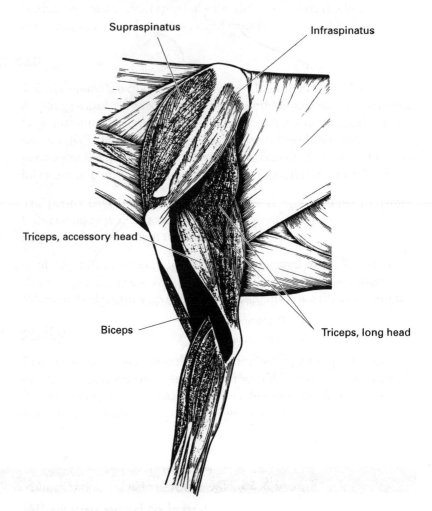

Figure 3.36 The deep muscles of the upper forelimb.

The deep muscles of the upper forelimb are the:

- infraspinatus (extends/flexes joint depending on position of joint, abducts shoulder, rotates limb laterally)
- supraspinatus (extends shoulder)
- biceps brachii (flexes elbow and extends shoulder)
- brachialis (flexes the elbow)
- extensors of carpus and digits
- flexors of carpus and digits.

The hindlimb muscles

Superficial muscles of the upper hindlimb

Lateral view

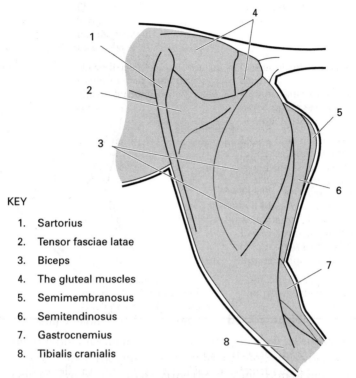

KEY
1. Sartorius
2. Tensor fasciae latae
3. Biceps
4. The gluteal muscles
5. Semimembranosus
6. Semitendinosus
7. Gastrocnemius
8. Tibialis cranialis

Figure 3.37   The superficial muscles of the hindlimb (lateral view).

The superficial muscles of the hindlimb are the:

- gluteals (extend hip, abduct limb)
- tensor fascia latae (tenses fascia lata, flexes hip, extends stifle)
- gastrocnemius (extends the hock and flexes the stifle)
- tibialis cranialis (flexes the hock)
- digital flexors
- digital extensors.

Hamstring muscles

The hamstring muscles are the:

- biceps femoris (extends hip, stifle and hock)
- semitendinosus (extends hip, flexes stifle, extends hock)
- semimembranosus (extends hip).

The tendon of the hamstring and the gastrocnemius muscles inserts on the calcaneus and is often called the **calcanean** or **Achilles tendon**.

Medial view

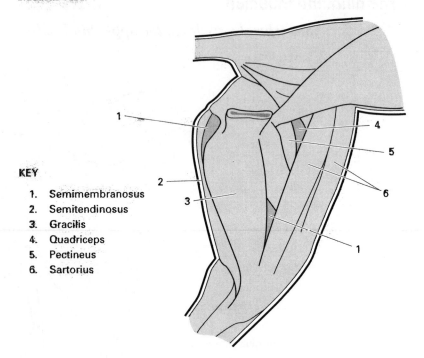

KEY

1. Semimembranosus
2. Semitendinosus
3. Gracilis
4. Quadriceps
5. Pectineus
6. Sartorius

Figure 3.38 The muscles of the hindlimb (medial view).

- sartorius (flexes the hip)
- quadriceps femoris (extends the stifle, flexes the hip)
- pectineus (adducts the limb)
- gracilis (adducts the limb).

2.3.14 Hair and skin

What you need to learn

🐾 You need to be able to describe the structure and functions of the skin, dermal glands, hair and hair growth in different species, including for dogs and cats:

  🐾 sebum
  🐾 cerumen
  🐾 tail and anal glands.

🐾 Explain the functions of different types of hair, such as covering or guarding hairs, vibrissae and eyelashes.

Functions of the skin

- Skin is a barrier against physical and chemical agents.
- It prevents viral, bacterial and fungal infections.
- It provides thermoregulation.
- It allows sensory perception of the environment.
- It stores nutrients, particularly fat but also electrolytes, water and vitamins.
- It allows communication via excretions, eg pheromones, anal gland secretions.
- It produces vitamin D through the action of sunlight.
- It contains pigment which protects from harmful UV light.

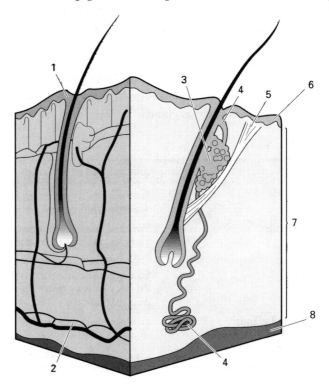

KEY

1.	Hair follicle	5.	Erector pili muscle
2.	Arterial networks	6.	Epidermis
3.	Sebaceous gland	7.	Dermis
4.	Sweat gland	8.	Subcutis

Figure 3.39   The basic structure of skin.

Structure of the skin

Epidermis

- Epidermis is keratinised stratified squamous epithelium.
- It varies in thickness from thin over the haired areas to very thick on the pads of the feet.
- It contains melanocytes in pigmented skin.
- It is anchored to the dermis by the basement membrane.
- Claws are modified epidermis.

Dermis

- Dermis is composed of connective tissue.
- It contains nerves and blood-vessel networks.
- It is thicker than epidermis, providing most of the elasticity and strength.
- It is responsible for repair of damaged skin.
- It contains hair follicles and **arrector pili** muscles.
- It contains various glands.

Table 3.7

Gland	Location and function
Sebaceous glands	Produce an oily secretion, *sebum*, which waterproofs the coat.
Sudorific (sweat) glands	Sweating is a minor route of heat loss in dogs and cats, most of the sweat glands are in the feet.
Ceruminous glands	Found in the outer parts of the ear canal. Produce earwax or *cerumen* which prevents dust reaching the inner parts of the ear.
Peri-anal, anal and tail glands	Produce pheromones which identify the animal to others within its territory.
Mammary glands	Produce milk which nourishes offspring.

Subcutis (hypodermis)

- The subcutis consists of loose connective tissue and fat.
- It varies in thickness.

Hair

- Each hair has a cortex, a medulla and a cuticle.
- Hairs arise from hair follicles within the dermis.
- Each hair has a sebaceous gland associated with its follicle.
- Each hair has an arrector pili muscle adjacent to the follicle which

erects the hair in cold weather so that air can be trapped, thereby conserving heat (this also occurs during stimulation of the sympathetic nervous system).
- **Primary** or **guard hairs** are long and coarse.
- **Secondary hairs** are shorter and softer and make up the undercoat. These tend not to have erector muscles.
- **Vibrissae are touch sensitive or tactile** hairs. They occur on the face and on the palmar surface of the carpus. The vibrissae found on the muzzle are called whiskers.
- **Eyelashes** or **cilia** protect the cornea from dust and foreign material.

The hair cycle

- **Anagen:** hair grows from the follicle.
- **Catagen:** the follicle atrophies.
- **Telogen:** hair is displaced by a new hair developing in the follicle, old hair is lost and anagen begins again.

The hair cycle is affected by season, nutrition, hormones (sex hormones, thyroxine and cortisol), health status and genetics. Hair coats can be **short** (eg Jack Russell terrier, boxer, etc), **intermediate** (eg Labrador) or **long** (eg Afghan hound, cocker spaniel, etc).

Coarse hair coats (eg Border terrier) have greater proportion of primary hairs than those with **fine** coats (eg saluki).

Thermoregulation

1 Hair traps air under the coat using the arrector pili muscles and conserves heat.
2 Subcutaneous fat provides effective insulation.
3 Alteration of blood flow to the skin can either reduce or increase heat loss:

- The autonomic nervous system controls the blood flow to the dermis. If body temperature is raised vasodilation occurs bringing blood closer to the body surface to allow cooling. If body temperature drops vasoconstriction occurs to restrict the amount of blood close to the body surface.
- Numerous arteriovenous anastomoses (AVAs) exist within the dermis. If the body temperature drops these shunt blood directly from the arterioles to the venules preventing it from entering the capillary beds near the surface where it will lose heat.

4 Sweating provides heat loss through evaporation.

2.3.15   Nervous system – general

What you need to learn

* You need to be able to define terms associated with the nervous system and describe its functions. Terms are:
  * central nervous system (CNS)
  * peripheral nervous system (PNS)
  * autonomic nervous system (ANS)
  * sensory and motor fibres
  * somatic and visceral fibres
  * afferent and efferent fibres
  * intercalated neuron
  * synapse
  * ganglion.

The nervous system allows the body to react to its environment. It does this by receiving and interpreting internal and external stimuli and then reacting appropriately. It is the most complex system in the body.

The nervous system can be divided into two main parts:

• the central nervous system (CNS): brain and spinal cord.
• the peripheral nervous system (PNS): cranial, spinal and autonomic nerves.

Neurones which carry impulses towards the brain and spinal cord are called **afferent** neurones. In the PNS these are called **sensory** neurones. Neurones which carry impulses away from the brain and spinal cord are called **efferent** neurones. In the PNS these are called **motor** neurones.

The part of the nervous system responsible for voluntary actions such as locomotion is called the **somatic system**. The part of the nervous system responsible for involuntary actions such as regulation of the internal organs (eg smooth muscle, cardiovascular system, endocrine system) is called the **visceral system**.

The neurones supplying the visceral system are called the autonomic nervous system (ANS) so the ANS controls the regulation of the internal organs. The ANS provides innervation of the viscera with two sets of nerves – the **sympathetic** and **parasympathetic** divisions. The actions of these two divisions are usually antagonistic (opposite).

The basic structure of a nerve cell was described on page 44.

The meninges and brain (also see 2.3.16)

The meninges

These are membranes which suspend and protect the brain and spinal cord. Inflammation of the meninges is called **meningitis.**

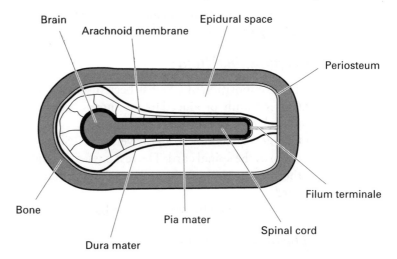

Figure 3.40 Schematic representation of the meninges surrounding the brain and spinal cord.

1 Epidural space

- This is a virtual space in the brain filled with fat and blood vessels.
- The space is wider in the spine where it is filled with loose areolar tissue and vessels, and is often used as site for injection of local anaesthetics.

2 Dura mater

- This is the outermost membrane.
- It is made of dense connective tissue.

3 Subdural space

- This is a virtual space but it can become enlarged following injury – subdural haemorrhage.

4 Arachnoid

- This is a delicate, avascular membrane.
- Its inner surface has fine filaments joining to the pia mater.

5 Subarachnoid space

- This space contains CSF.

- It widens at the **cisterna magna** (between atlas and skull) and **lumbar cistern** (Dog: L5–L6, Cat L6–L7), where it can be used to sample CSF.

6 *Pia mater*

- This is the innermost membrane covering the brain and spinal cord.
- It is highly vascular.

Cerebrospinal fluid

- The composition of CSF has been discussed on page 53.
- CSF is mainly produced by the **choroid plexuses** which are located in each of the ventricles of the brain.
- CSF flows caudally from the ventricles. Some enters the central canal of the spinal cord. The rest passes through small channels into the subarachnoid space and circulates around the brain and spinal cord.
- CSF is removed by drainage into blood and lymphatic vessels.

The blood–brain barrier

The permeability of the capillaries in the nervous tissue is greatly reduced. This prevents many molecules from diffusing from the blood to the brain and spinal cord. Many antibiotics are unable to cross this blood–brain barrier, making the treatment of CNS infections difficult.

2.3.16   Brain

What you need to learn

- You need to be able to describe the structure and functions of the brain and define associated terms. These include:
  - fore, mid and hindbrain
  - medulla oblongata
  - cerebellum
  - cerebral hemispheres
  - optic chiasm
  - olfactory bulbs
  - cranial nerves.
- Describe the function of the ventricular system of the brain.
- Describe the structure, location and function of the meninges (see 2.3.15).
- Describe the circulation and function of CSF (see 2.3.15).
- List the cranial nerves and their function.

The brain is divided into the forebrain, midbrain and hindbrain.

The forebrain: cerebrum, thalamus and hypothalamus

Cerebrum

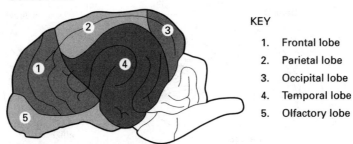

KEY

1. Frontal lobe
2. Parietal lobe
3. Occipital lobe
4. Temporal lobe
5. Olfactory lobe

Figure 3.41   The cerebral cortex.

• This is the centre for the higher functions such as sensation, olfaction (smell), vision and hearing.
• It is divided into two **cerebral hemispheres** separated by the **longitudinal cleft** or **fissure**.
• It is separated into lobes: the **frontal** lobe, **parietal** lobe, **occipital** lobe and **temporal** lobe.
• The left cerebral hemisphere controls the right side of the body and vice versa.

Thalamus

• This receives sensory input (except olfaction) and relays it to the relevant part of the brain (usually the cerebral cortex).

Hypothalamus

• This is concerned with thermoregulation, emotion and control of the autonomic nervous system and pituitary gland.
• The **optic chiasm** is the place where crossing over of nerves involved with vision occurs. It lies on the ventral surface of the forebrain.

The midbrain

• The midbrain sits between the thalamus and the pons.
• It contains the **aqueduct** which connects the third and fourth ventricles.
• It passes information regarding vision and hearing to the forebrain.

The hindbrain: pons, medulla oblongata and cerebellum

Pons

The pons is continuous with the medulla oblongata and shares many functions.

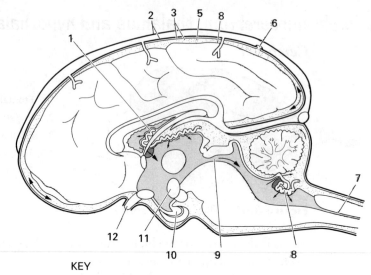

KEY

1. Choroid plexus, lateral ventricle
2. Dura
3. Arachnoid membrane and trabeculae
4. Subarachnoid space
5. Pia
6. Arachnoid villus
7. Central canal
8. Choroid plexus, fourth ventricle
9. Mesencephalic aqueduct
10. Hypophysis
11. Hypothalamus
12. Optic nerve

Figure 3.42 The sagittal section of the brain.

Medulla oblongata

- The medulla oblongata controls involuntary actions such as respiration, heart rate and digestion.
- It contains nuclei of some of the cranial nerves.
- It is continuous with the spinal cord.

Cerebellum

- The cerebellum is separated into two hemispheres – the cerebral hemispheres.
- It controls balance and co-ordination of posture and locomotion.
- The left hemisphere controls the left side of the body and vice versa.

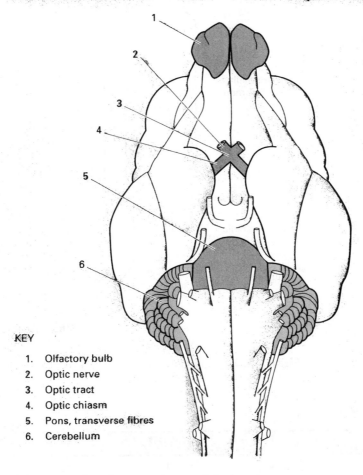

KEY

1. Olfactory bulb
2. Optic nerve
3. Optic tract
4. Optic chiasm
5. Pons, transverse fibres
6. Cerebellum

Figure 3.43 The ventral view of the brain.

The ventricles of the brain

- The ventricles are four connected cavities within the brain.
- They contain CSF.
- The lateral ventricles are within the cerebral hemispheres.
- The third ventricle surrounds the thalamus.
- The fourth ventricle lies between the cerebellum and the brainstem and continues as the central canal of the spinal cord.

See Figure 3.44.

The blood supply to the brain

- The blood supply to the brain is provided by the internal corotid arteries and the occipital arteries.
- These vessels branch and join together in a circular formation called the circle of Willis.
- Blood eventually drains into the jugular vein.

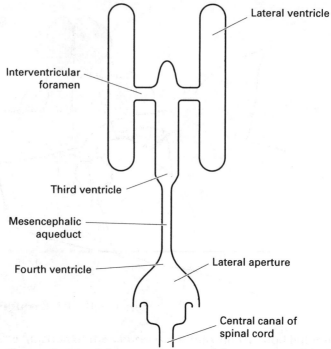

Lateral ventricle

Interventricular foramen

Third ventricle

Mesencephalic aqueduct

Fourth ventricle

Lateral aperture

Central canal of spinal cord

Figure 3.44 Schematic diagram of the ventricles of the brain.

Table 3.8

Nerve	Name	Sensory function	Motor function
I	Olfactory	Smell	
II	Optic	Vision	
III	Oculomotor	Eyeball muscles	Eye muscles and iris
IV	Trochlear	Eyeball muscles	Eyeball muscles
V	Trigeminal	Most facial structures	Masticatory muscles
VI	Abducens	Eyeball muscles	Eyeball muscles
VII	Facial	Taste	Facial, scalp and neck muscles Lacrimal/salivary glands
VIII	Vestibulocochlear	Hearing and balance	
IX	Glossopharyngeal	Taste	Swallowing
X	Vagus	Organs supplied by motor fibres	Respiratory tract, gastrointestinal tract
XI	Accessory	Muscles supplied by motor fibres	Pharynx, larynx and palate
XII	Hypoglossal	Tongue muscles	Tongue muscles

The cranial nerves

> • The 12 pairs of cranial nerves arise directly from the brain.
> • They are numbered from cranial to caudal (see Table 3.8).

2.3.17   Spinal cord

What you need to learn

❦ You need to be able to describe the structure, location and function of the spinal cord.

❦ Describe the structure of the cauda equina and state the site where it is found.

❦ Describe the structure of a typical spinal nerve, list the branches of which it is comprised and outline its function.

❦ Describe a simple reflex arc, a spinal reflex and state the nerve pathways involved in these. This includes simple and complex reflexes.

The posterior portion of the CNS is located within the vertebral canal of the bony spinal column. It starts from the foramen magnum at the back of the skull and extends caudally, terminating in the **cauda equina**. It is continuous with the medulla oblongata. The spinal cord is shorter than the vertebral canal, ending between L6–7 in the dog and between L6–S3 in the cat. The caudal spinal nerves travel together down the remainder of the vertebral column before emerging from their foramina. This bundle of spinal nerves is called the cauda equina. Every segment's paired spinal nerves pass out of the vertebral column through the intervertebral foramina.

A transverse section of the spinal cord is shown in Figure 3.45.

• The grey matter contains the cell bodies of the neurones.
• It is divided into three horns: the **dorsal horn** receives sensory inputs; the **lateral horn** contains both sensory and motor fibres; the **ventral horn** contains motor fibres.
• The **white matter** contains myelinated fibres in bundles called **tracts**.
• Afferent nerves enter the spinal cord through the **dorsal root**. The **dorsal root ganglion** contains the cell bodies of these nerves.
• Efferent nerves leave the spinal cord through the **ventral root**.
• The afferent and efferent nerves merge a short distance from the spinal cord creating the **spinal nerve**.

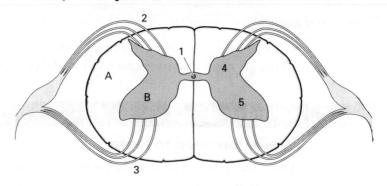

KEY

A. White matter   B. Grey matter

1. Central canal   4. Dorsal horn

2. Fibres of the dorsal root   5. Ventral horn

3. Fibres of the ventral root

Figure 3.45 Transverse sections of the spinal cord.

Stimulus response activity

The five basic elements necessary for a response to a stimulus to occur are:

1 a **receptor** receives the stimulus
2 an **afferent neurone** carries the impulse to the brain/spinal cord
3 a **synapse** occurs across the bridge between the afferent and efferent neurones
4 an **efferent neurone** carries an impulse back from the CNS to the PNS
5 an **effector**, this is usually a muscle or gland, responds to the impulse.

Simple reflex arc: the patellar reflex

There are five elements to the patellar reflex (see Figure 3.46):

1 **receptor:** stretch receptors on the patellar tendon
2 **afferent neurone:** afferent sensory fibres within the femoral nerve
3 **synapse** within the spinal cord
4 **efferent neurone:** efferent motor fibres within the femoral nerve
5 **effector:** muscle fibres within the quadriceps femoris are stimulated causing muscle contraction.

• Most reflexes are more complex than this, involving stimulation

and inhibition of numerous neurones to allow fine control.
- Further neurones can be stimulated which travel to the brain, making the animal conscious of the reflex.
- In these cases there are smaller **interneurones** between the afferent and efferent neurones.
- An example is a noxious stimulus such as a burn or pinprick (see Figure 3.47):

1 **Receptor:** pain receptor in the skin.
2 **Afferent neurone:** sensory neurone within local nerve.
3 **Synapse:** synapses (in the spinal cord) with a number of interneurones which pass impulses cranially to the brain, and across to the opposite limb so the animal can adjust its position to move away from the noxious stimulus. There is also a synapse directly with the efferent neurone.

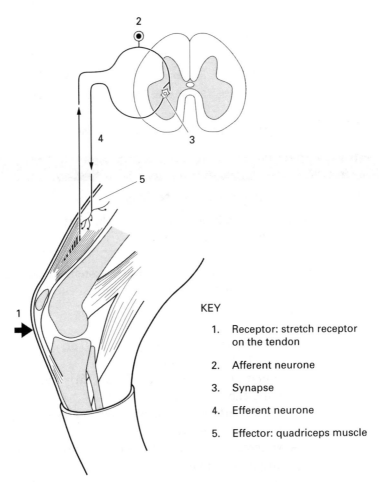

KEY

1. Receptor: stretch receptor on the tendon

2. Afferent neurone

3. Synapse

4. Efferent neurone

5. Effector: quadriceps muscle

Figure 3.46 A simple reflex arc: the patellar reflex.

4 **Efferent neurone:** motor neurone within local nerve as well as various neurones from the brain and in other limbs.
5 **Effector:** the brain and various muscles.

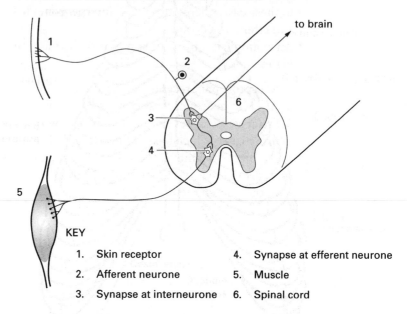

KEY

1.	Skin receptor	4.	Synapse at efferent neurone
2.	Afferent neurone	5.	Muscle
3.	Synapse at interneurone	6.	Spinal cord

Figure 3.47 A reflex chain involving an interneurone.

2.3.18 Peripheral nervous system

What you need to learn

☙ You need to be able to describe the anatomy and function of the peripheral nerve pathways.

The PNS consists of the nervous system outside the CNS, ie the cranial, spinal and autonomic nerves.

There are four types of neurones:

1 **somatic afferent (sensory) fibres** – carry information from skin, muscle, bone and joints
2 **somatic efferent (motor) fibres** – carry motor output to skin, muscle, bone and joints
3 **visceral afferent (sensory) fibres** – carry sensory information from the organs (viscera)
4 **visceral efferent (motor fibres)** – motor output to viscera, glands and smooth muscle

• The connective tissue surrounding each nerve fibre is called the **endoneurium**.
• The connective tissue surrounding bundles of nerve fibres is called

the **perineurium**.
- The connective tissue which surrounds the whole nerve is called the **epineurium**.
- **Receptors** are modified nerve cells which can detect a stimulus. Examples are stretch receptors in muscles and tendons; rod and cone cells in the retina; and pain, heat and pressure receptors within the skin.
- Receptors which monitor the internal environment (blood pressure, temperature, carbon dioxide and oxygen levels in the blood etc) are called **interioreceptors**.
- Receptors which monitor the external environment (the five senses) are called **exterioreceptors**.

Examples of important spinal nerves include the:

- **radial nerve** which is an important nerve in the forelimb
- **femoral nerve** and the **sciatic nerve** are important nerves in the hindlimb.

2.3.19   Autonomic nervous system

What you need to learn

- You need to be able to explain the differences in structure and function between sympathetic and parasympathetic fibres.
- Explain the control of heart rate, blood pressure, gastrointestinal motility, respiratory function, fight or flight response.

The neurones supplying the visceral system are called the autonomic nervous system (ANS) and control the regulation of the internal organs. The ANS provides innervation of the viscera with two sets of nerves – the **sympathetic** and **parasympathetic** divisions. The actions of these two divisions are usually antagonistic (opposite).

- The sympathetic nervous system prepares the body for action, it is the **'fight or flight'** part of the peripheral nervous system.
- Mass sympathetic response is activated when **adrenaline** is released from the brain.
- Sympathetic fibres use **noradrenaline** as the neurotransmitter.
- The ganglia of the sympathetic nervous system forms the **sympathetic trunk** which runs the length of the spine.
- The parasympathetic nervous system is the **'rest and digest'** part of the PNS.
- The actions of the parasympathetic system tend to be more specific and discrete than those of the sympathetic system.
- Parasympathetic fibres use **acetylcholine** as the neurotransmitter.
- The ganglia of the parasympathetic nerves are located on the target

organ. Many of the parasympathetic fibres are carried in the **vagus nerve** (cranial nerve X) which runs with the sympathetic trunk and is then called the **vagosympathetic trunk**.

2.3.20   Special sense organ – eye

What you need to learn

❋ You need to be able to describe the anatomy and function of the eyelids and lacrymal apparatus:
  ❋ conjunctiva
  ❋ third eyelid
  ❋ lacrymal apparatus
  ❋ meibomian gland
  ❋ lateral and medial canthus.
❋ Describe the anatomy and function of the eye and define associated terms:
  ❋ sclera
  ❋ uvea
  ❋ retina
  ❋ cornea
  ❋ choroids
  ❋ iris
  ❋ rods

Table 3.9

Target organ	Sympathetic effect	Parasympathetic effect
Iris	Dilation of pupil	Constriction of pupil
Heart	Increased cardiac output (heart rate and strength of contraction)	Decreased cardiac output (heart rate and strength of contraction)
Blood vessels	Increased blood flow to muscles Decreased blood flow to skin and gastrointestinal tract	Decreased blood flow to muscles Increased blood flow to gastrointestinal tract
Salivary glands	Decreased secretion	Increased secretion
Gastrointestinal tract	Decreased peristalsis Decreased secretions of digestive enzymes	Increased peristalsis Increased secretion of digestive enzymes.
Bladder	Sphincter constricts Bladder wall relaxes	Sphincter relaxes Bladder wall constricts
Bronchi	Relaxation	Constriction
Erector pili muscles	Constrict (hair stands up)	No action
Erectile tissue		Vasodilation of erectile tissue

* cones
* ciliary body
* anterior chamber
* posterior chamber
* aqueous humour
* vitreous humour
* pupil
* biconvex lens
* limbus
* tapetum
* suspensory ligament
* optic nerve.
* Describe how an image is formed.

The eye is the organ of vision. It consists of the eyeball (globe) which sits in the orbit on a pad of periorbital fat. The supportive structures, known collectively as the **adnexa**, are the:

* ocular muscles (controlled by cranial nerves III, IV and VI)
* eyelids (**palpebrae**)
* Lacrimal (tear-producing) apparatus.

The eyelids

* Each eyelid is supported by a fibrocartilage plate called the **tarsal plate**.
* The outer surface of the eyelid is covered with haired skin.
* The inner surface of the eyelid is lined with mucous membrane called the **conjunctiva**.
* The edge of the eyelid is lined by the openings of the **tarsal or meibomian glands** which contribute to the tear film.
* Just in front of the tarsal glands are the eyelashes (**cilia**).
* At the medial **canthus** (where the upper and lower lids join) the eyelids are firmly anchored, whereas at the lateral canthus they are more mobile.
* At the medial canthus is the protective third eyelid (**nictitating membrane**). This is a fold of conjunctiva supported by a T-shaped piece of cartilage.

The lacrimal apparatus

* The apparatus includes the lacrimal glands, the conjunctival sac and the lacrimal passages.
* This provides the **tear film** which lubricates, protects and nourishes the cornea.

See Figure 3.48.

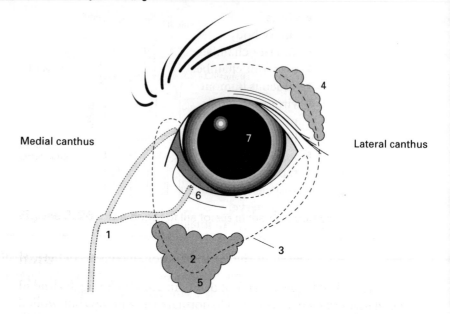

Medial canthus   Lateral canthus

KEY

Left eye of dog showing third eyelid and lacrimal apparatus

1. Nasolacrimal duct
2. Deep gland of the third eyelid
3. Third eyelid
4. Lacrimal gland
5. Gland of the third eyelid
6. Punctum lacrimale
7. Pupil

Figure 3.48   The third eyelid and lacrimal apparatus.

The globe

See Figure 3.49.

- The **outer coat** is composed of the **sclera** (tough white outer coat) and the **cornea**. The cornea and sclera meet at the **limbus**.
- The **cornea** is transparent because of the lack of blood vessels, the regular arrangement of the substance of the cornea (stroma), and because it contains very little water. The cornea is highly sensitive.
- The **middle layer** is composed of the **choroid,** the **ciliary body,** and the **iris** with its supporting structures. Together these structures are called the **uvea.**
- The iris is pigmented and contains circular and radial smooth muscle fibres. These muscle fibres alter the diameter of the aperture within the iris – the **pupil.**
- The choroid is a pigmented layer which lines the internal surface of

the sclera. This layer contains blood vessels. Part of this layer has a reflective surface, the **tapetum lucidum**.

- The ciliary body is between the iris and the choroid and contains muscles. **Suspensory ligaments** attach these muscles to the **lens** so that the shape of the lens can be altered.
- The **inner layer** is composed of the **retina** and its associated blood vessels and nerves.
- The retina is made up of ten layers of cells which can be separated into a layer of nervous tissue, and a layer of retinal pigment epithelium which overlies the choroid.

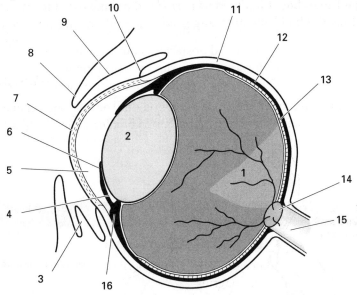

KEY

1. Tapetum lucidum
2. Lens
3. Third eyelid
4. Posterior chamber
5. Anterior chamber
6. Iris
7. Cornea
8. Superior eyelid
9. Palpebral conjunctiva
10. Bulbar conjunctiva
11. Sclera
12. Choroid
13. Retina
14. Optic disc
15. Optic nerve
16. Ciliary body

Figure 3.49 Cross-section of the globe and associated structure.

- The retina contains the **photoreceptor cells** (**rods** and **cones**) which receive light and convert it to electrical impulses. These travel through the optic chiasm and to the brain through the **optic nerve** (cranial nerve II) and images are perceived in the **visual cortex** of the cerebrum.

- The rods are sensitive to different **intensities** of light and are responsible for night vision.
- The cones are sensitive to different **wavelengths** of light and are responsible for colour vision.
- The blind spot is the optic disc where the optic nerve leaves the eye. There are no photoreceptor cells in the blind spot.
- The fovea (or yellow spot) is the area of the retina with the most acute vision. It contains many cone cells.

The lens and humors

- The iris divides the space between the lens and the cornea into the **anterior** and **posterior chambers**. Both of these chambers are filled with watery fluid, the **aqueous humor**.
- The rest of the globe is filled with a more viscous liquid, the **vitreous humor**.
- The lens is a fairly solid structure which changes shape to focus the image onto the retina. This is called **accommodation**. The lens is **biconvex**.

2.3.21   Special sense organ – ear

What you need to learn

- You need to be able to describe the structure of the ear and define associated terms:
  - external, middle and inner ear
  - pinna
  - external auditory meatus
  - tympanic membrane
  - auricular and annular cartilages.
- Explain the function of the ear and of its individual components that allows the detection of sound and balance. This includes:
  - auditory ossicles (malleus, incus and stapes)
  - oval window
  - round window
  - bony and membranous labyrinth
  - ventricle
  - saccule
  - semicircular canals
  - perilymph
  - endolymph
  - auditory or eustachian tube
  - organ of Corti.

The ear has two functions: hearing and balance.

The auditory (hearing) system consists of the external ear, the middle ear, and the cochlear part of the inner ear. The vestibular (balance) system consists of the **utricle**, the **saccule** and the **semicircular canals**.

The auditory system

Sound waves cause vibrations in the air which are detected by the auditory system and converted to electrical impulses. These impulses travel through the vestibulocochlear nerve (cranial nerve VIII) to the auditory areas of the cerebral cortex and are perceived as sounds.

- The **external ear** consists of the **pinna**, the **external auditory meatus** or **canal** and the **tympanic membrane**.
- The pinna varies greatly in shape and, in some species, can be moved to collect sounds (eg Alsatians.) The supporting cartilages of the pinna (**auricular cartilages**) determine its shape.
- The external auditory meatus is supported by encircling cartilage – the **annular cartilage**.
- The tympanic membrane separates the external ear from the middle ear.

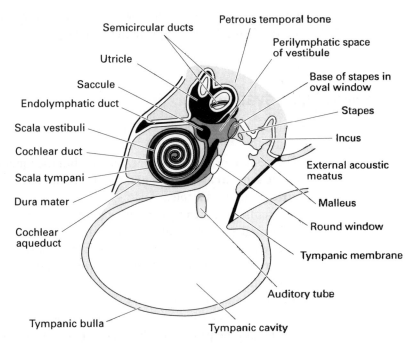

Figure 3.50 The middle and inner ear.

- The **middle ear** is an air-filled cavity within the temporal bone. The bony case is called the **typmanic bulla**.
- A tube called the **auditory** or **eustachian tube** communicates with

the nasopharynx. This ensures that the pressure in the middle ear remains the same as the outside air pressure.

- Three tiny bones (auditory ossicles), the **malleus** (hammer), **incus** (anvil) and **stapes** (stirrup) transmit the sound-wave vibrations across the inner ear and onto the **vestibular window** (oral window).
- The vestibular window transmits vibrations into the inner ear. A second window, the **cochlear window** (round window), leads to the cavity of the cochlea.
- The function of the middle ear is to amplify the sounds.
- The **inner ear** consists of a bony labyrinth which is in two parts which form the vestibular and cochlear systems.
- Inside all the tunnels of the bony labyrinth is a fluid called **perilymph**. Within this cavity is a **membranous labyrinth** lined with a fluid called **endolymph**.
- The **cochlea** is a system of coiled tubes which resembles a snail's shell. It contains the **organ of Corti** which changes vibrations into electrical impulses.
- The organ of Corti consists of numerous hair cells which detect tiny changes in pressure in the perilymph (caused by vibrations from sound waves). The organ of Corti can detect sounds of different frequencies.
- Changes in pressure in the perilymph cause the cochlear window to bulge. This prevents damage to the delicate structures of the inner ear.

The vestibular system

- This system informs the CNS of the movement and position of the head.
- The vestibular system is contained within the inner ear. It consists of the **semicircular canals** and two bony sac-like structures, the **utricle** and the **saccule**.
- The semicircular canals are three loop-shaped canals arranged at right-angles to one another. They contain endolymph.
- The sensory receptors in the semicircular canals are hair cells which detect movement of the fluid within the canals. Because of the orientation of the canals they detect rotational acceleration and deceleration of the head.
- Similar sensory receptors within the utricle and saccule sense changes in the posture of the head. These sensory receptor cells convert the information to electrical impulses which travel through the vestibulocochlear nerve (cranial nerve VIII) to the cerebellum where balance and movement is controlled.

2.3.22   Circulatory system – blood

What you need to learn

❧ You need to be able to describe the types, structure, formation, functions and life span of cells that occur in blood:
  - ❧ erythocyte
  - ❧ neutrophil
  - ❧ eosinophil
  - ❧ basophil
  - ❧ lymphocyte
  - ❧ monocyte
  - ❧ thrombocyte
  - ❧ reticulocyte.

❧ State the value of a normal total erythrocyte and white blood cell count and their relative proportions.

❧ Define plasma and serum and outline their constituents.

❧ State sites in the body where myeloid tissue is found.

❧ Itemise and understand the functions of blood. Describe the processes of blood clotting and phagocytosis. This includes normal clotting times.

❧ Itemise and understand the factors which increase or decrease clotting times.

Functions of blood

- Blood is a transport system for distributing oxygen, nutrients and water to the tissues.
- It removes waste products from the tissues.
- It distributes hormones.
- It protects animals from infection (by transporting cells and substances of the immune system).
- It heals and repairs tissues (via the clotting cascade).
- It controls temperature (through dilation and constriction of surface blood vessels).

Blood makes up approximately 8%–10% of body mass.
Blood is made up various cells suspended in a liquid (**plasma**).

Cells

Red blood cells: erythrocytes

These cells are specialised for carrying oxygen. They do not possess a nucleus, mitochondria or ribosomes. For this reason they are unable to regenerate or repair and so have a short life span (about 4 months).

They are biconcave to increase surface area for oxygen–carbon dioxide exchange. This shape also makes the erythrocyte flexible so it can squeeze through gaps in capillaries. Approximately 95% of the inside of the cell is made from haemoglobin – a protein which contains iron and carries oxygen molecules. Where oxygen levels are low (eg an exercising muscle) some oxygen diffuses from the haemoglobin molecule into the tissue. The oxygen is replaced by a carbon dioxide molecule from the tissues. This returns with the blood to the lungs and is breathed out.

The production of erythrocytes (**erythropoiesis**) occurs in the liver and spleen in the foetus. In the adult, erythropoiesis occurs only in the bone marrow. Old or damaged erythrocytes are removed from the circulation by the spleen. Erythrocyte production is stimulated by a hormone called **erythropoietin** which is produced in the kidney and released when blood oxygen levels drop.

Immature red blood cells are called **reticulocytes**. They often have visible remnants of the nucleus. Reticulocytes are seen in greater numbers when the body is regenerating erythrocytes, eg after blood loss.

The proportion of the blood which is made up of red blood cells is called the **packed cell volume (PCV)** or **haematocrit**. It is expressed as

Table 3.10

Type of Cell	Function	Other details
Neutrophil (See Figures 3.51 and 3.52).	Phagocytosis and destruction of bacteria. Immature (band) neutrophils are released in acute inflammatory processes (*shift to the left*).	~60% of WBC count Life span ~8h. Never return to circulation once they have left. Produced in the bone marrow.
Eosinophil	Increase in numbers with allergic processes and parasite infestations.	~5% of WBC count Life span ~30 min. Cytoplasmic granules inactivate histamine. Produced in the bone marrow.
Basophil	Behave like mast cells, releasing histamine in allergic reactions.	~0%–1% of WBC count Rarely seen. Produced in the bone marrow.
Lymphocyte	Important component of immune response. Production of antibodies. NB not capable of phagocytosis.	~20%–30% of WBC count Produced in bone marrow and lymph nodes (and the thymus gland in young animals).
Monocyte	Leave the blood and enter the tissues as macrophages. Phagocytose pathogens. Involved in immune response. Destroy tumour cells.	~5% of WBC count. Can move freely among the tissues. Long lived.

a percentage. Normal values are 40%–45% in the dog and 35%–40% in the cat.

A decrease in the number of circulating erythrocytes is called **anaemia**. It can be caused by blood loss, increased destruction of erythrocytes or decreased production by the bone marrow.

White blood cells: leucocytes

There are five types of white blood cells and they can be divided into two groups (see Table 3.10):

• granulocytes (cytoplasm contains granules) – neutrophils, eosinophils, basophils
• agranulocytes (no granules in cytoplasm) – lymphocytes and monocytes.

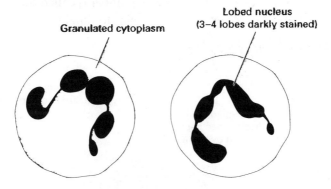

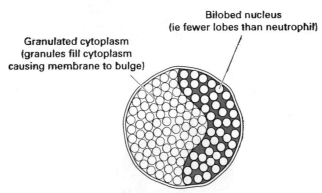

Figure 3.51 White blood cells.

Platelets (thrombocytes)

• Platelets are small cellular fragments derived from **megakaryocytes** in the bone marrow.
• They form plugs to help repair damaged vessels. When they form

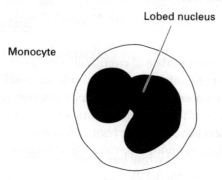

Figure 3.52 Platelets.

plugs platelets release chemicals which cause vasoconstriction, thereby reducing the size of the damaged vessel.
• A decrease in thrombocyte number is called thrombocytopaenia and can result in spontaneous bleeding.

Production of blood cells

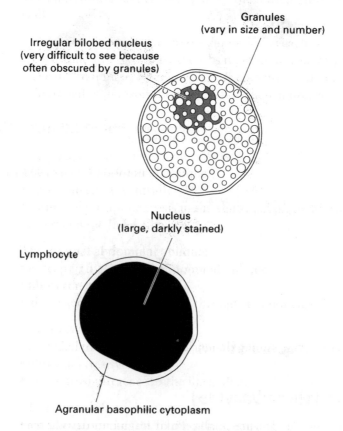

Figure 3.53 Blood cell production.

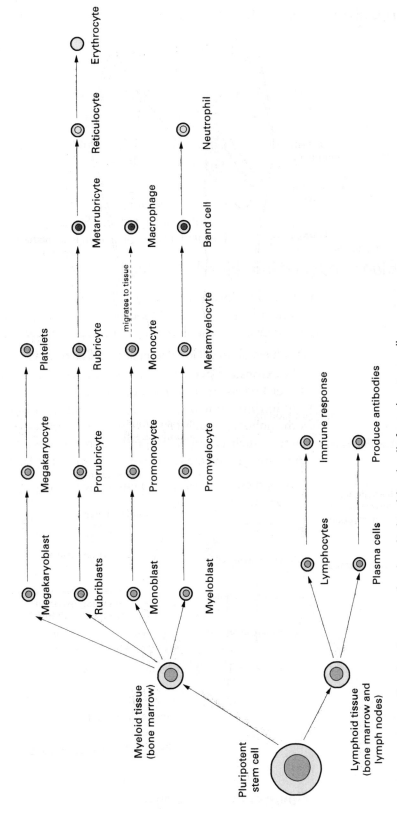

Figure 3.54 The development of red and white blood cells from the stem cell.

Plasma

Plasma is the liquid in which the cells are suspended. Plasma contains:

- plasma proteins (mainly albumin and globulin)
- clotting proteins (such as fibrinogen)
- hormones
- metabolic substrates and products (lipids, carbohydrates such as glucose, vitamins, amino acids, etc)
- water.

When blood has clotted the clotting proteins have all been used up. The liquid remaining is called **serum**. (Serum therefore contains all the same things as plasma except clotting proteins.)

Blood coagulation (blood clotting)

If there is damage to a blood vessel it is vital that a clot forms to prevent a large volume of blood being lost with potentially fatal consequences. For a blood clot to form two pathways must be activated:

- **The extrinsic system:** damaged cells in the tissues (outside the blood vessels) release tissue thromboplastin.
- **The intrinsic system:** damage to the lining of the blood vessel causes a thrombocyte plug to form. This reacts with a number of blood factors (such as von Willebrand's factor, vitamin K and calcium ions) stimulating the release of more thromboplastin.

If both these systems are activated, the clotting cascade is triggered (Figure 3.55).

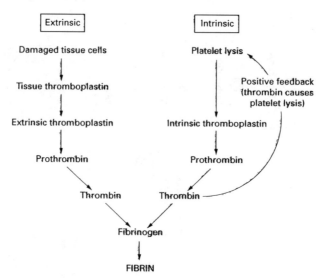

Figure 3.55 The clotting cascade.

Factors causing an increased clotting time (see Table 3.11):

Table 3.11

Cause	Action	Symptoms
Thrombocytopaenia	Lack of thrombocytes prevents plugs from forming in damaged blood vessels	Petechiae/ecchymoses on skin and mucous membranes.
Rodenticide poisoning, eg warfarin	Blocks vitamin K action in clotting cascade	Haemorrhage. Can be treated by supplementing vitamin K.
Deficiency of blood factors	Eg Von Willebrand's disease in Dobermans.	Haemorrhage. Disease is hereditary.
Overdose of anti-coagulant	EDTA scavenges calcium ions, heparin locks up thrombin.	Haemorrhage.
Disease	Eg disseminated intravascular coagulation (DIC). Clotting factors are all used up forming millions of microthrombi.	Haemorrhage results from lack of all clotting components – usually fatal condition.

2.3.23 Heart

What you need to learn

❧ You need to be able to describe the function and location of the heart.
❧ Describe the basic anatomy of the heart:
  ❧ endocardium
  ❧ myocardium
  ❧ epicardium
  ❧ pericardium
  ❧ atria
  ❧ ventricles
  ❧ atrioventricular valves
  ❧ chordae tendineae
  ❧ papillary muscles
  ❧ pulmonic and aortic semilunar valves
  ❧ Purkinje fibres.
❧ Explain systole and diastole and the method of control of cardiac contraction.
❧ Describe the cardiac cycle and explain the origin of the sounds heard on auscultation.
❧ Outline the control of blood pressure and explain the difference between diastolic and systolic pressures.
❧ Define functional terms related to the heart, pulse rate, rhythm and volume).

The heart is the organ which contracts rhythmically to pump blood around the body. It is located within the thorax.

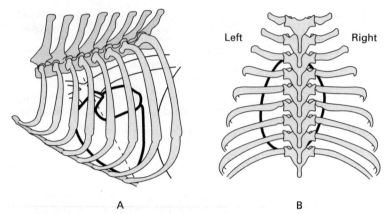

Figure 3.56 The location of the heart within the thorax.

The structure and general position of the heart is the same in all mammals. The regulation of the rate and strength of the heart beats ensures that sufficient blood is delivered to the rest of the body.

Anatomy of the heart

- The heart sits within the **pericardium,** a closed sac of serous membrane. A small amount of **pericardial fluid** allows the heart to move easily within the pericardium. The heart and pericardium sit within the mediastinum.
- The **epicardium** is the outer surface of the heart.
- The **myocardium** is the muscular wall of the heart.
- The **endocardium** is the layer lining the inner walls of the heart.
- The heart is divided into four chambers: the right atrium, left atrium, right ventricle and left ventricle.
- The left and right atria are separated by a **septum,** as are the left and right ventricles.
- The atrium and ventricle of each side communicate through a large opening, the **atrioventricular valve.** (NB The left atrioventricular valve is sometimes called the bicuspid or mitral valve; the right atrioventricular valve is sometimes called the tricuspid valve.)
- The right atrium receives deoxygenated blood from the body and the right ventricle pumps this blood out to the lungs.
- The left atrium receives oxygenated blood back from the lungs and the left ventricle pumps this blood out to the rest of the body.
- The myocardium of the left ventricle is therefore thicker and stronger than that of the right ventricle.
- Blood flows into the atria from the body. When the atria contract the blood flows into the ventricles.

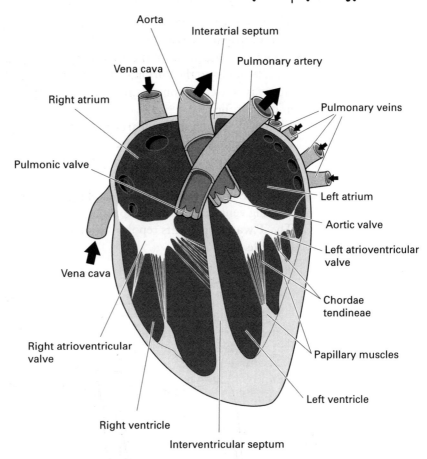

Figure 3.57 The internal structure of the heart.

- The atrioventricular valves are a series of thin **leaflets** which are anchored by fibrous strands (**chordae tendineae**) to the **papillary muscles**. The function of these valves is to close when the ventricles contract so that blood cannot flow back into the atria.
- The blood leaves the heart when the ventricles contract. It passes through another set of valves which close after the contraction to prevent blood flowing back into the ventricles. On the right side of the heart the valve is called the **pulmonic valve**. On the left side it is called the **aortic valve**. (NB These valves are sometimes called semilunar valves.)

The electrical activity of the heart

- The rhythmic beating of the heart is controlled by a pacemaker – the **sinoatrial node** which is located in the wall of the right atrium. Impulses from this node cause the atria to contract together.

- The impulse then passes towards another pacemaker node – the **atrioventricular node**.
- Excitation spreads from the atrioventricular node through the Bundle of His to the **Purkinje fibres** in the walls of the ventricles. In this way muscular contraction of both ventricles is co-ordinated and controlled.
- Electrical activity in the heart can be measured using an **electrocardiograph (ECG) machine**.
- The **P wave** represents depolarisation of the atria, causing atrial contraction.
- The **QRS complex** represents depolarisation of the ventricles causing ventricular contraction.
- The **T wave** represents repolarisation of the ventricles during diastole.

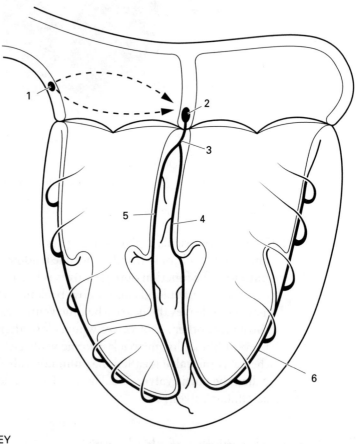

KEY

1.	Sino-atrial node	4.	Left bundle	the Purkinje system
2.	Atrio-ventricular node	5.	Right bundle	
3.	Bundle of His	6.	Purkinje fibres	

Figure 3.58 The conduction pathways within the heart.

Electrical activity

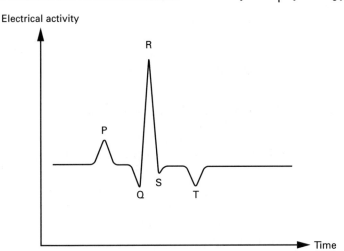

Figure 3.59 An ECG trace.

The cardiac cycle

- The **cardiac cycle** describes the mechanical activity of the heart during one heartbeat.
- The relaxation period between beats is called **diastole**. This is the longest phase of the cardiac cycle. The atrioventricular valves are open but the aortic and pulmonary valves are closed. The ventricles fill with blood.
- When an electrical impulse arrives in the ventricles contraction of the ventricular myocardium begins. This contraction phase is called **systole**.
- The increase in pressure in the ventricle during systole forces the atrioventricular valves to close. At this point the **first heart sound** (**lub**) can be heard using a stethoscope.
- The increasing pressure then forces the aortic and pulmonic valves open and the blood is ejected from the heart. The aortic and pulmonic valves close and the **second heart sound** is heard (**dup**).
- The pressure in the ventricles falls as the myocardium relaxes. When atrial pressure exceeds ventricular pressure the atrioventricular valves reopen and the cycle starts again.

Blood pressure

- The pressure of the blood in the arteries after ejection from the ventricles is called **systolic pressure.** It is relatively high.
- The pressure of the blood in the veins which fill the relaxed heart is called **diastolic pressure**. It is relatively low.
- Blood pressure is measured by stretch receptors (baroreceptors) in the aortic arch and carotid sinus. When blood pressure changes an appropriate response occurs.

- An example is when an increase in blood pressure is detected by the receptors. The medulla oblongata co-ordinates a response to reduce blood pressure (reduction in cardiac output, dilation of blood vessels, reduction in circulating blood volume).

Functional terms related to the heart

- **Heart rate** is the number of heartbeats per minute.
- **Heart rhythm** is the spacing between beats. It is normal for the heart rate to increase slightly during inspiration and slow down during expiration. This variation is called **sinus arrhythmia**. Abnormal alterations in rhythm are called **dysrhythmias**.
- **Stroke volume** is the volume of blood ejected from the heart with each heartbeat.
- **Cardiac output** is the volume of blood ejected by the heart every minute. It can be calculated:

> cardiac output = stroke volume × heart rate

- A **pulse:** can be felt with the fingertips when the peripheral arteries expand slightly as the pressure wave from a heartbeat passes. Palpating the pulse can help assess heart rate and rhythm, and gives a guide to stroke volume. If the heart is ejecting less blood (eg a diseased heart) the pulse will feel weak.

2.3.24 Blood circulation

What you need to learn

- You need to be able to describe the cardiac, pulmonary and systemic circulation of blood.
- Describe the hepatic portal circulation and explain its function.

Here is a summary of the blood flow:

- Freshly oxygenated blood travels in the pulmonary vein to the left side of the heart and is pumped out via the aorta to supply the body tissues with oxygen.
- Blood which has passed through the gut is rich in nutrients and is diverted through the liver so that these nutrients can be utilised. This is called the **hepatic portal system.**
- Blood passes into the veins, eventually draining into the **vena cava.** It is now carrying less oxygen and more carbon dioxide. The blood from the vena cava enters the right side of the heart and is pumped into the pulmonary artery. This carries the blood back to the lungs where carbon dioxide diffuses out and oxygen diffuses in.

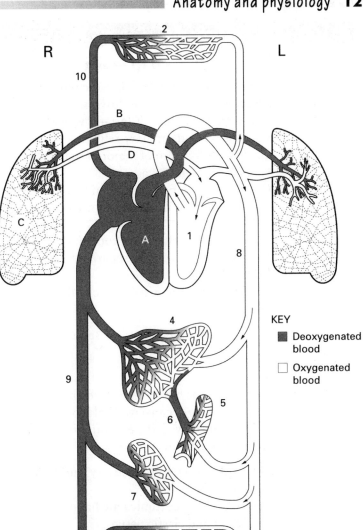

R L

KEY

■ Deoxygenated blood

□ Oxygenated blood

KEY

Systemic circulation

1.	Left side of the heart	6.	Hepatic portal vein
2.	Vessels in the cranial part of the body	7.	Kidneys
3.	Vessels in the caudal part of the body	8.	Aorta
4.	Liver	9.	Caudal vena cava
5.	Intestines	10.	Cranial vena cava

Pulmonary circulation

A.	Right side of the heart	C.	Lung
B.	Pulmonary artery	D.	Pulmonary vein

Figure 3.60 Schematic diagram of the circulation of blood through the body.

2.3.25   Blood vessels

What you need to learn

☙ You need to be able to define the terms artery, vein and capillary.
☙ Describe the structure of different types of blood vessels and explain their different functions (artery, vein and capillary).
☙ State the normal capillary refill time.
☙ Identify the location of major blood vessels:
  ☙ aorta and vena cava
  ☙ carotid, axillary, brachial and femoral arteries
  ☙ cephalic, superficial saphenous, coccygeal and jugular veins.

The cardiovascular system consists of the heart and the blood vessels. The blood vessels can be separated into three groups:
• arteries
• microcirculation (arterioles, capillary network and venules)
• veins.

The structure of the blood vessels varies according to their function.

Arteries

Arteries are the blood vessels which receive blood from the heart and deliver it to the organs. Arterial blood is oxygenated and is bright red in appearance (with the exception of the deoxygenated blood in the pulmonary arteries).

• The inner surface of the artery (**tunica interna**) is lined with endothelium.
• The middle layer (**tunica media**) is the thickest and consists of muscular and elastic tissues.
• The outer surface (**tunica adventitia**) is made of fibrous tissue which prevents excessive expansion of the artery.
• Arteries which receive blood under the highest pressure (such as the aorta) contain more elastic in their walls to absorb some of the pressure.
• Further away from the heart the blood pressure is slightly less and the arteries become more muscular (smooth muscle).
• Towards the capillary beds the arteries become very small and contain very little muscle in their walls. These small arteries are called **arterioles**. They are important in regulating resistance to blood flow and therefore blood pressure.

Small vein (x 400%)

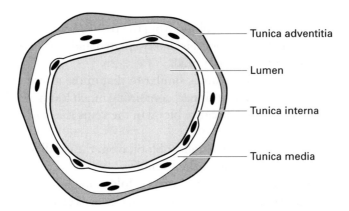

Tunica adventitia

Lumen

Tunica interna

Tunica media

Arteriole

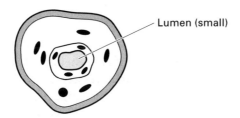

Lumen (small)

Almost no elastic fibre.
High resistance pathway

Venule

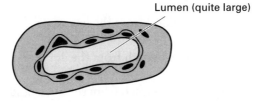

Lumen (quite large)

These merge with
surrounding connective
tissue. Their great
compliancy makes them
blood reservoirs
(no tunica media)

Small artery

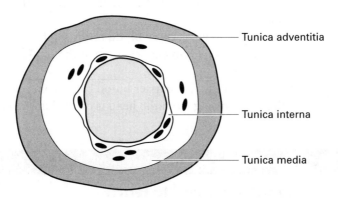

Tunica adventitia

Tunica interna

Tunica media

Figure 3.61 Blood vessels.

Veins

Veins receive the blood from the tissues and transport it back to the heart. Venous blood is deoxygenated and dark red in colour (except in the pulmonary veins).

The basic structure is similar to that of the arteries but the walls of veins are much thinner, containing much less muscular and elastic tissue. This is because blood in the veins is at low pressure.

- The veins which collect blood from the capillary network are very small. These are called **venules**.
- The tunica interna of veins is folded in places to form **valves**. These prevent blood from flowing backwards (arteries do not need valves because of the high pressure of the blood).
- Movement of the body muscles helps push blood through the veins.

Capillaries

Capillaries are narrow tubes of endothelium. The walls are only one cell thick. They are the exchange vessels where fluid passes into the tissues, nutrient and metabolite exchange occurs, then some of the fluid is reabsorbed into the capillary network.

Some major blood vessels

- The aorta carries blood from the left ventricle. It is the biggest artery.
- The carotid arteries branch from the aorta and carry blood to the head.
- The axillary arteries branch from the aorta and carry blood to the front legs. These arteries travel down the legs becoming the brachial arteries.
- The femoral arteries branch from the aorta and carry blood down the hindlimbs.
- The cephalic veins carry blood returning from the front legs.
- The saphenous vein carries some of the blood returning from the hindlimbs.
- The coccygeal vein carries blood back from the tail.
- Blood returning from the head is carried in the jugular veins.

2.3.26   Lymphatic system

What you need to learn

- You need to be able to describe the functions and the composition of lymph.

❧ Describe the structure of lymphatic vessels and state the differences between them and blood vessels.

The lymphatic system consists of:

• lymphatic vessels (capillaries and veins)
• lymph nodes (aggregates of lymphoid tissue spread throughout the body).

Fluid (known as tissue fluid) passes from the blood capillaries into the tissues. Not all of this fluid can be reabsorbed by the capillary network. The excess fluid is collected by the lymphatic capillaries and is called lymph.

The lining of the gut contains many lymph vessels (called lacteals) which absorb fats from the digestive process. Once absorbed this fluid is called chyle. Lymphatic vessels from the gut and caudal part of the body converge to form the cisterna chyli. Fluid from the lymphatic circulation drains back into the blood through the thoracic duct.

Lymphatic vessels are similar in structure to veins but the walls are much thinner. Lymph vessels have valves. Lymph capillaries are more permeable than blood capillaries.

Lymph nodes

Lymph nodes are firm, bean-shaped structures with an outer capsule. All lymph passes through at least one lymph node before returning to the blood. As it passes through the lymph node:

• phagocytic cells remove any unwanted particles or micro-organisms
• lymphocytes are added to the fluid
• if the lymph node detects an infection an immune response is mounted.

Lymph nodes swell when they are active, ie during an infection. They act as a barrier to tumour cells and therefore swell if a tumour starts to metastasise (spread).

Examples of superficial lymph nodes

• Lymph nodes are examples of lymphoid tissue.
• Lymphoid tissue is also present in the **tonsils**, the **spleen** and the **thymus** gland.
• The thymus is a gland in the cranial thorax. It is large in young animals but atrophies with age. By the time an animal reaches maturity the thymus has almost disappeared. The function of the thymus is to produce lymphocytes (specifically T-cell lymphocytes).

Lymphocytes produced in the thymus migrate into the lymph nodes and multiply.

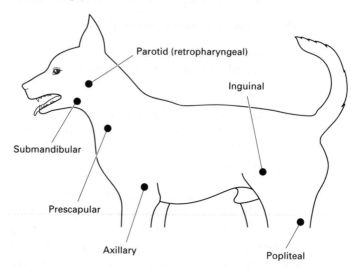

Figure 3.62 The position of the main palpable superficial lymph nodes.

2.3.27 Immune system

What you need to learn

❧ You need to be able to describe the basic cellular and humoral components of the immune system.

❧ Describe where lymphoid tissue is found:
  ❧ lymph nodes
  ❧ tonsils
  ❧ spleen thymus

❧ Describe the structure and function of a lymph node.

❧ Name and list sites where superficial lymph nodes might be found.

❧ Describe the circulation of lymph.

❧ Describe the structure, location and functions of the spleen. (Also see 2.3.26).

- **Immunity** is the ability of the body to resist disease.
- **Passive immunity** relates to the antibodies received by a foetus or young animal from its mother. It is short lived.
- **Active immunity** is when the immune system of an animal has learnt to recognise and destroy foreign material which is presented to the lymph node. This kind of immunity is acquired.
- **Antigens** are substances which stimulate a response from the immune system. They are usually proteins on the surface of a cell or micro-organism.

- The immune system normally recognises its own antigens and does not mount an immune response.
- Lymphocytes are the most important cells in the immune system. There are two types:
  1 T-cells (from the thymus). These travel to the lymph nodes and mature.
  2 B-cells (from the bone marrow). These circulate in the blood and are present in lymph nodes.

Cellular immune response

- Antigens enter the lymph nodes through the lymphatic system.
- T-cells recognise the antigen as foreign and stimulate an immune response.
- The foreign antigens are damaged and phagocytosed by various white blood cells.
- Special **memory T-cells** remember the antigen so that a similar response can be mounted quickly if the antigen is encountered in the future.

Humoral immune response

- Antigens enter the lymph nodes through the lymphatic system.
- B-cells recognise the antigen. The B-cells multiply and swell, becoming **plasma cells.**
- Plasma cells produce special proteins called antibodies.
- Antibodies attach to the foreign antigen and make it an easy target for phagocytosis.
- Special memory T-cells remember the antigen so that a similar response can be mounted quickly if the antigen is encountered in the future.

Spleen

- The spleen is found in the cranial abdomen on the left side. It is joined to the greater curvature of the stomach by the greater omentum.
- The capsule which surrounds the spleen is muscular, allowing the spleen to swell.
- The spleen consists of two main types of tissue: the *red pulp* and the *white pulp*.
- Red pulp consists of blood vessels, stored blood products and sometimes haemopoietic tissue.
- White pulp consists of lymph nodules which are capable of phagocytosis and immune response.

Functions of the spleen

There are five functions:

1. Blood storage: the spleen contracts to increase the circulating blood volume. This occurs during exercise (causing pain known as a 'stitch') or during haemorrhage.
2. Removal of worn out and damaged erythrocytes.
3. Removal of other particles such as cellular debris from the blood.
4. Production of lymphocytes and monocytes.
5. Haemopoiesis in the foetus. This function can return in adult life if necessary (production of blood cells and platelets).

How much have you learnt?

1   Describe the structure of a simple cuboidal epithelial cell. Where might a cell like this be found?

2   Name three long bones. Draw a diagram of the basic structure of one of these.

3   Which structures pass through the diaphragm?

4   Describe the structure of the sternum.

5   Explain the structure and function of the various hairs on the face.

6   Explain which parts of the nervous system make up the *central* and *peripheral* nervous systems.

7   What are cranial nerves? What are the functions of cranial nerve V?

8   What are rods and cones? How do they differ from one another?

9   Explain the difference between the auditory and vestibular systems.

10 Describe the path taken by an erythrocyte from joining the vena cava to leaving the aorta.

The answers can be found within this unit, up to page 128.

2.3.28 Respiration

What you need to learn

- You need to be able to describe the anatomical structures involved in the process of respiration and their physiological function. These include:
  - intercostal muscles
  - diaphragm
  - abdominal muscles.
- Describe the process of respiration (sequence of inspiration and expiration).
- Define associated terms:
  - tidal air
  - tidal volume
  - residual volume
  - minute volume
  - total lung capacity
  - vital capacity
  - functional residual capacity
  - respiratory rate
  - anatomical and functional dead space. ·
- Describe the structures which make up the respiratory dead space.
- Describe the exchange of gases in the lung and the principles of tissue respiration.
- Explain the ways that respiration is controlled including neural factors and factors influencing the the respiratory centre (chemoreceptors).
- Explain factors that will reduce vital capacity.

Respiration is the process of gas exchange between an organism and the environment. Internal (tissue) respiration is the intracellular transfer of oxygen (oxygen) and carbon dioxide. External respiration is transfer of oxygen and carbon dioxide between the blood and the external environment. This section deals with external respiration. The organs of respiration are the lungs and the passages between the lungs and the outside (including nasal cavity, pharynx, larynx, trachea, bronchi and bronchioles).

The respiratory cycle

- The diaphragm contracts. This lowers the pressure within the thorax.
- At the same time the intercostal muscles contract, this swings the ribcage upwards and outwards, lowering the pressure in the thorax.

- Air flows into the respiratory tract from the atmosphere until the air pressure outside the body is equal to the pressure within the thorax. This is **inspiration** and it is an active process.
- At this point the muscles relax. This reduces the volume of the thorax, raises the pressure and pushes air out. This is **expiration** and it is a passive process.

Terms associated with respiration

- **Tidal air** is the air which passes in and out of the lungs with each breath.
- **Tidal volume** is the volume of gas inspired with each breath during normal respiration.
- **Functional residual capacity** is the reservoir of gas in the lungs after normal expiration. This reservoir allows oxygenation of the blood to continue in between breaths.
- **Total lung capacity** is the volume of gas in the lung after maximal inspiration.
- **Residual volume** is the volume of gas left in the lungs after maximal expiration.
- **Vital capacity** is the maximal volume of gas that can be expired after a maximal inspiration. It can be reduced if the respiratory muscles become weakened; if the muscles are unable to contract normally because of the body position, or if the lungs are unable to expand.

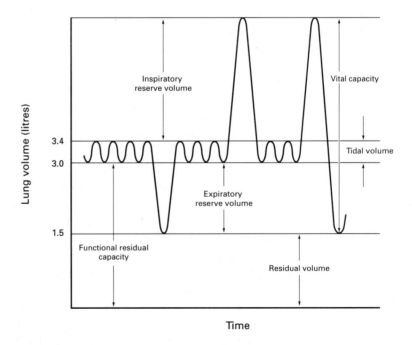

Figure 3.63   The various lung volumes.

• **Respiratory rate** is the number of breaths taken per minute. It varies with the body's oxygen requirement. (Resting respiratory rate is 10–30 breaths per minute for the dog, 20–30 per minute in the cat.)
• **Minute volume** is the volume of gas inhaled during 1 minute.

Respiratory dead space

The parts of the upper respiratory tract which are filled with air during respiration but which do not take part in oxygen exchange are called **anatomical dead space**. The structures which make up this dead space are the nasal passages, pharynx, trachea, bronchi and bronchioles.

Parts of the lung which are less well perfused with blood, (eg the dorsal lobes of the lung are less well perfused because of the effects of gravity) can also act as dead space because oxygen exchange is reduced. This dead space is called **functional dead space**.

Gas exchange in the lung

• An air molecule passes through the upper airways, into the trachea, and down the bronchi into the lung.
• The bronchi divide into **bronchioles**.
• These divide further. Some bronchioles (called respiratory bronchioles) have alveoli lining the walls.
• The bronchioles terminate in **alveolar ducts**. These ducts lead to **alveolar sacs** which are lined with alveoli.
• Gas exchange occurs at the alveolus.
• The alveoli are surrounded by a very rich capillary bed.
• Blood reaching these capillary beds is deoxygenated blood from the pulmonary artery. It also contains a lot of oxygen.
• Oxygen is at a high concentration in the air within the alveolus but is at a low concentration in the deoxygenated blood in the capillary. Oxygen molecules cross from the alveolus into the capillaries by diffusion.
• Oxygen molecules then bind to haemoglobin in the erythrocytes.
• At the same time as this the oxygen from the blood diffuses across into the alveolar air so that it can be breathed out.
• Blood leaving the capillary beds rejoins the pulmonary vein and returns to the heart.
• The opposite exchange to this occurs in the tissues. Oxygen diffuses out of the erythrocytes and into the tissues and carbon dioxide (produced during tissue respiration) diffuses into the blood. Most carbon dioxide is dissolved in the plasma as a bicarbonate ion. Some carbon dioxide is carried by the erythrocytes.

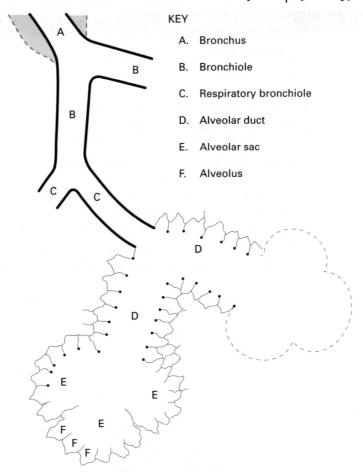

KEY

A. Bronchus

B. Bronchiole

C. Respiratory bronchiole

D. Alveolar duct

E. Alveolar sac

F. Alveolus

Figure 3.64 The lower airways.

Neural control of respiration

- The **respiratory centre** in the medulla oblongata co-ordinates the actions of the respiratory muscles.
- **Chemoreceptors** in the aortic and carotid body monitor oxygen levels in the blood. When oxygen levels rise these receptors send information to the respiratory centre which stimulates an increase in respiratory rate to remove the excess oxygen.
- Mechanoreceptors measure the tension in the lung tissues. When there is an increase in tension (during inspiration) impulses are transmitted to the respiratory centre. The respiratory centre then inhibits inspiration so that expiration can occur. This mechanism prevents overstretching of the lungs.

2.3.29   Nasal cavity

What you need to learn

☙ You need to be able to describe the basic anatomy and function of the nasal cavity.
☙ Describe turbinate bones and state their functions.
☙ Describe the location and functions of the sinuses.

- The haired skin meets the mucous membrane of the nose at a mucocutaneous junction.
- Inside the nostrils are the openings of the nasolacrimal duct. Secretions from this duct keep the nasal cavity moist.
- The nasal cavity is separated from the oral cavity by the hard palate.
- The caudal part of the nasal cavity contains the nasal turbinate bones. These are delicate scrolls of bone covered by mucous membrane.
- The function of the turbinate bones is to moisten and warm air before it travels to the lower airways. They also trap small particles of dust, ensuring that air travelling to the lungs is as clean as possible.

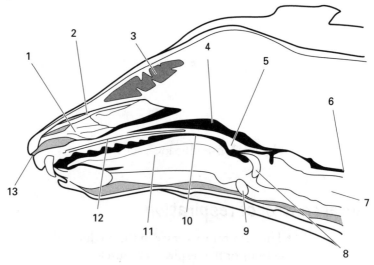

KEY

1.	Ventral nasal concha	6.	Oesophagus	10.	Oropharynx
2.	Dorsal nasal concha	7.	Trachea	11.	Tongue
3.	Front sinus	8.	Epiglottis	12.	Hard palate
4.	Nasopharynx	9.	Basihyoid	13.	Right nostril
5.	Soft palate				

Figure 3.65   Transverse section of the head showing the nasal cavities.

• The ethmoid turbinate bones sit behind the nasal turbinates. These are covered with olfactory mucosa. This detects chemicals in the air and sends information through the **cribriform plate** to the olfactory centre in the brain (cranial nerve I). These organs therefore constitute the sense of smell and are highly developed in the dog. The anatomy of the paranasal sinuses has already been discussed on p. 64.

2.3.30 Pharynx

What you need to learn

🐾 You need to be able to describe the anatomy and structure of the pharynx and its functions (see also p. 150).

The pharynx connects the oral cavity and nose with the oesophagus and trachea (windpipe).
• The pathways of air and ingesta cross in the pharynx.
• During swallowing the soft palate lifts to divide the pharynx into the **oropharynx** and the **nasopharynx**. In this way inhalation of food particles is prevented.
• The auditory tubes (from the middle ear) open into the dorsal pharynx.

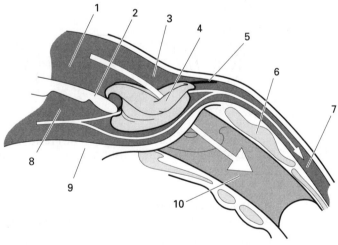

KEY

1. Nasal cavity
2. Soft palate
3. Nasopharynx
4. Larynx (protruding through pharyngeal floor)
5. Palatopharyngeal arch
6. Cricoid cartilage
7. Oesophagus
8. Oral cavity
9. Root of tongue
10. Trachea

Figure 3.66 Schematic diagram of the pharynx.

• The pharynx also contains the **tonsils** which are areas of lymphoid tissue in the palatoglossal arch.

2.3.31 Larynx

What you need to learn

❧ You need to be able to describe the structure and functions of the larynx. These include:
  ❧ epiglottis
  ❧ glottis
  ❧ vocal ligament
  ❧ the anatomy of the larynx
  ❧ vocal cord.
❧ Explain the function of the hyoid apparatus and state how it is related to the larynx.

The larynx connects the nasopharynx to the trachea. It is suspended from the base of the skull by a series of bones – the **hyoid apparatus**. It consists of a number of adjoined pieces of cartilage.

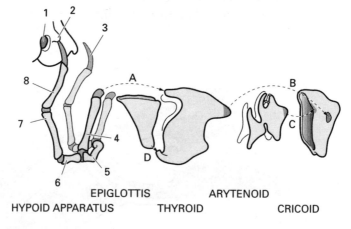

KEY

A.	Thyrohyoid articulation	C.	Cricoarytenoid articulation
B.	Cricothyroid articulation	D.	Thyroepiglottic attachment

1.	External acoustic meatus	5.	Basihyoid
2.	Mastoid process of skull	6.	Ceratohyoid
3.	Tympanohyoid	7.	Epihyoid
4.	Thyrohyoid	8.	Stylohyoid

Figure 3.67 The thyroid apparatus and larynx.

- The **epiglottis** is the most rostral cartilage.
- The **thyroid** cartilage forms the floor of the larynx.
- The **arytenoid** cartilage holds the attachment for the vocal folds.
- The **cricoid** cartilage is the most caudal cartilage and joins on to the first tracheal rings.
- The lumen of the larynx is called the **glottis**. It is bounded by the arytenoid cartilages and vocal folds.

The functions of the larynx are:

- **Vocalisation.** Sound is made from the vibration of the air column as it passes through the glottis. The vocal folds modify the sound.
- **Prevention of inhalation of food particles.** Contact of solid particles with the mucosa of the larynx elicits the cough reflex.
- **Control of air flow into the respiratory tract.**

The hyoid apparatus

This consists of a series of adjoined bones which suspend the tongue and larynx from the skull.

- The **stylohyoid** bones articulate with the mastoid process on the temporal bone of the skull.
- A number of muscles are attached to the hyoid bones. These muscles move the hyoid (and therefore the tongue and larynx) during swallowing.

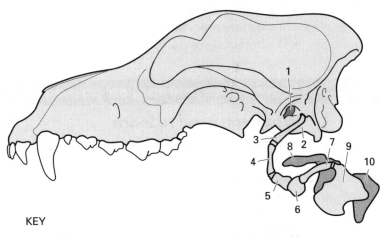

KEY

1. External acoustic meatus	6. Basihyoid
2. Tympanic bulla	7. Thyrohyoid
3. Styohyoid	8. Epiglottic cartilage
4. Epihyoid	9. Thyroid cartilage
5. Ceratohyoid	10. Cricoid cartilage

Figure 3.68 The hyoid apparatus.

2.3.32   Trachea

What you need to learn

🐾 You need to be able to describe the location, structure and function of the trachea.

The trachea and bronchi carry air from the larynx to the lower airways. The trachea enters the mediastinum at the **thoracic inlet**. The trachea consists of C shaped cartilaginous rings joined by elastic connective tissue. The lumen is lined with ciliated pseudostratified epithelium.

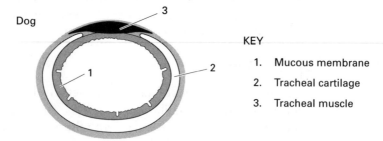

Dog

KEY

1.   Mucous membrane
2.   Tracheal cartilage
3.   Tracheal muscle

Figure 3.69   Cross-section of the trachea.

- The rigid structure prevents the trachea from collapsing.
- The trachea forks at the distal ends into the bronchi, which divide further into bronchioles.
- The branching of the bronchi is called the **bronchial tree**.

2.3.33   Bronchi and terminal air passages

What you need to learn

🐾 You need to be able to describe the structure and function of the bronchial tree.

🐾 Describe and state the functions of the bronchi and terminal air passages:
  🐾 bronchi
  🐾 bronchioles
  🐾 terminal bronchioles
  🐾 respiratory bronchioles
  🐾 alveolar ducts
  🐾 alveolar sacs and pulmonary alveoli

See 2.3.28 Gas Exchange in the Lungs.

2.3.34   Lungs and pleural cavity

What you need to learn

🐾 You need to be able to describe the structure, position and the functions of the lungs and pleural cavity:
- 🐾 mediastinum
- 🐾 pleural
- 🐾 parietal
- 🐾 visceral pleura.

The lungs are the site of gaseous exchange. This occurs within the alveoli. Most of the lung tissue is composed of small airways, pulmonary vessels and connective tissue. The lungs sit within the pleurae. Their size and shape changes with the phase of respiration. The lungs are divided into lobes. The left lung is divided into the cranial and caudal lobes; the right lung is divided into the cranial, middle and caudal lobes.

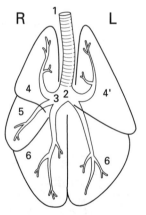

KEY
1. Trachea
2. Birfurcation of trachea
3. Right mainstem bronchus
4. Right cranial lobe
4'. Left cranial lobe
5. Middle lobe
6. Caudal lobes

Figure 3.70   The lung lobes of the dog.

2.3.35   Digestive system

What you need to learn

🐾 Outline the structure and function of the digestive system of:
- 🐾 carnivores
- 🐾 omnivores
- 🐾 herbivores
- 🐾 reptiles
- 🐾 fish.
🐾 Define terms associated with digestion (see terms on p. 395):
- 🐾 digestion

* deglutition
* peristalsis
* absorption
* catabolic reaction
* anabolic reaction
* basal metabolic rate
* enzyme
* protein
* polypeptide
* peptide
* amino acid
* carbohydrate
* polysaccharide
* disaccharide
* monosaccharide
* polymerisation
* fatty acid.

The digestive system breaks down ingesta into its component molecules so that they can be absorbed and utilised by the body. The digestive system is basically a tubular tract extending from the mouth to the anus. It also includes a number of glands which open into the tract.

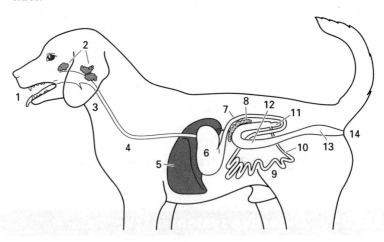

KEY

1. Mouth	6. Stomach	11. Caecum
2. Salivary glands	7. Duodenum	12. Colon
3. Pharynx	8. Pancreas	13. Rectum
4. Oesophagus	9. Jejunum	14. Anus
5. Liver	10. Ileum	

Figure 3.71 Diagram of the digestive system.

- The digestive system and its contents are continuous with the outside of the body.
- The digestive tract is divided into parts, each of which has a particular function.
- Cats and dogs eat meat (they are **carnivores**). Meat is digested by **chemical digestion** (action of **enzymes**).
- Carnivores eat a diet consisting wholly of meat.
- Herbivores eat a diet consisting wholly of vegetation.
- Omnivores eat a mixture of meat and vegetation.

Herbivorous mammals include the lagomorphs and most rodents as well as larger mammals such as cattle and horses. Herbivores have a digestive system which allows grinding and fermentation of the food, this releases the nutrients which are locked in the cells. Herbivores often have an enlarged caecum which serves as a fermentation and mixing bag.

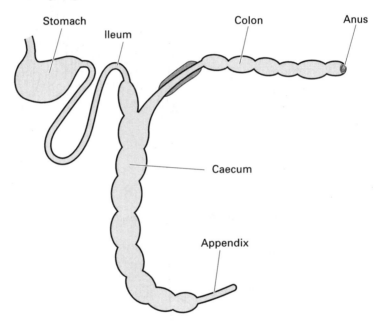

Figure 3.72 Schematic diagram of the digestive system of a rabbit.

Lagomorphs produce pellets of partly digested food called **caecotrophs**. These are immediately consumed again and pass through the gut a second time. They emerge this time as firm dry droppings.

Omnivores include animals such as some birds, most reptiles, hedgehogs, primates and pigs. Rats and mice will eat a varied diet and are often given titbits of meat.

In the bird there is often a distensible sac associated with the distal oesophagus called the **crop** which stores food before digestion. The glandular stomach is called the **proventriculus.** The muscular, grinding part of the stomach is called the **gizzard** or **ventriculus.** This is important in birds because they are unable to mechanically reduce food through mastication. The caecum, when present, varies greatly in size and shape between species. The gastrointestinal tract terminates in the **cloaca** which receives the excreted products of the urinary and digestive tracts.

Domestic chicken (*Gallus gallus*, var. domesticus)

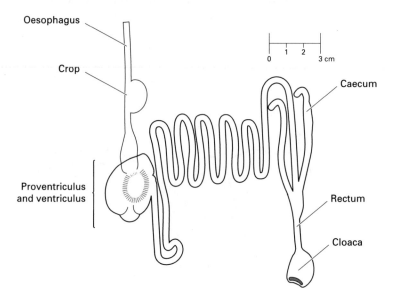

Budgerigar (*Melopsittacus undulatus*)

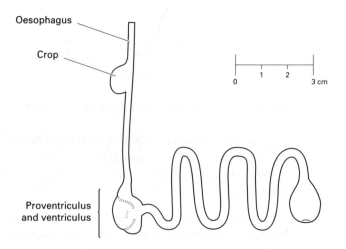

Figure 3.73 Diagram of the digestive systems of two species of bird.

Reptiles have a fairly simple gastrointestinal tract. The stomach is a short tube. A short caecum is often present. The gastrointestinal tract terminates in the cloaca which receives the excreted products of the urinary and digestive tracts.

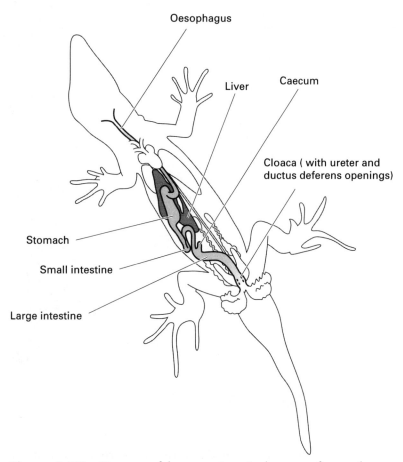

Oesophagus

Liver

Caecum

Cloaca (with ureter and ductus deferens openings)

Stomach

Small intestine

Large intestine

Figure 3.74 Diagram of the gastrointestinal system of a reptile.

The gastrointestinal system of the fish is broadly similar to other animals and varies depending on the food eaten.

2.3.36 Oral cavity

What you need to learn

☙ You need to be able to explain the basic anatomy and functions of the oral cavity.

The oral cavity is responsible for receiving food and mechanically reducing it to smaller particles through the action of the teeth (called chewing or **mastication**). The first stage of the chemical digestion process begins in the mouth with the addition of saliva. Action from the cheek and tongue muscles forms the chewed food into a **bolus** which is moved to the back of the oral cavity and swallowed.

KEY

1. Hard palate
2. Canine tooth
3. Soft palate
4. Palatine tonsil
5. Vestibule
6. Tongue
7. Sublingual caruncle
8. Frenulum
9. Palatoglossal arch

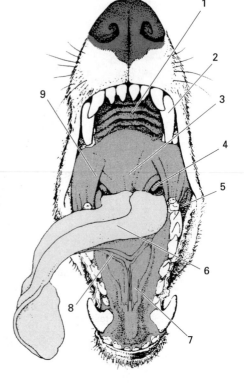

Figure 3.75 The oral cavity.

The lips are used to form a seal around the teat in the new-born mammal but have little function in the digestive process in the adult.

2.3.37 Teeth

What you need to learn

☙ You need to be able to describe the structure, function and location in the jaw of different types of teeth:

☙ incisor

☙ canine

☙ pre-molar and molar teeth

☙ enamel

☙ dentine

☙ pulp

* cement
* periodontal ligament.
* State the bones in which the alveoli of the teeth are located:
    * maxilla
    * mandible
    * incisive.
* Define deciduous and permanent dentition.
* Enumerate differences in the structure of teeth in different species:
    * cat
    * dog
    * rabbit
    * guinea pig
    * rodent
    * chelonian.
* State the dental formulae for deciduous and permanent dentitions:
    * cat
    * dog
    * exotics (rodents and lagomorphs).

Mammalian teeth

The basic structure of all the teeth is similar although the shape and function of different teeth vary greatly.

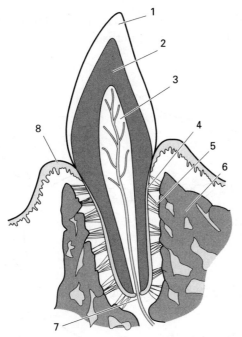

KEY

1. Enamel
2. Dentine
3. Pulp
4. Cement
5. Periodontal ligament
6. Socket (alveolus)
7. Apical foramen
8. Gum

Figure 3.76 A cross section of a tooth.

- The part of the tooth above the gum line is called the **crown**. It is coated with **enamel** – a very hard calcified material.
- The part of the tooth below the gum line is called the **root** and is not covered with enamel. Instead the root is coated in **cement**. Cement has a similar structure to bone but is very resistant to wear.
- Beneath the enamel is the **dentine** layer which forms the substance of the tooth. The structure of dentine is similar to bone.
- The **pulp cavity** runs down the centre of the dentine. Pulp is a soft material made from connective tissue. The pulp cavity contains nerves, blood vessels and lymphatics. It is very sensitive.
- Each tooth is implanted in a bony socket (**alveolus**).
- The alveolar bone is covered in a thick layer of mucus membrane – the **gingiva** or **gums**.
- The tooth is anchored to the socket by the **periodontal ligament**.

Teeth are classified into groups depending on their structure, function, and position in the mouth.

- Incisors are the most rostrally placed teeth. They have a single root and are mainly used for nibbling and for grooming in cats and dogs.
- Canine teeth are well developed in the dog and cat. They have a large single root, a pointed crown, and are used for piercing flesh and holding prey.
- Pre-molar teeth have multiple roots which provide firm anchorage in the jaw. The crowns have cusps which create a serrated edge for cutting flesh.
- Molar teeth also have multiple roots. The crowns have a broader surface and are designed for crushing.

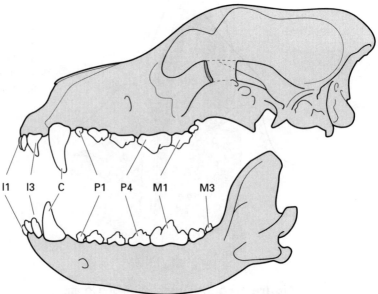

Figure 3.77 Lateral view of the teeth of the dog.

NB In the carnivores the upper pre-molar 4 and lower molar 1 are enlarged. The rostral surface is designed for cutting while the caudal surface is designed for crushing. These teeth are called the **carnassials**.

The first set of teeth which erupt are the **deciduous** teeth. These are lost as the animal grows and are replaced by the **permanent** teeth. The dental formula lists the number of each kind of tooth for each species. The type of tooth is represented by its initial (eg incisors: I, canines: C); the teeth in each side of the upper jaw are listed above the teeth in each side of the lower jaw (see Table 3.12).

Table 3.12

Species	Deciduous teeth	Permanent teeth
Dog	I3 C1 P3 I3 C1 P3	I3 C1 P4 M2 I3 C1 P4 M3
Cat	I3 C1 P3 I3 C1 P2	I3 C1 P3 M1 I3 C1 P2 M1

Exotics

Rodents and lagomorphs have teeth which have open roots and erupt continually. The incisor teeth are used for gnawing and cutting. Molar teeth are used for grinding. The gap between the incisors and molars is called the **diastema**. Dental disease is extremely common in pet rodents and rabbits.

The dental formula of the guinea-pig is: $I\frac{1}{1} C\frac{0}{0} PM\frac{1}{1} M\frac{3}{3}$

Lagomorphs are distinguished from rodents because they have a pair of incisors on the upper jaw – the **peg** teeth.

The dental formula of rabbits is: $I\frac{2}{1} C\frac{0}{0} PM\frac{3}{2} M\frac{3}{3}$

Chelonians and birds possess a horny beak rather than teeth. In birds the shape and function of the beak depends on the lifestyle and diet of the species. Some carnivorous reptiles such as crocodilians possess teeth which are used for slicing prey. In snakes the teeth are often modified to inject venom into prey and can sometimes be retracted.

2.3.38   The tongue

What you need to learn

☙ You need to be able to describe the structure and function of the tongue.

The tongue is suspended from the skull by the hyoid apparatus. It is a very muscular organ and its tip is freely mobile. It has a number of functions including:

- licking and tasting food
- lapping liquid
- manipulating food within the oral cavity
- grooming
- vocalisation
- heat loss (especially in the dog).

- The tongue is attached to the floor of the oral cavity by the **frenulum.**
- The dorsal surface of the tongue is covered with **papillae** made from modified mucosa (stratified squamous epithelium). The papillae have various shapes:
  - **Filiform papillae** are the soft papillae that cover most of the tongue. In the cat these are modified in places to form rasp-like instruments.
  - **Fungiform, foliate** and **vallate** are other examples of papillae. These help to move the bolus caudally, aid in grooming and also contain taste buds.
- The sublingual vein and artery provide the blood supply to the tongue. A pulse can be palpated in the lingual artery on the ventral surface of the tongue.

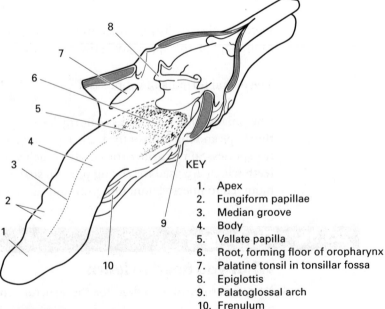

KEY

1. Apex
2. Fungiform papillae
3. Median groove
4. Body
5. Vallate papilla
6. Root, forming floor of oropharynx
7. Palatine tonsil in tonsillar fossa
8. Epiglottis
9. Palatoglossal arch
10. Frenulum

Figure 3.78 The tongue.

2.3.39   Salivary glands

What you need to learn

❧ You need to be able to describe the function of the salivary glands and identify their location.

❧ Describe the functions and constituents of saliva and the factors which stimulate salivation.

There are four pairs of salivary glands:

• **parotid** glands
• **submandibular** glands
• **zygomatic** glands
• **sublingual** chain of salivary glands.

The salivary glands produce saliva. This has a number of functions:

• lubricating and softening food
• dissolving soluble parts of food
• moistening the oral mucosa
• heat loss through evaporation
• aids in cleaning the coat.

Saliva is a watery mucous solution. It is alkaline and does not contain digestive enzymes in the dog and cat. A small amount of saliva is produced continuously. The parasympathetic and sympathetic branches of the nervous system have some control over the production of saliva. When an animal anticipates food or starts to eat the salivary glands are stimulated to produce more saliva.

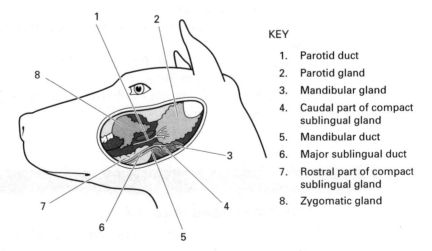

KEY

1. Parotid duct
2. Parotid gland
3. Mandibular gland
4. Caudal part of compact sublingual gland
5. Mandibular duct
6. Major sublingual duct
7. Rostral part of compact sublingual gland
8. Zygomatic gland

Figure 3.79 The salivary glands.

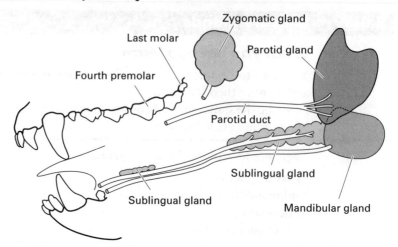

Figure 3.80 The salivary glands.

What you need to learn

☙ You need to be able to describe the structure and function of the hard and soft palates.

- The **hard palate** forms the roof of the oral cavity. It is a thick mucosa overlying the palatine bones (incisive, maxillary and palatine). It is firm and immobile.
- The mucosa of the hard palate forms ridges (**rugae**) which help direct the food caudally.
- The caudal border of the hard palate is continuous with the **soft palate**.
- The soft palate is a mobile muscular flap which is covered with a smooth mucous membrane.
- The soft palate lifts during swallowing to divide the pharynx into the nasopharynx and oropharynx.

What you need to learn

☙ You need to be able to describe the structure and functions of the pharynx.
☙ Describe the mechanisms of swallowing.

See 2.3.30 Pharynx, pp. 135–6.

Swallowing (deglutition)

After the food has been mechanically reduced by mastication the process of deglutition begins. This occurs in three phases:

1 **Oral phase:** this is a voluntary phase. The food is pressed onto the hard palate by the tongue forming a bolus. As the jaw closes the bolus is pushed into the oropharynx.

2 **Pharyngeal phase:** the pressure of the bolus on the pharyngeal mucosa initiates the swallowing reflex. The action is now involuntary. The soft palate is raised dividing the oropharynx from the nasopharynx. The hyoid apparatus swings forward so that the epiglottis shields the opening of the larynx. Contraction of smooth muscles in the oropharynx draws the bolus caudally towards the oesophagus.

3 **Oesophageal phase:** waves of contractions of the oesophageal smooth muscle push the food distally towards the stomach. These waves of contractions are called **peristalsis**. The soft palate and hyoid apparatus return to the resting position.

2.3.42   Oesophagus

What you need to learn

❧ You need to be able to explain the structure, anatomy and function of the oesophagus.

- The oesophagus (or **gullet**) is a muscular tube which conveys food from the pharynx to the stomach.
- The cervical part of the oesophagus runs along the left side of the trachea down the neck. It passes into the thorax at the thoracic inlet.
- The thoracic part of the oesophagus lies within the mediastinum. It runs dorsally past the aortic arch and passes through the diaphragm at the **oesophageal hiatus**.
- The outer layer of the oesophagus is called the **serosa**.
- Circular and longitudinal muscle fibres beneath the serosa make up the **muscular layer**.
- The **submucosa** contains blood vessels and nerves.
- The **mucosa** is lined with stratified squamous epithelium.

LONGITUDINAL VIEW   TRANSVERSE SECTION

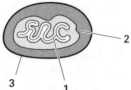

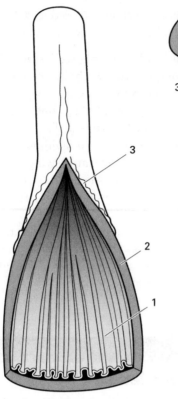

KEY

1. Mucosa
2. Muscular layer
    (longitudinal and circular)
3. Serosa

Figure 3.81 The oesophagus.

2.3.43   Stomach

What you need to learn

🐾 You need to be able to explain the structure, anatomy and functions of the stomach and the composition of the gastric secretions.

🐾 Explain the mechanisms of vomiting.

🐾 Define chyme and explain how it is produced.

The stomach is a dilation of the gastrointestinal tract between the oesophagus and small intestine. It lies on the left side of the abdomen adjacent to the diaphragm.

Functions of the stomach

• The stomach in carnivores is the site of the first stages of chemical digestion.

• The ingesta are ground by the action of the muscular wall.

• The stomach acts as a storage vat controlling the rate of delivery of ingesta to the small intestine.

The oesophagus opens into the stomach at the **cardia**. The **fundus** acts as a storage vat. The **antrum** mixes the gastric secretions with the ingesta. The antrum grinds and sieves the ingesta. It ensures that food particles are a suitable size for digestion in the small intestine. The **pylorus** and **pyloric sphincter** also control the passage of particles to the small intestine.

EXTERIOR

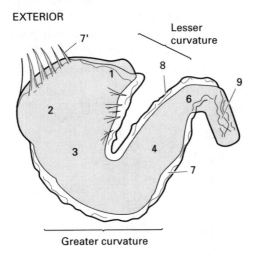

KEY

1.	Cardia	6.	Pylorus
2.	Fundus	7.	Greater omentum
3.	Body	7'.	Gastrosplenic ligament
4–6.	Pyloric part	8.	Lesser omentum
4.	Pyloric antrum	9.	Mergence of attachment
5.	Pyloric canal		of greater and lesser omenta

INTERIOR

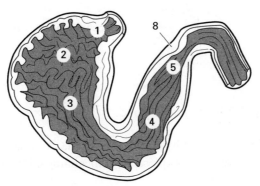

Figure 3.82 The stomach.

- The stomach wall has three layers:
- mucosa
- muscle (longitudinal, circular and oblique)
- serosa.

The folds in the stomach wall are called **rugae**.

- Peritoneum makes up the serosa. At the greater curvature this is reflected to create the greater omentum.
- The gastric mucosa is modified to produce the gastric secretions.
- The mucosa is lined with columnar epithelium.
- Numerous **gastric glands** within the **gastric pits** (folds of mucosa) secrete **gastric juice**. This consists of hydrochloric acid (from **parietal** or **oxyntic**) cells and **pepsinogen** (from **peptic** or **chief cells***).

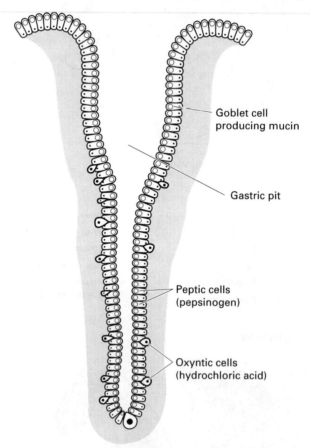

Goblet cell producing mucin

Gastric pit

Peptic cells (pepsinogen)

Oxyntic cells (hydrochloric acid)

Figure 3.83 A gastric gland.

Mucous is secreted by **goblet cells** in the mucosa. The layer of mucus protects the mucosa from mechanical injury and the actions of digestive enzymes.

Chemical digestion

- **Hydrochloric acid** keeps the contents of the stomach acidic. This kills any harmful microbes which may have been ingested and provides optimal conditions for the digestive enzymes.
- **Pepsinogen** is converted to **pepsin** by the action of an enzyme. Pepsin is an enzyme which breaks down peptide linkages in proteins producing polypeptides.
- **Gastrin** is a hormone secreted when food is detected in the mouth or stomach (via the action of the parasympathetic nervous system). It enhances gastric motility and stimulates the production of gastric juice.
- After a few hours the stomach contents are a liquid mixture of gastric juice and partially digested ingesta. This material is called **chyme**.
- Liquid meals are processed quickly in the stomach (< 30 mins). Solid meals take 3–4 hours in the stomach and meals with a high fat content take even longer.

Vomiting (emesis)

Vomiting is the passage of stomach contents through the oesophagus to the exterior. It is a protective reflex to remove toxins or foreign bodies from the gastrointestinal tract. It is caused in one of two ways:

1 **Peripheral stimulation:** tension and chemoreceptors in the stomach and duodenum.
2 **Central stimulation:** drugs or toxins affect the **chemoreceptor trigger zone (CTZ)** in the brainstem.

Vomiting is a complex procedure:

- Salivation occurs to protect the mucous membranes from the acidic stomach contents.
- An involuntary deep breath is taken.
- The glottis and nasopharynx are closed and an expiratory movement is made. Because the glottis is closed air can't be breathed out. This has the effect of increasing intrathoracic pressure (this is called the **Valsalva manoeuvre**).
- The abdominal muscles and diaphragm contract simultaneously.
- The oesophagus and body of the stomach relax.
- The pylorus closes firmly (to prevent chyme moving into the small intestine).
- The increased pressure pushes the stomach contents up the oesophagus and the contents are propelled out of the mouth.
- With prolonged vomiting the pylorus may open causing flow of duodenal contents into the stomach.

2.3.44   Small intestine

What you need to learn

❧ You need to be able to describe the structure, anatomy and the functions of the small intestine.
  ❧ duodenum
  ❧ jejunum
  ❧ ileum
  ❧ bile
  ❧ pancreatic juice
  ❧ intestinal juice
  ❧ villae
  ❧ intestinal glands.
❧ Describe the motility, digestion and absorption of carbohydrates, fats and proteins.

The small intestine extends from the pylorus to the ileocaecocolic junction. It has three main parts:

• duodenum
• jejunum
• ileum.

The functions of the small intestine are further chemical digestion of food and the absorption of the products of digestion. A hormone called cholecystokinin is produced in the small intestine when chyme is present. Cholecystokinin stimulates the release of pancreatic juice and bile. Most of the small intestine is surrounded and supported by the mesentery, a folded layer of peritoneum. Numerous lymph nodes are associated with the mesentery.

Peristalsis occurs along the whole of the gastrointestinal tract to move ingesta distally. The outer layers of the small intestine are similar to the rest of the gastrointestinal tract. The mucosa is highly folded into **villi.** This has the effect of increasing the surface area available for the absorption of nutrients.

Between the villi lie crypts (the crypts of Lieberkühn). Cells in these crypts secrete a large volume of alkaline fluid into the small intestine. Brunner's glands and goblet cells secrete mucus which protects the villi. The surface of the small intestine is lined with simple columnar epithelium. Digestion occurs at this surface. Areas of the mucosa are rich in lymphoid tissue. These patches are sometimes visible and are called **Peyer's patches.**

The duodenum is quite short, extending from the pylorus to the point where the small intestine enters the mesentery. Bile (from the liver) enters the duodenum through the bile duct. Bile is involved with

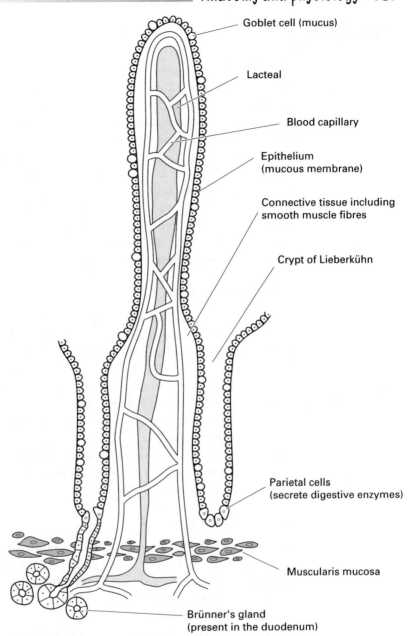

Goblet cell (mucus)

Lacteal

Blood capillary

Epithelium
(mucous membrane)

Connective tissue including
smooth muscle fibres

Crypt of Lieberkühn

Parietal cells
(secrete digestive enzymes)

Muscularis mucosa

Brünner's gland
(present in the duodenum)

Figure 3.84 A small intestinal villus.

emulsification of fats. Pancreatic juice (a mixture of pancreatic enzymes) enters the duodenum from the pancreatic duct.

The jejunum and ileum make up the rest of the small intestine. The junction is not well demarcated. The proximal portions are responsible for digestion while the distal portions are responsible for absorption of water, electrolytes and products of digestion. The ileum joins the large intestine (colon) at the ileocaecocolic junction.

Digestion

Fat digestion

- **Bile** comes from the liver. It contains bile acids which emulsify fats, providing a larger surface area for the action of enzymes.
- **Lipases** are enzymes which come from the pancreas. They break fats into their constituent parts (**fatty acids and glycerol**)
- Fatty acids form into **micelles** which are soluble in water. Micelles also contain cholesterol and fat-soluble vitamins. They are transported into the cells of the intestinal wall.
- Di- and tri-glycerides are then formed inside the epithelial cells. These are incorporated into envelopes called **chylomicrons** which are absorbed through the **lacteal** of the intestinal villus. This liquid is chyle. Do not confuse with chyme.

Protein digestion

Proteins are made up of chains of **polypeptides** joined by **peptide bonds**. Polypeptides are made up of chains of **amino acids**.

- Protein digestion begins in the stomach with the action of **pepsin**. Pepsin breaks the peptide bonds in proteins reducing them to polypeptides and free amino acids. Enzymes which break down proteins are called **proteolytic** enzymes.
- Enzymes in the pancreatic juice (**trypsin** and **chymotrypsin**) break down proteins in a similar way in the small intestine.
- Intestinal enzymes in the epithelial cell complete the breakdown of proteins into free amino acids. The amino acids are then absorbed into the blood vessels of the villi.

Carbohydrate digestion

- Individual sugar molecules are called monosaccharides. These can be effectively absorbed in the small intestine. Most are joined into multiple molecules, di- and polysaccharides.
- An enzyme in the pancreatic juice called **amylase** converts polysaccharides into monosaccharides.
- Most carbohydrate digestion occurs in the jejunum.
- Monosaccharides are absorbed into the blood vessels of the villi. This movement is **against** the concentration gradient and requires the input of energy. This is called **active transport**.

2.3.45   Large intestine

What you need to learn

- 🐾 You need to be able to describe the structure, anatomy and function of the large intestine:

❧ colon
❧ caecum
❧ rectum
❧ anal canal.
❧ Describe the motility, microbial fermentation, role of fibre, water absorption and defecation.

The large intestine consists of the caecum, the colon, and the rectum and anus.

The caecum

This is a blind-ending section of gut at the junction between the ileum and the colon. It has little function in the dog and cat.

The colon

- The colon extends from the ileocaecocolic junction until it leaves the abdominal cavity and becomes the rectum.
- Carnivores do not rely on bacterial fermentation products and so the colon is relatively simple.
- The action of bacteria in the colon produces vitamin K.
- The main function of the colon is the reabsorption of water and electrolytes. This occurs mainly in the proximal colon. The distal colon stores and periodically expels faeces.
- The structure of the walls of the colon is similar to the rest of the gastrointestinal tract except that there are no villi. The mucosa does have crypts of Lieberkühn.
- The epithelial cells secrete mucus which is rich in bicarbonate.
- Waves of peristalsis stimulated by the presence of material in the colon move the faeces distally.
- Fibre in the faeces absorbs water and swells, stimulating peristalsis. This reduces the length of time the faeces remains in the colon. Fibre also binds some of the fatty acids and carbohydrates in the diet, preventing their absorption.

The rectum

The rectum is the most dorsal organ in the pelvis. Most of it is outside the abdominal cavity and is not covered with peritoneum. The rectum joins the colon to the anus.

The anus

The short anal canal joins the colon to the exterior at a mucocutaneous junction. The folds of the mucosa are pressed together to help prevent incontinence. There are two muscles, the internal and external anal sphincter muscles, which keep the anus closed.

The anal glands (or sacs)

These paired glands lie ventrolaterally ('twenty to four' clockface position) between the internal and external anal sphincters just inside the anus. They secrete strongly smelling fluid which contains pheromones and is used for scent marking.

Defaecation

- The internal anal sphincter consists of smooth muscle. It is not under voluntary control.
- The external anal sphincter consists of striated muscle and is under voluntary control.
- Distension of the rectal walls with faeces stimulates a wave of peristalsis.
- As the wave of peristalsis approaches the anus the constriction of the internal anal sphincter muscles is inhibited.
- If the animal relaxes the external sphincter muscle faeces will be ejected.
- This process is aided by the animal raising the pressure in the abdomen through contraction of the abdominal muscles, and performing the Valsalva manoeuvre (expiration against a closed glottis).
- Defaecation can be blocked by voluntary contraction of the external sphincter muscles.

2.3.46   Liver

What you need to learn

- You need to be able to describe the anatomy, structure and functions of the liver.
- Describe the hepatic portal circulation and explain its functions.

The liver occupies the cranial part of the abdomen adjacent to the diaphragm. It is divided into lobes. The lobes are divided further into lobules. The liver has a dual blood supply. It is supplied by the hepatic artery **and** the hepatic portal vein. The hepatic portal vein carries nutrient-rich blood from the gastrointestinal tract to the liver so that metabolism can take place.

The liver has a number of functions which are now listed.

1 Metabolism of proteins

- Proteins which are old or damaged are **deaminated** (amino groups are removed, ammonia is produced).
- The amino groups are used to provide energy for tissue respiration.
- The ammonia is toxic and is converted to the less toxic **urea**.

2 Metabolism of carbohydrates

- Carbohydrates absorbed in the gut usually arrive in the liver as glucose.
- Excess glucose is converted to glycogen (by the action of insulin) and stored in the liver.

3 Metabolism of fats

- Fats are also converted to glycogen and stored in the liver.

4 Protein synthesis

- Proteins are not stored in the body.
- The liver acts as an amino acid pool and synthesises plasma proteins such as albumin, and clotting proteins such as fibrinogen.

5 Detoxification

- Toxic substances in the blood are modified by the liver and excreted.
- The liver also breaks down hormones such as insulin and sex hormones.

6 Metabolism of haemoglobin

- Phagocytic cells called **Küpffer cells** remove old or damaged erythrocytes from the circulation.
- The haemoglobin is split into amino acids (from the globin protein), iron and the **haem** pigment.
- The haem is converted to **bilirubin** and other bile pigments which are excreted in the bile. These pigments are excreted in the faeces, giving them their characteristic colour.
- Iron is transported to the bone marrow or stored in the liver.

7 Vitamin storage

- The fat soluble vitamins (D, A, K and E) are stored in the liver.

8 Heat production

• The numerous chemical reactions occurring within the liver produce a large amount of heat.

9 Cholesterol synthesis and excretion

• Cholesterol is an important constituent of cell membranes.
• If there is insufficient cholesterol it can be synthesised by the liver.
• Excess cholesterol is excreted in the bile.

2.3.47 Gall-bladder

What you need to learn

☙ You need to be able to describe the structure, function and position of the gall-bladder and common bile duct.

Bile made in the liver is stored in the **gall-bladder**. After a meal the gall-bladder contracts, expelling the bile through the **bile duct** and into the gut. Contraction of the gall bladder is stimulated by a hormone called **cholecystokinin**. Bile contains bile salts, haem pigments and sometimes cholesterol.

2.3.48 Pancreas

What you need to learn

☙ You need to be able to define the term mixed gland and explain the anatomy and function of the pancreas in digestion.

The pancreas is a **mixed** gland which lies between the greater curvature of the stomach and the duodenum. A mixed gland is one which has both endocrine and exocrine functions (see p. 43). The **exocrine** part of the pancreas produces pancreatic juice consisting of digestive enzymes (including amylase, trypsin, chymotrypsin and lipases) and bicarbonate. Pancreatic juice is released into the duodenum through two **pancreatic ducts**. The release of pancreatic juice is stimulated by cholecystokinin.

2.3.49 Urinary system

What you need to learn

☙ You need to be able to describe the anatomy and functions of the urinary system.

The urinary system consists of the kidneys, ureters, bladder and urethra. (See sections 2.3.50 to 2.3.53.) The functions of the urinary system are excretory and homeostatic.

2.3.50   Kidneys

What you need to learn

☙ You need to be able to explain the anatomy and functions of the kidneys and its blood supply. This includes:
  ☙ glomerular capsule (the Bowmann's capsule)
  ☙ glomerulus
  ☙ renal corpuscle
  ☙ proximal convoluted tubule
  ☙ ascending and descending parts of the loop of Henlé
  ☙ distal convoluted tubule
  ☙ renal pelvis.
☙ State the main constituents, pH and specific gravity of urine, of various animals including cats and dogs.

The two kidneys:
• lie on either side of the vertebral column pressed to the dorsal wall of the abdominal cavity
• lie outside the peritoneum (**retroperitoneal**), with the right kidney lying more cranially than the left
• are surrounded by a protective fat pad.

The kidney is organised into three regions: the **cortex**, the **medulla** and the **renal pelvis**. The kidney is supplied by the **renal artery**. This branches within the kidney to become several **interlobar** arteries. These branch again to form the **arcuate arteries,** then **interlobular arteries** which supply the individual nephrons. Where the blood vessels and ureter attach to the kidney there is an indentation – the **hilus**.

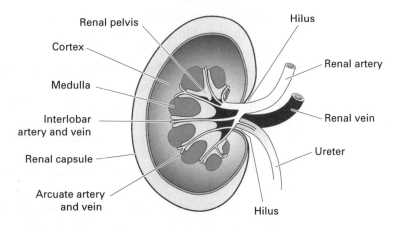

Figure 3.85   Transverse section of a kidney.

The nephron

Each kidney contains almost a million urinary tubules called **nephrons**. These are the functional units of the kidney.

- A cluster of blood vessels (the **glomerulus**) sits within a cup-shaped region at one end of the nephron (**Bowmann's capsule**). The glomerulus and capsule form the **renal corpuscle**. This part of the nephron lies within the renal cortex.
- The rest of the nephron is in the form of a long tubule.
- The **proximal convoluted tubule** leads from Bowmann's capsule to a loop of tubule which sits in the medulla (the **loop of Henlé**).
- The **distal convoluted tubule** leads from the loop of Henlé to the **collecting tubule**.

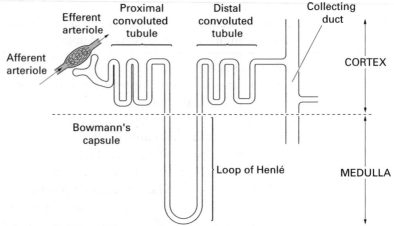

Figure 3.86 Schematic diagram of a nephron.

- The walls of the glomerulus are made up of a semi-permeable basement membrane.
- Blood enters the glomerulus at quite high pressure so that some of the fluid from the blood passes through into the tubule.
- Plasma proteins and erythrocytes are too large to pass through the membrane. Glomerular filtrate is therefore similar to plasma without the plasma proteins.
- Water and electrolytes are selectively reabsorbed as this fluid passes along the tubule.
- Urea (the waste product from protein metabolism) is excreted into the tubule.
- When the fluid from the tubule reaches the collecting duct it is called **urine.**
- A pituitary hormone acting on the kidney (**anti-diuretic hormone** or **ADH**) determines how concentrated the urine is, depending on the amount of water in the body.

• The collecting ducts join together to form the **renal pelvis.**

Other kidney functions include the following:

• the regulation of the acid base balance in the body
• production of the hormone **erythropoietin** which stimulates synthesis of erythrocytes in the bone marrow
• production of **renin** which is an important hormone in the regulation of blood pressure
• conversion of vitamin D.

Specific gravity is a measure of how concentrated the urine is. The higher the specific gravity, the more concentrated the urine. Normal urine can have a specific gravity of 1.016–1.060 in the dog and 1.020–1.040 in the cat.

The pH of urine is related to the diet; in the dog and cat it is usually between 5 and 7. Urine does not normally contain blood, protein, amino acids, glucose, bile, ketones or solid material such as crystals and casts. The presence of these suggest an underlying disease process. Dogs produce 20–80 ml/kg of urine daily, cats produce 10–15 ml/kg daily.

2.3.51 Ureters

What you need to learn

❧ You need to be able to describe the anatomy and functions of the ureters.

The ureters are tubular structures which arise from the renal pelvis. They carry urine from the kidneys to the bladder.

They are lined with transitional epithelium. The walls of the ureters contain smooth muscle. Waves of peristalsis push the urine distally to the bladder.

2.3.52 Bladder

What you need to learn

❧ You need to be able to describe the anatomy and functions of the bladder and define associated terms, including urine, micturition and trigone.

• The bladder is a distensible organ which stores urine.
• The ureters enter the bladder at an oblique angle near the neck of the bladder. This helps to prevent urine flowing back up the ureters from the bladder.

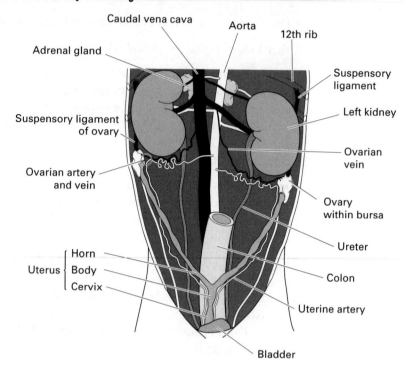

Figure 3.87 The urinogenitary tract within the abdomen.

KEY

1. Ureter
2. Bladder lumen
3. Bladder wall
4. Bladder neck

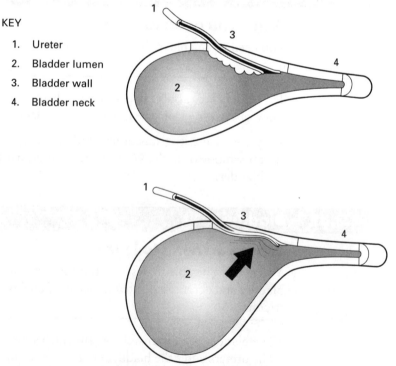

Figure 3.88 Diagram showing how increased pressure in the bladder prevents backflow of urine into the ureters.

- The **urethra** leaves the bladder close to the paired ureter openings. The triangle formed by these three openings is called the **trigone**.
- The bladder is lined with transitional epithelium. The bladder wall contains layers of smooth muscle. Together these allow the bladder to expand when it fills with urine.

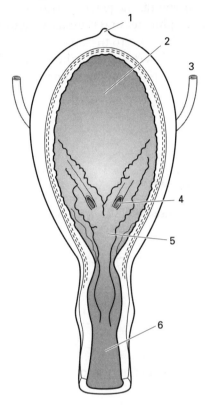

KEY

1. Scar of urachus
2. Bladder
3. Ureter
4. Ureter orifice
5. Trigone of bladder
6. Urethra

Figure 3.89 The bladder.

- When the bladder is full stretch receptors in the bladder wall send information to the brain. This makes the animal aware of its full bladder.
- If the animal chooses to urinate the smooth muscle wall of the bladder contracts expelling the urine. This is urination or **micturition**.
- There is no sphincter in the bladder.

2.3.53   Urethra

What you need to learn

❧ You need to be able to describe the anatomy and function of the urethra for both males and females.

- The urethra runs from the neck of the bladder to the outside of the body.
- Smooth muscle in the urethral wall functions as a sphincter. Control of this sphincter is **involuntary**. During micturition the urethra becomes shorter and wider.
- Striated muscle surrounds the pelvic portion of the urethra. This also functions as a sphincter and is under **voluntary** control.
- In the male the urethra runs to the tip of the penis.
- In the female the urethra opens onto the floor of the **vestibule**. The vestibule is a common tube leading from the vagina to the vulva.

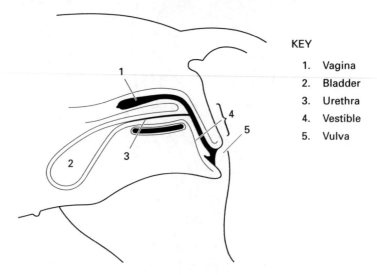

KEY

1. Vagina
2. Bladder
3. Urethra
4. Vestible
5. Vulva

Figure 3.90 The lower urinary tract in the bitch.

How much have you learnt?

1 Describe the journey of an inspired oxygen molecule from the atmosphere until it reaches an erythrocyte.

2 Name four types of teeth and explain how their shape suits their function.

3 List the functions of the tongue in a dog.

4 What is the pharynx?

5 How does food pass from the mouth to the stomach?

6 How is protein digested and what are the end products?

7 What is the hepatic portal system?

8 What features prevent a) urinary and b) faecal incontinence?

9 Why is the pancreas described as a mixed gland?

10 Draw a labelled diagram of a kidney.

The answers can be found within this unit, up to page 168.

2.3.54   Endocrine system

What you need to learn

* You need to be able to describe the functions of the endocrine system and define associated terms, including endocrine gland and hormone.
* Outline the process of normal metabolism.

The endocrine system co-ordinates and controls many functions of the body. Endocrine glands synthesise and secrete **hormones** directly into the blood stream (compare with exocrine glands). Hormones are chemical messengers which travel in the blood stream to **target organs**. At the target organ the hormone binds to receptors and causes a response. In some places the cells of the endocrine cells are not organised into glands, but act as individual cells, eg gastrin secretion in the gastrointestinal tract.

2.3.55   Pituitary gland

What you need to learn

* You need to be able to describe the anatomy and function of the pituitary gland and define the associated terms:
  * **Hypophysis**
  * adenohypophysis and the suffixes -trophic or -trophin
  * **Anterior** hypophysis
  * growth hormone
  * thyroid stimulating hormone
  * adrenocorticotrophic hormone
  * follicle stimulating hormone
  * prolactin
  * **Posterior** hypophysis
  * oxytocin
  * anti-diuretic hormone
  * pineal gland.

The pituitary gland lies on the ventral surface of the midbrain. It is connected to the hypothalamus. The hypothalamus receives information from the body and organises the appropriate response from the endocrine system. The hypothalamus secretes a number of **releasing hormones** which all act on target cells in the pituitary gland. The pituitary gland is separated into two lobes called the **anterior hypophysis** (or **adenohypophysis**) and the **posterior hypophysis** (or **neurohypophysis**).

The two lobes secrete different hormones: (see Table 3.13).

Tabel 3.13

Hormone	Hypophysis	Target cells	Action
Adrenocorticotrophic hormone (ACTH)	Anterior	Adrenal cortex	Cortisol synthesis
Growth hormone (GH) (sometimes called somatotrophin)	Anterior	All tissues	Stimulates growth and repair of tissues, and speeds the breakdown of fat stores.
Follicle stimulating hormone (FSH)	Anterior	Ovary, testes	Maturation and growth of ovarian follicles and spermatozoa.
Luteinising hormone (LH)	Anterior	Ovary, testes	Induces ovulation, stimulates formation of oestrogen and testosterone.
Prolactin (sometimes called luteotrophic hormone)	Anterior	Mammary glands	Increased milk synthesis.
Thyroid stimulating hormone (TSH)	Anterior	Thyroid glands	Stimulates thyroid function.
Oxytocin	Posterior	Mammary glands, uterus	Milk release, uterine contraction, prostaglandin secretion.
Anti-diuretic hormone (ADH) (sometimes called vasopressin)	Posterior	Kidney (collecting ducts)	Increased water reabsorption.

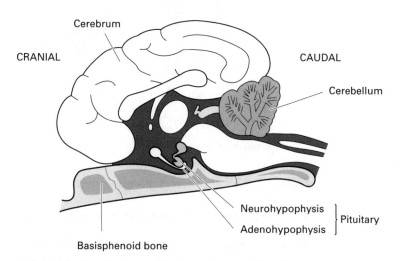

Figure 3.91   Diagram showing the position of the pituitary gland.

- Follicle stimulating hormone and luteal hormone are known as the **gonadotrophins**.
- The **pineal gland** is a small gland on the ventral surface between the cerebral hemispheres and the cerebellum. It produces the hormone

melatonin. The pineal gland functions as a biological clock, affecting the production of the gonadotrophins. It regulates gonadal activity throughout the day and also through the seasons.

2.3.56   Thyroid gland

What you need to learn

❧ You need to be able to describe the anatomy and function of the thyroid gland:
  ❧ thyroxine
  ❧ calcitonin
  ❧ triiodothyronine.

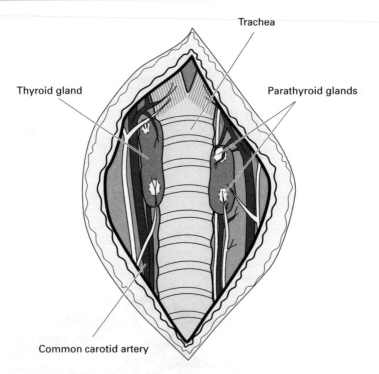

Figure 3.92 The thyroid glands, ventral view.

The paired thyroid glands lie on either side of the trachea.

They are composed of **follicles** of cuboidal epithelial cells which secrete the thyroid hormones. The thyroid hormones are called **triiodothyronine** (T3) and **tetraiodothyronine** (T4) which is better known as **thyroxine**. T3 is the active form of the hormone. Synthesis of the thyroid hormones requires iodine. Thyroid-stimulating hormone (TSH) released from the pituitary gland causes an increase in the production of thyroid hormones.

Control of the plasma levels of thyroid hormones is through **negative feedback**:

• the hypothalmus detects the increase in plasma T3 and T4, and releases thyrotrapin releasing hormone (TRH) which stimulates the pituitary to release thyroid stimulating hormone. The TSH then acts on the thyroid gland to stimulate production of T3 and T4.

The thyroid hormones affect all the body tissues and have two main actions:

• **Metabolic:** thyroid hormones control the **basal metabolic rate (BMR)**. This is the rate at which energy must be used to maintain vital functions such as respiration, heartbeat, peristalsis and biosynthesis (construction of proteins and other molecules). The BMR is high in young animals to allow for growth. It levels off in mature animals and then declines with old age.
• **Growth and development:** thyroid hormones are involved with the growth and development of tissues such as the skeleton, central nervous system, reproductive system and hair cycle.

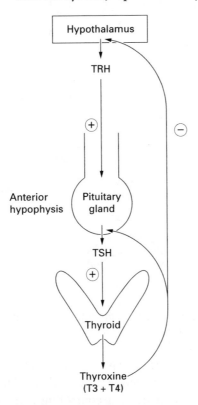

Figure 3.93 Diagram showing the control of thyroid hormones.

Remember: Thyroid hormones are important during metamorphosis in amphibians. Axolotls are the larval stage in the development of the salamander. Treating Axolotls with thyroid hormones can stimulate them to develop into mature salamanders.

A group of cells called **C-cells** within the thyroid gland secrete the hormone **calcitonin**. This hormone causes calcium to be deposited in the bones. Calcitonin therefore has a role in calcium homeostasis.

2.3.57 Parathyroid gland

What you need to learn

☙ You need to be able to describe the anatomy and function of the parathyroid glands, including the parathyroid hormone.

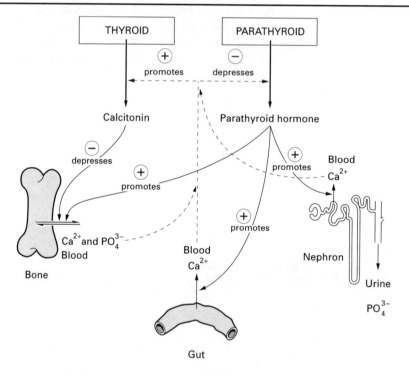

Figure 3.94 Diagram showing the effects of parathyroid hormone and calcitonin on blood calcium levels.

The parathyroid glands are closely associated with the thyroid gland. They synthesise and secrete the **parathyroid hormone**. Parathyroid hormone is involved in controlling calcium distribution in the body. Calcium (Ca^{2+}) is a very important ion. It is involved in muscle contraction, blood clotting and nerve impulse conduction, as well as providing teeth and bone structure. Calcium levels are very tightly controlled.

The main actions of parathyroid hormone are:

- increasing absorption of Ca^{2+} from the gut
- stimulating reabsorption of Ca^{2+} through the proximal convoluted tubule in the kidney
- promoting movement of Ca^{2+} from the skeleton into the plasma

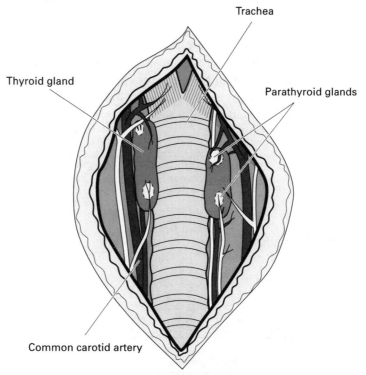

Figure 3.95 The parathyroid glands, ventral view.

2.3.58   Pancreas

What you need to learn

☙ You need to be able to explain the endocrine function of the pancreas:
  - ☙ insulin
  - ☙ glucagon
  - ☙ somatostatin.
☙ Describe the actions of the individual hormones produced by the pancreas.

The anatomy and exocrine function of the pancreas is discussed on page 162. Within the pancreas are islands of endocrine tissue called the **islets of Langerhans**. These areas contain three types of cells: **alpha** (α), **beta** (β) and **delta** (δ) cells.

Beta cells secrete **insulin** when blood glucose levels rise, eg after a meal. It performs two functions:

• Insulin stimulates synthesis of **glycogen** which is a polymer of glucose. Glycogen can be stored in the liver and skeletal muscle cells.
• Insulin aids the transport of glucose **from** the blood **into** respiring cells.

Alpha cells secrete **glucagon** when blood glucose levels decrease. Glucagon has the opposite effect to insulin. It stimulates the conversion of glycogen back to glucose, thereby raising blood glucose levels. Delta cells produce **somatostatin**. Somatostatin reduces gut motility and inhibits secretion of pancreatic and gastric secretions.

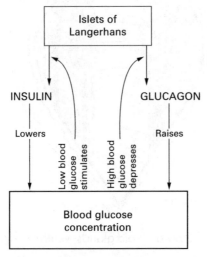

Figure 3.96 Diagram summarising the effects of insulin and glucagon on blood glucose levels.

2.3.59 Adrenal glands

What you need to learn

☙ You need to be able to describe the anatomy and function of the adrenal glands. These include:
  ☙ cortex:
  ☙ mineralocorticoids
  ☙ glucocorticoids
  ☙ sex steroids.
☙ Differentiate between the cortex and medulla of the adrenal glands and describe the functions of the hormones produced:
  ☙ **medulla:**

* adrenaline
* noradrenaline
❧ Describe the factors that control the production of the individual adrenal hormones.

The adrenal glands lie just cranial to the kidneys. They are retroperitoneal. Each adrenal gland is divided into two independent parts:

• the outer **cortex**
• the **medulla**.

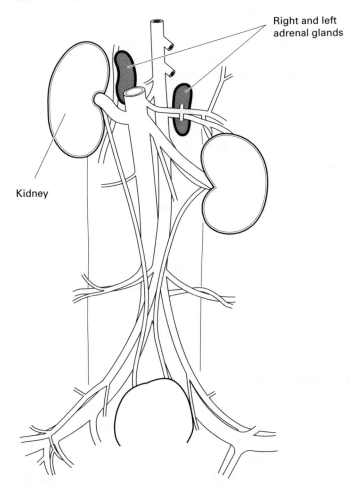

Right and left adrenal glands

Kidney

Figure 3.97 Diagram showing the position of the adrenal glands.

The adrenal cortex

The adrenal cortex produces **steroid** hormones. The release of these hormones is controlled by adrenocorticotrophic hormone from the pituitary gland and is regulated by negative feedback mechanisms.

The three main groups of hormones produced are the:

• **mineralocorticoids** (aldosterone)
• **glucocorticoids** (eg cortisol, cortisone)
• **sex hormones** (steroids) (progesterone, testosterone, oestrogen).

Glucocorticoids are very important in allowing animals to cope with physical and mental stress. Glucocorticoid levels are much higher in stressed animals. They have numerous functions:

• **Carbohydrate metabolism:** glucocorticoids raise blood glucose levels and stimulate the release of glucose from glycogen stores. (These effects are opposite to those of insulin.) They also stimulate the mobilisation of fats from adipose tissue.
• **Protein metabolism:** glucocorticoids promote conversion of amino acids into glucose (this process is called **gluconeogenesis**).
• **Immune suppression:** glucocorticoids cause eosinopenia and lymphopenia.
• **Anti-inflammatory effect:** glucocorticoids can delay wound healing.

Mineralocorticoids regulate the concentrations of sodium (Na^+) and potassium (K^+) ions in the body. The most important mineralocorticoid is **aldosterone.** Low sodium levels in the plasma stimulate aldosterone release. Aldosterone has various effects:

• aldosterone stimulates reabsorption of sodium in the kidney, this in turn causes water retention at the kidney
• uptake of sodium suppresses potassium reabsorption at the kidney resulting in decreased potassium levels.

The sodium : potassium ratio is tightly controlled. The production of sex hormones in the adrenal cortex is of minor importance.

The adrenal medulla

• The functions of the adrenal medulla are related to the sympathetic nervous system (fight or flight response).
• Two hormones are produced in the medulla: **adrenaline** and **noradrenaline**. These hormones have similar effects.
• Stimulation of the adrenal medulla by sympathetic nerves causes release of these hormones.
• The effects adrenaline and noradrenaline are shown in Figure 3.98:

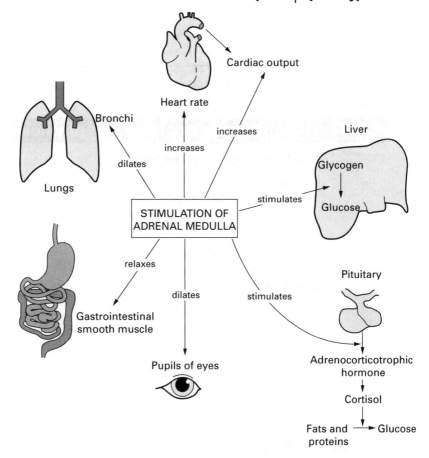

Figure 3.98 Summarising the actions of adrenaline and noradrenaline.

2.3.60   Body cavities

What you need to learn

❧ You need to be able to describe the basic anatomy and functions of the body cavities:
  - ❧ thorax
  - ❧ abdominal and pelvic cavities
  - ❧ mediastinum
  - ❧ diaphragm
  - ❧ omentum
❧ Define these associated terms:
  - ❧ parietal
  - ❧ mediastinal
  - ❧ diaphragmatic
  - ❧ costal pleural
  - ❧ mesentery

* peritoneal fluid
* State the sites where pleural and peritoneal fluid is found and describe their function.

See 2.3.02 Basic tissue types, pp. 51–52.

2.3.61 Comparative anatomy and physiology

What you need to learn

* You need to be able to outline the gross anatomy of mammals, birds, reptiles and chelonia commonly kept as pets. This includes:
  * teeth
  * digits
  * digestive system
  * sexing.
* Outline the nutritional requirements of animals and birds commonly kept as pets. This includes:
  * common foods
  * feeding methods
  * quantity.
* Describe the dentition of rodents and rabbits:
  * normal dentition
  * common abnormalities.

Exotics – sexing

Birds

In some species there are obvious physical differences between the male and female of the species. This is known as sexual dimorphism. Examples of sexual dimorphism are:

• In the cockatiel the males lose the horizontal bars on the ventral aspect of the tail at approximately 1 year of age.
• In the budgerigar the male has a blue cere while the female has a brown cere.
• In some cockatoos (white and pink) the iris is dark brown or black in the male but red in the female.
• In many species the male is more brightly coloured than the female.

In species which are not sexually dimorphic the sex of the bird can be determined through endoscopy (visualisation of the reproductive organs using an endoscope) or through examining DNA from a blood sample.

Rodents and lagomorphs

In mature animals sexing is usually simple because of the presence or absence of testicles. Sexing of younger animals is more difficult as testicles can be undescended or extremely small. Sex determination in these young animals is often based on the distance between the openings of the genito-urinary tract and the anus. In female animals the distance is shorter in nearly all species.

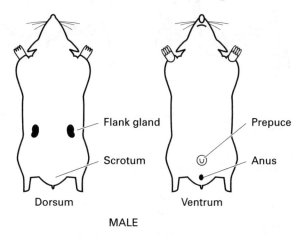

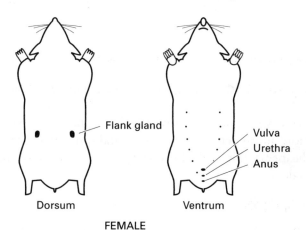

Figure 3.99 Sexing rodents (in this case hamsters).

Reptiles

Snakes can be sexed using a lubricated probe which is inserted caudally into the cloaca. The probe will penetrate 8–16 scale lengths in the male, but only 2–6 in the female. Chelonians are sexually dimorphic. The male has a longer, wider tail than the female. In some species the plastron is more concave in the male. In the red-eared terrapin the front claws are longer in the male than in the female.

MALE   FEMALE

Testudo hermanni (Herman's tortoise)

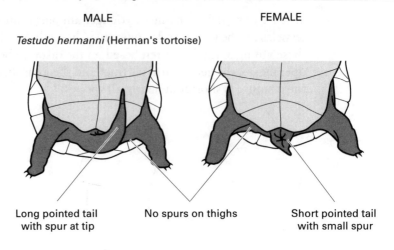

Long pointed tail   No spurs on thighs   Short pointed tail
with spur at tip   with small spur

Testudo graeca (Spur-thighed tortoise)

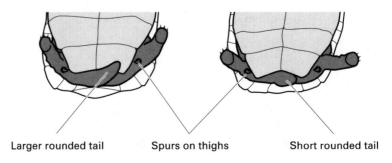

Larger rounded tail   Spurs on thighs   Short rounded tail

Figure 3.100 Diagram showing the difference in sexes in tortoises.

Lizards are sometimes sexually dimorphic, with the males carrying more adornments (such as horns and spurs) than the female. Pores in the medial thigh called **femoral pores** are often more developed in the male.

Exotics – nutrition

All animals must be provided with fresh water daily. The water should be provided in a suitable receptacle with which the animal is familiar.

Birds

Diet varies greatly depending upon the species encountered. Anyone considering owning a bird should obtain as much information regarding the diet and husbandry of the species as possible. All birds need to eat fragments of grit and other abrasive materials. These fragments pass into the gizzard where they help to grind food.

Caged birds are often divided into **hardbills** and **softbills**.

Hardbills (most of the parrot-like birds and finches) remove the outer husk to reach the nutritious kernel from seeds and nuts. Their beaks are specially adapted for this purpose. Softbills eat food such as fleshy fruit, invertebrates (eg many garden birds including blackbirds and tits), or pollen and nectar (eg hummingbirds, lorikeets).

The distinction is not always clear cut. Psittacines will eat fruit and some softbills will eat seed as a supplement to their diet.

Water fowl, including ducks, geese and swans, will often eat bread, mixed corn and water plants. Birds such as swans often prefer the food to be fed in a bowl of clean water. Some water birds such as seabirds and herons are fish eaters. Care should be taken when feeding birds on whitefish as it contains an enzyme which causes thiamine deficiency. Captive fish-eating birds should therefore be provided with a vitamin B supplement.

Birds of prey such as eagles, hawks, falcons and owls require a carnivorous diet. **Whole** animals should be fed to provide a balanced diet. Day-old chicks, or dark mice (as wild birds will often not recognise white mice as food) fed with a vitamin and mineral supplement will usually suffice. Larger birds can be fed on pigeons and rabbits.

NB It is illegal to offer live vertebrate food.

Rodents

Omnivores such as rats, mice and hamsters can be fed with well-balanced, commercially available diets. Food should be stored in a cool dry place to prevent spoiling. Treats such as raw fruit and vegetables can be offered. Chocolate and sweet treats should be fed only very occasionally as they can cause obesity.

Gerbils can be fed on well-balanced, commercially available diets but these should be supplemented with seeds, fruits and leafy vegetables. Guinea-pigs are naturally herbivorous. They can be fed with well-balanced, commercially available diets which have been **specifically** designed for guinea-pigs. Guinea-pigs, like humans, are unable to synthesise vitamin C and therefore obtain it from the diet. Many commercial rodent foods lack sufficient vitamin C and contain too much vitamin D for guinea-pigs. The diet of a guinea-pig should be supplemented with good quality hay and grass, along with a variety of fruit and vegetables.

Chinchillas may be fed with a well-balanced, commercially available diet. Pelleted food can be supplemented with a small amount of fresh or dried fruit and vegetables. Fresh, good quality hay should be available.

Rabbits

Rabbits are grazing animals. Their natural diet is grass and hay. The digestive system of rabbits is designed to digest this high-fibre, low-protein diet. Commercial diets are usually too low in fibre and too high in protein which results in digestive and dental disorders. Many rabbits will eat their commercial diets selectively so that much of the fibre is ignored in favour of the grains and pulses. This leads to obesity and, because of the low calcium content, problems with the teeth and bones. An ideal diet for a rabbit consists of good quality grass and hay. A small amount of a good quality commercial diet should be fed only as a supplement. A suitable commercial diet would be one which consists of just one type of pellet thereby avoiding selective feeding.

Reptiles

A balanced diet is essential in keeping a reptile healthy. Most of the disorders encountered in reptiles are a direct result of improper feeding and husbandry. Reptiles are cold blooded and will eat more when they are warm. Obesity and anorexia are both common problems in reptiles. The weight of an animal should be monitored if the animal is not feeding properly. Great care should be taken to make sure that the diet contains sufficient calcium and phosphorous to prevent metabolic bone disease. The actual diet fed depends upon the species. Anyone considering owning a reptile should obtain as much information regarding the diet and husbandry of the species as possible.

Chelonians

Tortoises are mainly herbivorous although there are some species which occasionally eat meat or insects. A variety of fruit and vegetables should be offered.

NB It should be noted that lettuce contains very little in the way of nutrients and should be avoided because it is often eaten preferentially by tortoises.

Lizards

Some lizards, such as geckos, are insectivorous and should be fed on locusts, crickets and occasional mealworms. The feed should be dusted with a vitamin and mineral supplement. It is important to also feed the locusts well as an undernourished locust will provide little nourishment for the lizard.

Larger lizards such as iguanas are predominantly herbivorous and should be fed a wide variety of fruit and vegetables. Water dragons are insectivorous when very young but become omnivorous as they age. Carnivorous lizards can be fed on mice. The whole animal, rather than pieces of meat, should be fed to provide a balanced diet. Chameleons are difficult to feed as they are very fastidious, preferring a variety of winged insects, caterpillars and crickets.

Snakes

All snakes are carnivorous although the kind of meat they eat varies between species. Most species will eat small mammals. The whole animal, rather than pieces of meat, should be fed to provide a balanced diet. **Pinkies** are bald baby mice and can be fed to small snakes. **Fuzzies** or **furries** are young mice with a fine coat.

Adult mice and rats can also be fed. The size of the snake determines the size of food which should be provided. A small snake will refuse food which is too big to swallow whole. A large snake will often refuse prey which is too small, or lose weight because it will often only eat one animal at each feeding time.

Some snakes are fish eaters (eg garter snakes). Fish should be fed whole to provide a balanced diet. Care should be taken when feeding snakes on whitefish as it contains an enzyme which causes thiamine deficiency.

Some snakes are cannibalistic or eat prey such as lizards. Owners should be advised to obtain all the necessary information before deciding to take on these species.

Amphibians

Almost all adult amphibians are carnivorous. Anyone considering owning an amphibian should obtain as much information regarding the diet and husbandry of the species as possible. Aquatic species can usually be fed on mealworms or earthworms. **Terrestrial** (land-living) species can usually be fed on maggots, crickets or small mice. **Arboreal** (tree-living) species can be fed on flies such as fruit flies.

Fish

Fish can be herbivorous, carnivorous or omnivorous. Most commonly kept fish can be fed with a well-balanced, commercially available diet. These are usually in the form of pellets or flakes. Live foods such as daphnia and blood worms are available but care should be taken when feeding these as they can introduce parasites to the pond or aquarium. Care must be taken not to overfeed fish as the tank can become polluted with rotting surplus food. If an owner is considering keeping fish such as Koi carp or discus on a larger scale they should be advised to obtain as much information regarding the diet and husbandry of the species as possible.

Dentition in rodents and rabbits

The dental formula of the guinea-pig is: $I\frac{1}{1}C\frac{0}{0}PM\frac{1}{1}M\frac{3}{3}$

The dental formula of the rabbit is: $I\frac{2}{1}C\frac{0}{0}PM\frac{3}{2}M\frac{3}{3}$

Incisors are used for nipping off the grass or plant food. Only the anterior surface of the incisors is covered with enamel. This means that the posterior surface wears away more quickly, creating the chisel shape of the incisors. Molars are used for grinding the food to increase the surface area available for digestion. The teeth have open roots and erupt continuously. This ensures that the teeth are not worn away by the constant grinding of fibrous food. The premolars and molars sit in a group which is separated from the incisors by a gap called the **diastema**. Lagomorphs (rabbits and hares) are distinguished from rodents because they have a third pair of incisors on the upper jaw – the **peg** teeth.

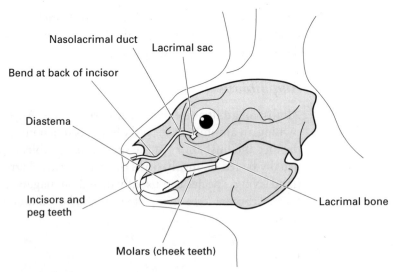

Figure 3.101 Diagram showing the teeth and nasolacrimal system in the lagomorph.

Dental disease is common in rodents, particularly the rabbit. Failure of the teeth to meet properly is called **malocclusion**. Malocclusion of the incisors is very common. Because the teeth are not wearing against each other they grow too long and can cause injury to the soft tissue of the face. Malocclusion can result in an animal being unable to eat. Malocclusion of the molars causes eating difficulties and often causes incisor malocclusion.

If the teeth are not able to grow into the mouth the roots grow backwards into the bone. This is known as reverse eruption. In the upper incisors this can cause obstruction of the nasolacrimal duct resulting in infection and inflammation (**dacryocystitis**). In the molars the impacted roots can cause pain, infection and eventually abscessation.

2.3.62   Reproductive system

What you need to learn

* You need to be able to describe the anatomy and function of the female and male reproductive tracts.
* Describe how the sex of exotics is determined and indicate knowledge of sexing sexually dimorphic avian species:
   * exotics
   * budgerigars
   * tortoises
   * snakes
   * reptiles.
* Describe the hormonal control of reproductive processes.

See pp. 180–182.

2.3.63   Female genital tract

What you need to learn

* You need to be able to describe the anatomy and functions of the tubular genital system:
   * fallopian tubes
   * uterus
   * cervix
   * vagina.
* Describe the structure and location of the uterine tubes and define associated terms including fimbrae and infundibulum.
* Describe the anatomy and functions of the uterus. Define associated terms:
   * horns
   * body
   * endometrium
   * myometrium

* broad ligament
* multiparous
* primigravid
* multigravid.

🐾 Describe the changes to the uterus which take place in pregnancy.
🐾 Explain why the bitch and the queen in cats and dogs have very long uterine horns.
🐾 Describe the location, structure and function of the cervix
🐾 Describe the location, structure and functions of the vagina and define associated terms.
🐾 Describe the structure and functions of the vulva and vulval labia:
  * vestibule
  * external urethral opening
  * clitoris.

The female reproductive organs

The female reproductive organs consist of the **tubular genital tract** and the paired **ovaries**.

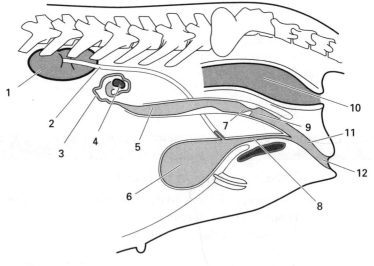

KEY

1.	Right kidney	7.	Cervix
2.	Ureter	8.	Urethra
3.	Uterine tube	9.	Vagina
4.	Ovary	10.	Rectum
5.	Uterine horn	11.	Vestibule
6.	Bladder	12.	Vulva

Figure 3.102 The urogenital tract of the female dog.

The tubular genital tract

The **uterine tubes** (these used to be called **oviducts** or **fallopian** tubes)

- The function of the uterine tubes is to receive the **ovum** after ovulation and convey it to the **uterus.**
- The entrance to the uterine tubes is called the **infundibulum.**
- The edges of the infundibulum are formed into finger-like projections called **fimbrae** which come into contact with the ovary.
- Fertilisation of the ovum with sperm occurs in the uterine tubes.
- The uterine tubes are lined with ciliated simple columnar epithelium. The cilia beat to move the ovum along the uterine tube towards the uterus.

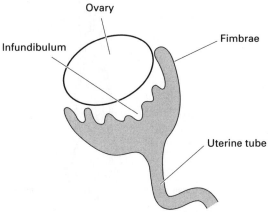

Figure 3.103 Schematic diagram of the ovary and uterine tube.

The uterus

- The function of the uterus is to carry and nourish embryos until they are ready for birth (**parturition**).
- In cats and dogs the uterus consists of paired uterine **horns** and a single short uterine **body** where the horns join close to the cervix.
- The uterine horns are long in these species because they need to be able to carry a number of foetuses.
- The outer surface of the uterus is called the **serosa** or **perimetrium.**
- The thick muscular layer of the uterine wall is called the **myometrium.**
- The inner surface of the uterus is called the **endometrium.** It is lined with simple columnar epithelium. Numerous glands open onto the surface of the endometrium,
- The uterus is suspended from the dorsal surface of the abdominal cavity by the **broad ligament** (or **mesometrium**). The broad ligament contains blood vessels and a variable amount of fat. Round ligament is a fibrous band in the lateral edge of broad ligament.

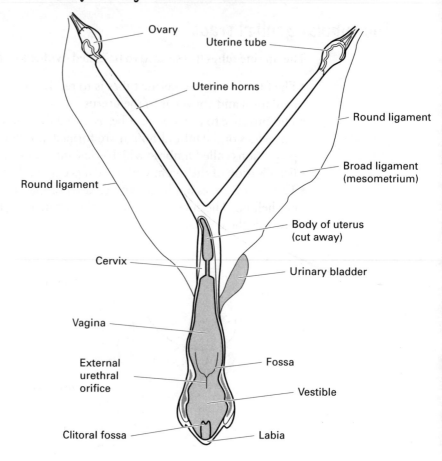

Figure 3.104 The uterus of the bitch.

- The uterus is capable of massive expansion during pregnancy.
- An animal which has not yet been pregnant is called **nulliparous**.
- When the animal carries its first pregnancy it is called **primiparous** or **primigravid**.
- An animal which has carried numerous pregnancies is called **multiparous** or **multigravid**.

The cervix

- The cervix is the thick-walled caudal segment of the uterus. It is a very short segment.
- It functions as a sphincter to prevent passage of material into and out of the uterus.
- The cranial end of the cervix is called the **internal cervical os** and communicates with the uterine body.
- The caudal end of the cervix is called the **external cervical os** and communicates with the vagina.

- The lumen of the cervix is constricted and almost occluded by folds of mucosa.
- The cervix is opened during parts of the reproductive cycle and during parturition.

The vagina

- The vagina is a thin-walled expandable tube. It is relatively long in the dog, but short in the cat.
- The cranial part of the vagina extends from the cervix to the urethral opening. This part has only reproductive functions.
- The caudal part of the vagina is called the **vestibule** and extends from the urethral opening to the vulva. This part has both reproductive and urinary functions.
- The reproductive functions of the vagina are to receive the sperm during copulation; and to expand, forming part of the birth canal during parturition.
- The folded mucosa of the vagina is lined with stratified squamous epithelium. The cranial part of the vagina is lined with glands which produce moisture.

The vestibule and vulva

- The vulva is the caudal part of the tract which communicates with the outside.
- The urethra opens onto the floor of the vestibule at the **external urethral orifice** (opening).
- The opening of the vulva is bounded by the **labia**.
- The **clitoris** is the female version of the penis. It consists of erectile and nervous tissue. It is often difficult to see because it is concealed in the **clitoral fossa**.
- The **vestibular glands** line the vestibule and secrete mucus.

2.3.64   Ovaries

What you need to learn

- ☙ You need to be able to describe the location and structure of the ovaries and define associated terms:
  - ☙ mesovarium
  - ☙ ovarian ligament
  - ☙ ovarian bursa
  - ☙ follicle
  - ☙ follicular fluid
  - ☙ ovulation.

❧ Explain the hormonal control of ovarian function.

❧ Describe the hormones produced by the ovary and explain the factors which influence the production of each ovarian hormone:

  ❧ relaxin

  ❧ progesterone

  ❧ oestradiol

  ❧ oestrogen.

❧ Describe how these hormones bring about the clinical signs shown in the various stages of the oestral cycle, ovulation, pregnancy, pseudo-pregnancy and parturition. This means knowing when to recognise a bitch is in season or a queen is calling.

❧ Describe the normal oestrus cycle of the bitch and queen, and show an understanding of the following terms:

  ❧ season

  ❧ hormones

  ❧ behavioural change

  ❧ frequency of the oestrus cycle.

❧ Outline medical and surgical methods for controlling oestrus, including hormonal methods and ovariohysterectomy.

❧ Explain the advantages and disadvantages of drugs used to control oestrus.

❧ Define misalliance.

❧ Describe the care of a female to prevent accidental matings.

❧ Explain the advantages and disadvantages of drugs used to prevent pregnancy after misalliance.

The ovaries

• The ovaries are the oval shaped, paired female gonads.

• They produce hormones and the female gametes (**ova** or **eggs**).

• The ovaries are found in the dorsal part of the abdomen near the caudal poles of the kidneys. They are suspended by the cranial part of the broad ligament – the **mesovarium**.

• The ovary sits within a fold of the mesovarium called the **ovarian bursa**.

• The **suspensory ligament** (also known as the ovarian ligament) of the ovary holds the ovary in position. It is cut during ovariohysterectomy. The suspensory ligament and the associated blood vessels are often called the **ovarian pedicle**.

• Within each ovary are thousands of immature ova, each of which is enclosed in a **follicle**.

• Under the action of various hormones a number of ova become mature. These are released from their follicles along with the follicular fluid. This process is called **ovulation**.

• The ova are caught by the fimbrae of the uterine tubes and pass into the infundibulum.

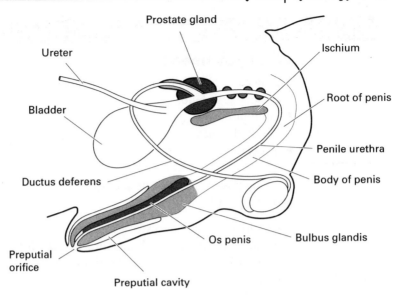

Figure 3.110 Cross-section of the urogenital tract of the dog.

In the cat the non-erect penis points caudally, with the preputial orifice lying beneath the testes. When the cat penis becomes erect it is directed cranially. The cat penis is covered with small barbs. These stimulate the female to ovulate during copulation. The os penis is very short in the cat.

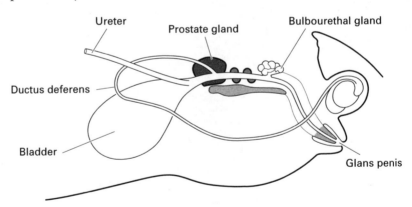

Figure 3.111 Cross-section of the urogential tract of the cat.

2.3.66   Male accessory glands

What you need to learn

* You need to be able to describe the functions and location of the accessory sex glands:
  * bulbourethral
  * seminal vesicle
  * prostate.

The dog possesses only one accessory sex gland. It is called the **prostate gland**.

There are two main accessory sex glands in the cat. These are the prostate gland and the **bulbourethral gland**. Note that neither the dog nor cat possesses a vesicular gland (originally called the seminal vesicle).

The prostate gland

The prostate gland surrounds the neck of the bladder and the proximal urethra. It is bi-lobed.

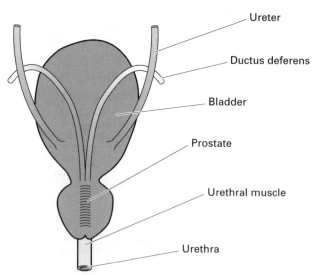

Figure 3.112   The position of the prostate gland in the dog. Ventral view.

The prostate gland produces **prostatic fluid** which carries and nourishes the sperm at ejaculation. Prostatic fluid passes into the urethra. It is weakly alkaline to neutralise the acidity of the male urethra. The prostate becomes larger in older entire animals. It is very small in castrated males.

The bulbourethral glands

These are paired glands which lie at the caudal end of the penis of the cat. They are approximately pea sized. These glands open into the urethra and contribute to the seminal fluid.

2.3.67   Testes

What you need to learn

* You need to be able to describe the location, structure and functions of the testes and define associated terms:
  * spermatic cord
  * vas deferens
  * tunica vaginalis
  * seminiferous tubule
  * efferent tubules
  * spermatozoa
  * Sertoli cells
  * cells of Leydig
  * spermatogenesis
  * monorchid
  * cryptorchid.
* Explain the hormonal control of testicular function.
* Describe the hormones produced by the testes and their functions.
* State the factors which control the production of these hormones.

The testes

* The testes are the male gonads.
* They are paired oval organs which have both endocrine and exocrine functions.
* Each testis is suspended in the scrotum by its **spermatic cord,** wrapped in the **tunica vaginalis.**
* The outer surface of each testis is covered with a fibrous capsule.
* Within the testis are many tiny tubules (**seminiferous tubules**) lying within supportive tissue (**interstitial** or **Leydig** cells).
* **Germ cells** within the seminiferous tubules are the site of sperm production (**spermatogenesis**). **Spermatozoa** are the male gametes.
* The walls of the seminiferous tubules are made up of **Sertoli cells** which support the tubules and also secrete hormones.
* The Leydig cells produce the male sex hormone – **testosterone.**
* Both ends of every seminiferous tubule drain into the **rete testis,** which in turn drains into the **efferent tubules.** These join to form the epididymis where sperm is stored.

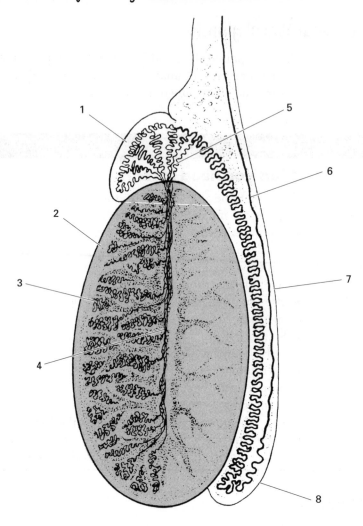

KEY

1. Head of epididymis
2. Fibrous capsule (tunica albuginea)
3. Seminiferous tubules
4. Rete testis
5. Efferent ductules
6. Deferent duct
7. Body of epididymis
8. Tail of epididymis

Figure 3.113 Schematic diagram of the testis and epididymis.

- In the foetus the testes are formed in a position just caudal to the kidneys (where the ovaries are in the female).
- During foetal development the testes descend caudally in the abdomen; then through a hole in the abdominal wall called the **inguinal ring,** and down into the scrotum.

- If the descent of the testes is not completed one or both testes may remain inside the abdomen, or outside the inguinal ring but not within the scrotum. The undescended testicle is called a **cryptorchid** testicle. The correct term for a single undescended testicle is **unilateral cryptorchidism**. If both testes are undescended the term is **bilateral cryptorchidism**.
- Testes which are within the abdomen are at a higher temperature than those within the scrotum. They are more likely to become cancerous. Abdominal testes are still capable of producing hormones but cannot produce viable sperm.

Remember: very rarely an animal can be born with a testicle missing completely. This is called a **monorchid** animal. The term monorchid should not be confused with unilateral cryptorchid.

Hormonal control of testicular function

- Luteinising hormone (LH) stimulates the Leydig cells to produce testosterone.
- Testosterone and other sex steroids have a number of functions. They are responsible for male sexual drive (**libido**) and aggression. They also promote growth and development of the reproductive organs. Testosterone also influences growth rate and body composition.
- Follicle stimulating hormone (FSH) promotes spermatogenesis by stimulating cells within the seminiferous tubules.
- LH and FSH are both released from the anterior pituitary gland.
- Libido is also affected by environmental factors. High temperature and humidity often lower libido.
- Production of testosterone and spermatogenesis starts when a male animal reaches puberty.

2.3.68   Genetics

What you need to learn

- You need to be able to describe common congenital defects associated with identified breeds:
  - dogs – hip dysplasia, cryptorchidism, eye defects, umbilical hernia, progressive axonopathy.
  - cats – Manx, polydactyly, deafness, folded ears.
- Outline the causes and implications of recessive and hereditary defects.
- Outline the elements of genetics and describe how this affects

development and breeding:
* gene
* homozygous
* heterozygous
* dominant
* recessive
* phenotype
* genotype
* in-breeding
* line breeding
* out-breeding
* hybrid.
* Outline the provisions of the British Veterinary Association and Kennel Club control schemes and voluntary breed schemes for:
  * hip dysplasia (HD)
  * progressive retinal atrophy
  * hereditary cataracts, etc.

Genetics is the study of how characteristics are inherited from generation to generation. An understanding of genetics is important in veterinary science because many domestic animals are bred to inherit certain traits, eg pedigree dogs and cats. If sufficient care is not taken when breeding animals, unwanted characteristics can be passed on to subsequent generations. Unwanted characteristics can be **traits** such as aggression, or hereditary defects.

Congenital and hereditary defects

> **Remember:** a **hereditary** condition is one which is passed on through the genes. A **congenital** condition is a condition which is present at birth. Congenital defects are often but not always hereditary (see Table 3.16).

* Congenital defects include **cleft palate** (where the hard palate fails to fuse in the midline) and heart abnormalities such as **persistent ductus arteriosus** (PDA) (where the blood vessel which allows blood to bypass the lungs in the foetus fails to close at birth).
* Some hereditary defects are harmless and even desirable (such as the polydactyly in Bernese mountain dogs).
* Some hereditary defects can cause problems in some but not all of the offspring (such as the Manx tail gene which causes short or absent tails in some kittens but can cause fatal defects similar to spina bifida in other kittens in the same litter).
* Some inherited defects always cause problems, eg the genes which cause deafness. Breeders try to ensure that these genes are not passed on to the next generation.

Table 3.16

Condition	Symptoms	Breeds commonly affected
Hip dysplasia	Loose, poorly fitting coxo-femoral (hip) joints. Affected animals usually develop osteoarthritis in later years.	Labrador, German shepherd, clumber spaniel.
Cryptorchidism	Unilateral or bilateral retained testicles.	Any breed, boxers.
Eye defects including:		
Entropion	In-turning of eyelids causing irritation of cornea by hair.	Shar-pei, chow, bulldog.
Collie eye anomaly	Underdeveloped choroid layer and retina.	Rough and smooth collie.
Retinal dysplasia	Folds and areas of non-attachment of retina.	CKCS, Rottweiler, English springer spaniel.
Umbilical hernia	Failure of umbilicus to close over after detachment of umbilical cord. Results in protrusion of omentum, fat and/or gut through hole.	Any breed.
Progressive axonopathy	Progressive nerve damage, starts as weakness in the hind limbs, eventually also affecting forelimbs. Untreatable.	Boxers.
Manx	Varying degrees of tail shortening. Can have a short tail or no tail at all.	Manx cats.
Polydactyly	Extra digits, usually in the front feet in cats. Often extra dew claws are seen in the Bernese mountain dog.	Bernese mountain dogs. Any breed of cat but most commonly the Maine Coone.
Deafness	Unilateral or bilateral deafness. Caused by defect in the auditory pathway (cochlea to auditory nerve).	Dalmatians, white boxers, white English bull terriers, white cats.
Folded ears	Folded ear tip	Scottish fold cat.

• An animal can carry and pass on genes for hereditary defects without showing outward signs. This makes selection of animals for breeding more difficult.

Terms used in genetics

• A **chromosome** is made from chromatin fibres which are highly folded strands of DNA. Each chromosome carries many thousands of genes. Chromosomes are found within the nucleus of a cell.
• The pair of chromosomes that is concerned with sex determination are called the **sex chromosomes.** Males have XY sex chromosomes whereas females have XX sex chromosomes. Characteristics which are carried on the sex chromosomes can therefore be linked to sex. For example the gene for coat colour in tortoiseshell cats is only expressed in females.
• All the other chromosomes are called **autosomal chromosomes.**
• A **gene** is part of the DNA molecule which carries the instructions for the synthesis of a polypeptide or protein.
• Each gene is composed of two **alleles.** The alleles can be identical (**homozygous**) or non-identical (**heterozygous**). One allele comes from each parent.
• Where an animal is heterozygous for a particular gene one of the alleles is usually **dominant** to the other, therefore masking the effect of the less dominant or **recessive** allele.
• The genetic make up of an animal is called its **genotype.**
• The physical appearance and characteristics of an animal are called its **phenotype.**
• **In-breeding** is where an animal breeds with an immediate relative (eg brother–sister or parent–offspring matings). It is used by breeders to pass on particularly good genes in show animals but there are great risks with in-breeding. Undesirable and harmful genes are often passed on and they become concentrated. Alleles which are recessive and normally masked can become expressed in the phenotype (there is increased homozygosity). In-breeding sometimes has to be used to preserve a rare breed or species.
• **Line breeding** is where an animal breeds with a more distant relative such as a grandparent or cousin. This is undesirable for similar reasons to in-breeding.
• **Out-breeding** is where an animal breeds with an unrelated animal. There is greater variety in the genes of the offspring and there is increased heterozygosity.
• A **hybrid** is a cross between two different species. An example is the mule which is a cross between a male donkey and a female horse.

Inheritance of a characteristic – Example black spot and liver spots in the Dalmatian

A capital letter denotes the dominant form of the gene (black spots in this case) while a lower-case letter denotes the recessive form of the gene (liver-coloured spots).

If a homozygous black spotted Dalmatian (BB) is mated with a liver-spotted (bb) Dalmatian the possible outcomes are shown below:

	B	B
b	Bb	Bb
b	Bb	Bb

- The first generation of offspring is called the **F1 generation**.
- The black form of the gene (B) is dominant so all of the offspring will have black spots. Therefore their **phenotype** is black spots.
- Although the parents were homozygous, the **genotype** of all the offspring will be heterozygous for the gene coding for coat colour.

If two of the F1 generation were mated the possible outcomes would be:

	B	b
B	BB	Bb
b	Bb	bb

- The second generation is called the **F2 generation**.
- The phenotype of three-quarters of the offspring will be black spots. Some will be homozygous (BB) and the rest will be heterozyygous (Bb).
- The phenotype of one quarter of the offspring will be homozygous recessive (bb) and their phenotype will be liver-coloured spots.

Schemes to assess breeding animals

- To avoid passing harmful traits on to future generations the British Veterinary Association (BVA) and the Kennel Club (KC) have devised schemes for screening potential breeding animals. These schemes are voluntary but are used by all responsible breeders.
- The **Hip Dysplasia Scheme** aims to select potential breeding animals which have little or no sign of hip dysplasia. Radiographs of the dogs' hips are taken under general anaesthesia and posted to the assessors at BVA/KC. Animals are scored out of 106. The fewer the signs of hip dysplasia that are evident, the lower the score is.

Each breed is given an average score. Only animals with a lower score than the breed average should be used for breeding.
- Various eye schemes are used to assess potential breeding animals for hereditary ocular disease. The animals are examined by an ophthalmologist and certified free of disease before breeding is allowed. Eye conditions which can be identified in this way are **collie eye anomaly** (rough and smooth collies, Shetland sheepdog), **progressive retinal atrophy** (Irish setters, miniature toy poodles, rough collies) and **hereditary cataracts** (golden retrievers and Afghan hounds).

2.3.69 Mating

What you need to learn

- You need to be able to outline the factors influencing the selection of a suitable male and female.
- Describe the normal mating process in dogs and cats.
- Explain the approximate time that a 'tie' lasts.
- Describe methods of assisting if difficulties arise during mating.

- When mating is planned the owner must select a suitable male and female animal.
- If the breed is known to suffer with a hereditary problem measures should be taken to ensure that the breeding animals are free of this condition.
- Dogs should be hip and eye scored if this is indicated by their breed.
- Pedigree animals should be good examples of their breed.
- The temperament of breeding animals should be taken into account as temperament is partly inherited. Aggressive or excessively fearful animals should not be bred.
- Breeding animals, particularly the female, should be in good condition so that a pregnancy will not cause undue stress. Over or underweight animals will reproduce less successfully.
- The male and female should be approximately matched in size to avoid problems with mating and parturition.
- Both animals should be fully vaccinated and free of parasites.

The mating process in dogs

- The dog is interested in the bitch during pro-oestrus. The bitch will only stand to allow mating during oestrus.
- There is usually little courtship between dogs. Usually the male will sniff or lick the vulva briefly and then will try to mount the bitch.
- The bitch will hold her tail to one side while the dog mounts. The presence of the os penis means that penetration occurs without the

dog's penis being fully erect. Penetration during mating is known as **intromission**.

- Once the penis is inside the vagina it becomes fully erect. The bulbus glandis becomes very swollen.
- The dog makes strong thrusting movements and **ejaculation** occurs (passage of sperm and prostatic fluid (**semen**) from the epididymis through the urethra and out of the urethral orifice).
- The dog dismounts by lifting his hind leg over the bitch. However, because of the engorged bulbus glandis the penis is locked in position in the vagina so the dogs end up **tied** together standing tail to tail.
- During the tie ejaculation of sperm-rich fluid continues.
- The tie can last from 5 minutes to 1 hour (usually about 20 minutes). The tie ends when the swelling of the bulbus glandis subsides.
- Inexperienced dogs often have difficulty achieving intromission and can be directed and aided by an experienced breeder.
- Inexperienced bitches can be frightened during the procedure and may need reassurance from an owner.
- Breeders often use an experienced dog with an inexperienced bitch and vice versa to help prevent problems.
- Occasionally there can be a size mismatch between the bitch and dog. Short-legged dogs can have difficulty achieving intromission with a long-legged bitch. In this case mating can take place on a small hill to make the process easier.

The mating process in cats

- The queen will allow mating during oestrus. She often crouches with her tail to one side to encourage mating. There is ventral curving of the spine (lordosis).
- The tom bites the back of the queen's neck and mounts her, holding on to her chest with his front legs.
- As the tom's penis becomes erect it points forwards. Intromission is brief and ejaculation occurs. As the penis is withdrawn the caudal-pointing barbs cause discomfort to the queen and she usually vocalises loudly. This process stimulates the LH surge which causes ovulation.
- The whole mating process usually takes less than 5 minutes in the cat.
- Mating is often repeated a few times.
- As with dogs mating is easier if an experienced tom is used.
- Some queens will reject certain toms but accept others.

2.3.70   Sire

What you need to learn

☙ You need to be able to describe the factors which influence the commencement of a dog's use at stud. This includes:
  ☙ onset of puberty
  ☙ use of the BVA and KC schemes for KC-registered dogs to reduce hereditary diseases
  ☙ moral and legal responsibilities of an owner.
☙ Explain how often a dog should be used as a stud.

Selection of a sire

• The male parent is called a **sire**.
• When mating is planned the owner must select a suitable sire.
• If the breed is known to suffer with a hereditary problem measures should be taken to ensure that the breeding animals are free of this condition.
• Dogs should be hip and eye scored if indicated by their breed.
• Pedigree animals should be good examples of their breed.
• The temperament of breeding animals should be taken into account as temperament is partly inherited. Aggressive or excessively fearful animals should not be bred.
• Male dogs are fertile from 8 or 9 months old. Most breeders prefer to wait until the dog is a little older before using him as a stud animal.
• A breeder has a moral responsibility to try to reduce the passage of undesirable genes to future generations.
• Irresponsible breeding including in-breeding is responsible for a great number of the breed-associated problems which are currently encountered. Often animals which have good show qualities are used for breeding regardless of the health problems from which they suffer. These include valvular heart disease in cavalier King Charles spaniels, allergic dermatitis in west highland white terriers as well as the numerous other conditions already mentioned.
• It is illegal for breeders to provide misleading information about their animals. This could include falsifying pedigree or health certificates, or deliberately misidentifying animals.
• Stud dogs should not be overused. Mating is tiring and sperm quality will be reduced if the dog is allowed to mate too frequently. Each bitch will usually be mated a few times over 3 or 4 days. The stud dog should be allowed to rest after this period.

2.3.71   Foetal development and neonatal anatomy

What you need to learn

* You need to be able to describe the process of fertilization and foetal development in different species and understand the terms:
  * zygote
  * conceptus
  * embryo
  * foetus.
* Describe the changes that occur in the zygote as it passes along the uterine tube to the uterus and the time after fertilisation that implantation takes place. This includes:
  * inner cell mass
  * trophoblast
  * embryo
  * ectoderm
  * endoderm
  * mesoderm.
* Describe the structure of the extra-embryonic membranes and use the associated terms:
  * amnion
  * yolk sac
  * chorion
  * allantois
  * villi.
* Describe the structure of the umbilical cord.

Foetal development

* Sperm is deposited in the proximal vagina during mating. The sperm must travel through the cervix and uterus, and then up the oviducts.
* Spermatozoa are mobile. Each spermatozoa has a tail which beats, driving it forwards. The journey of the sperm through the female genital tract is aided by the rhythmic contractions of the muscular tract and the movement of cilia within the uterine tubes.
* **Fertilisation** is the fusion of the male gamete (spermatozoon) with the female gamete (ovum). Fertilisation occurs in the uterine tubes. A fertilised ovum is called a **conceptus** until it is born.
* When fertilisation occurs the genetic information carried in the head of the spermatozoon enters the cytoplasm of the ovum. Once fertilisation has occurred the fused cell is called a **zygote**. The zygote is now a **diploid** cell because the ovum and spermatozoon each had the **haploid** number of chromosomes.
* The zygotes travel down the uterine tube towards the uterus. As

they travel they undergo divisions, first dividing into two cells, then four cells and so on. By the time the zygotes are ready to implant in the uterus each consists of a ball of 16 to 32 cells. The ball of cells is called a **morula**. Zygote to morula takes 5–8 days in the bitch and 3–5 days in the queen.

- Further cell divisions cause a space to develop within the ball of cells. The space becomes fluid filled. The conceptus is now called a **blastocyst**. In the blastocyst there is an **outer cell layer** and an **inner cell mass**.
- The outer cell layer of the blastocyst is called the **trophoblast layer** and will be responsible for attaching the blastocyst to the endometrium. Trophoblast and endometrial cells form the placenta and foetal membranes.
- The trophoblast layer exerts pressure on the endometrium and finger-like projections called **villi** push into the endometrium forming a firm attachment with a large surface area.
- The trophoblast layer forms the **chorion** which is part of the placenta.
- At 13 to 18 days after fertilisation the blastocysts are evenly spaced along the uterine horns and become implanted in the endometrium.
- The inner cell mass will develop into the **embryo**.

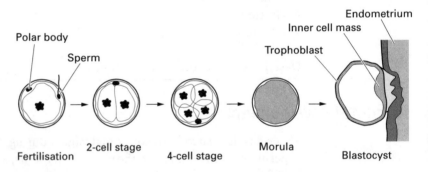

Figure 3.114 Diagram showing development from fertilisation to implantation.

- Part of the inner cell mass becomes organised into a single-cell layer called the **endoderm**. The endoderm grows around the inside of the trophoblast layer to form the yolk sac.
- The rest of the inner cell mass forms the **ectoderm**. Spaces form within the ectoderm which join to form the amniotic cavity.
- The embryo now consists of a double layer of cells called the **embryonic disc** (see Figure 3.115).
- After a few days the ectoderm folds inwards and creates another layer of cells between the endoderm and ectoderm which is called the **mesoderm**.

- The endoderm, mesoderm and ectoderm are the germ-cell layers which go on to create all of the structures of the body. Each layer produces different structures (see Table 3.17).

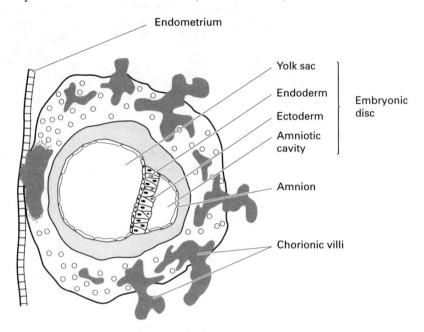

Figure 3.115 The embryonic disc.

Table 3.17

Endoderm	Mesoderm	Ectoderm
Respiratory tract	All connective tissues	Skin, hair and nails
Thyroid gland	including bone, muscle,	Central and peripheral
Thymus gland	lymphoid tissue, blood	nervous systems
Gastrointestinal tract	Cardiovascular system	Epithelia of sense organs,
Liver	Lymphatic system	mouth and skin
Pancreas	Urogenital tract	
	Adrenal cortex	

- At the edge of the embryonic disc the endoderm forms the pouch-like **allantois**.
- The allantois forms two layers. The inner layer lies against the amnion, while the outer layer lies against the chorion forming the **allantochorion**. This is the foetal part of the **placenta** (see Figure 3.116).
- The allantochorion is rich in blood vessels. These blood vessels pass into the chorionic villi deep in the endometrium. The blood supply from the mother and foetus are sufficiently close that exchange of materials such as oxygen, carbon dioxide, waste products and nutrients can occur.

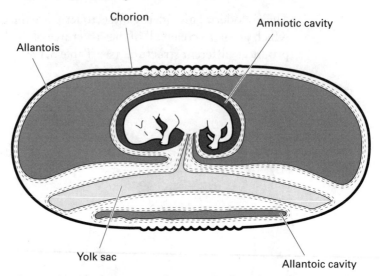

Figure 3.116 Diagram showing the foetal membranes of the dog.

- As well as providing exchange of substances the placenta is important in providing protection and lubrication of the foetus. The placenta also produces a number of hormones which are important during pregnancy and parturition.
- The blood vessels travel from the placenta in a tube of allantochorion into the developing embryo at the position which will become the umbilicus. This tube is called the **umbilical cord**.
- The umbilical cord contains the umbilical artery and vein. It also contains a vessel called the **urachus** which carries nitrogenous waste from the foetal bladder into the allantois. The urachus closes at birth.
- The umbilical artery carries **deoxygenated** blood from the foetus to the placenta. The umbilical vein carries **oxygenated** blood back to the foetus.
- The placenta of cats and dogs is described as **zonary**. This is because the chorionic villi are restricted to a band around the foetal membranes.

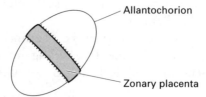

Figure 3.117 Schematic diagram of the zonary placenta of the dog and cat.

- When the major organs have developed the conceptus is called a **foetus**.

2.3.72 Normal pregnancy

What you need to learn

☙ You need to be able to describe the length of a normal pregnancy, the physical changes of pregnancy and the times that they occur.

☙ Explain how a veterinary surgeon would diagnose pregnancy. Tests include:
  ☙ radiography
  ☙ auscultation
  ☙ ultrasound
  ☙ abdominal palpation
  ☙ blood test.

☙ Describe the endocrine control that operates during pregnancy.

☙ Describe the care and feeding of the bitch throughout pregnancy.

☙ Describe abnormalities which may occur during pregnancy, eg abortion, resorption.

Duration of pregnancy and physical changes

Pregnancy lasts for 63–65 days in both dogs and cats. There is some variation in this as sperm can survive for up to 7 days in the reproductive tract of the bitch. During pregnancy the mother gains weight. Bitches usually gain approximately 35% of their body weight. Abdominal distension is usually obvious in the last third of pregnancy. Movement of the foetuses can be seen in the last week of pregnancy. Mammary development occurs in the second half of pregnancy. Secretions from the mammary glands may be present when birth is imminent. Some animals become more docile as pregnancy progresses.

Pregnancy diagnosis

Pregnancy diagnosis can be performed in a number of ways at different stages of pregnancy (see Table 3.18).

Hormonal control of pregnancy

• Hormone levels in pregnant bitches are similar to those during metoestrus (see Figure 3.118).

• Progesterone levels tend to stay at a steady plateau through pregnancy, declining suddenly at parturition.

• Oestrogen levels rise during the last third of pregnancy and decline suddenly at parturition.

• Prolactin levels increase as progesterone levels drop. Prolactin promotes milk production and levels continue to be raised until the offspring are weaned.

Table 3.18

Method	Stage of pregnancy	Comments
Abdominal palpation	3–4 weeks in dogs, slightly earlier in cats	Difficult in fat or tense animals.
Radiography	45 days	Only useful once foetal skeletons have become mineralised. Possible radiation risk to foetuses.
Ultrasound	3–4 weeks	Dependent on skill of operator.
Auscultation	8–9 weeks	Can only be used late in pregnancy. Foetal heart rate is more rapid than that of the dam.
Measurement of acute-phase proteins	4–5 weeks	Reliable. Requires blood sample. Not used in cats.

- Relaxin is a hormone produced by the placenta approximately 4 weeks after conception. It is not present in non-pregnant animals.

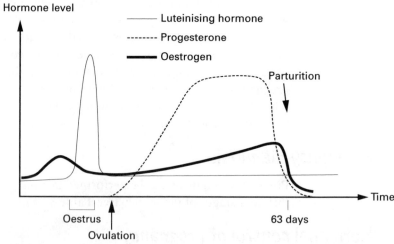

Figure 3.118 Diagram showing the hormonal changes during pregnancy in the bitch.

Care of the bitch during pregnancy

- Pregnant bitches should be fed a balanced, nutritious and highly digestible diet throughout pregnancy. It is important not to overfeed as obesity will cause problems during parturition.
- Vitamin and mineral supplementation are not usually necessary if a

good quality diet is provided. In particular, calcium supplements should be avoided until after parturition.
- The quantity of food required increases from week five of pregnancy. At the time of parturition the bitch will require 30% more food than when non-pregnant. At peak lactation the bitch will need three times the amount of food she needed when not pregnant. Meals should be fed little and often at this stage.
- Exercise should be continued to maintain the fitness of the bitch but strenuous exercise should be avoided.
- A worming programme should take place from mid-pregnancy up to parturition as some species of worm can infect foetuses across the placenta resulting in puppy worm burdens.
- A suitable area for parturition (whelping) should be provided 1 week before the expected whelping date.
- Great care must be taken when providing medication for pregnant bitches. For example steroids can cause abortion, and tetracycline antibiotics can cause tooth and bone discolouration.

Problems during pregnancy

- Problems can occur during foetal development which can result in loss of the pregnancy.
- Causes of pregnancy failure include foetal defects, trauma, infection, or abnormal maternal environment. In cats there are numerous viruses which can cause abortion or resorption.
- If the pregnancy fails early on the embryos will be resorbed with few outward signs. Hormone levels will return to normal although some bitches will suffer from a pseudopregnancy after resorption of embryos.
- If the pregnancy fails later on the foetuses will be aborted. This means that the uterus will contract and expel the foetuses and the foetal membranes. The bitch may be systemically ill and may require treatment with fluids and antibiotics.

2.3.73 False pregnancy (also known as phantom pregnancy or pseudopregnancy)

What you need to learn

- You need to be able to describe how false pregnancy arises and list its clinical signs.
- Describe the hormonal changes which lead to the condition of false pregnancy.
- Describe the different methods used to treat false pregnancy.
- Describe the nursing care for false pregnancy.

Signs of false pregnancy develop 3 to 4 weeks after oestrus and can persist for months. Clinical signs of false pregnancy include all the symptoms of pregnancy:

• behaviour changes such as restlessness and nesting
• mammary development and production of milk (lactation).

Some dogs in false pregnancy can have abdominal distension and even experience phantom parturition. False pregnancy is caused by the rising levels of prolactin which occur as progesterone levels fall when the corpora lutea regress during metoestrus. This situation can also be caused by spaying a bitch too soon after oestrus (ie surgically removing the corpora lutea). Treatment is not necessary in mild cases. If the bitch is distressed by the false pregnancy various treatments can be used:

• progestogens such as proligestone or megoestrol acetate
• androgen/oestrogen combinations such as testosterone/oestradiol
• prolactin-suppressing drugs such as cabergolamine are very effective
• antibiotics may be required if mastitis occurs.

Some bitches find false pregnancy very distressing. These dogs may require sedation. They should be housed somewhere quiet and dark. Affected bitches will often become calmer if they are allowed to nest or nurse toys.

2.3.74 Parturition

What you need to learn

☙ You need to be able to describe the hormonal control of parturition and list the changes brought about by the individual hormones involved.
☙ Describe the stages of labour and their normal duration.
☙ Describe the signs of imminent parturition.
☙ Describe the average length of time that straining normally takes place for the birth of a puppy litter and explain when veterinary assistance should be sought.
☙ Describe the monitoring and care of an animal in labour.

• It is thought that parturition (**birth, whelping**) is stimulated by a series of hormonal changes. It is likely that the whole process of parturition is brought about by **cortisol** release from the maturing foetus.
• Levels of **progesterone**, which has helped to sustain pregnancy, start to decrease. Progesterone inhibits uterine contractions.

- **Oestrogen** levels start to rise. Oestrogen helps to co-ordinate contraction of the muscular uterine wall (myometrium).
- The placenta produces a hormone **prostaglandin F2α (PGF2α).** This causes the corpus luteum to regress. It also stimulates production of the hormone **relaxin.**
- Relaxin causes relaxation of the pelvic ligaments and aids in dilation of the cervix.
- This combination of hormones initiates the uterine contractions.
- Stretching of the cervical region stimulates release of **oxytocin** from the pituitary gland. Oxytocin promotes uterine contraction.

Parturition is described in three stages:

- **Stage one:** uterine contractions and cervical relaxation and dilation cause the foetus to move into the pelvic canal. The head is engaged in the cervix. This stage lasts about 4 hours but in primigravid bitches it can last for 24–36 hours.
- **Stage two:** the expulsion of the foetus by involuntary contractions of the myometrium and voluntary contractions of the maternal abdominal wall. The duration of this stage varies considerably. As a general rule the bitch should strain for no more than 30 minutes before passing a puppy, but will take breaks for up to 4 hours between puppies. The bitch should be examined by a vet if she is taking more than 6 hours between puppies or is straining unproductively for more than 30 minutes. Large litters can take more than 24 hours to be born.
- **Stage three:** separation and expulsion of the placentas. In polytocous species such as dogs and cats the expulsion of each foetus is followed by the expulsion of a placenta. The mother will often eat the placentas as they are expelled.

Bitches show a number of signs when parturition is imminent. These include:

- A drop in body temperature to 37–38 °C. This is not a consistent sign as the temperature can be lower for the last week of pregnancy.
- Seeking dark quiet areas for nesting occurs 2 to 3 days before parturition.
- Food is often refused for 24–48 hours before parturition.
- Milk usually (but not always) is produced in the mammary glands.
- The vulva becomes slightly swollen and a slight vaginal discharge is seen just before parturition.

Bitches should be allowed peace and quiet during parturition although it is necessary to occasionally check the bitch carefully and quietly to ensure that parturition is progressing normally. Veterinary attention should be sought if parturition is not progressing as described.

Dystonia = difficulty in giving birth
Maternal = problem with mother (uterine inertia; small birth canal)
Foetal = problem with foetus (oversize, malpresentation).

2.3.75 Mammary glands

What you need to learn

☙ You need to be able to describe the structure, location and function
of the mammary glands and define associated terms. These include:
  ☙ gland sinus
  ☙ teat sinus
  ☙ teat canal
  ☙ teat orifice
  ☙ numbers of glands.

- The mammary glands are modified sweat glands. The secretion
  from the mammary gland nourishes the offspring.
- There are usually five pairs of mammary glands in the dog, and four
  pairs in the cat. The glands are spread along the ventral aspect of the
  trunk.
- The two cranial pairs are called **thoracic** mammary glands. The
  next two pairs are the **abdominal** mammary glands and the caudal
  pair are called the **inguinal** mammary glands.

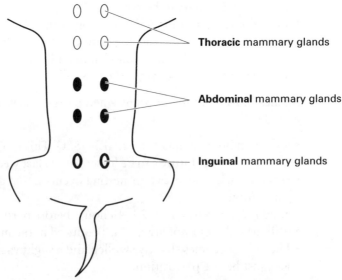

Figure 3.119 Schematic diagram of the mammory glands of the dog.

- The glandular tissue of the mammary glands is arranged into
  lobules. The milk produced here passes along a duct system until it
  arrives at the lactiferous sinus which stores the milk.

- The lactiferous sinus is described as two compartments – the gland sinus, and the teat sinus which extends into the teat.
- Milk travels through the **teat canal** from the teat sinus to the **teat orifices**. In the dog there are 8–20 orifices per teat, in the cat there are 4–7 orifices per teat.

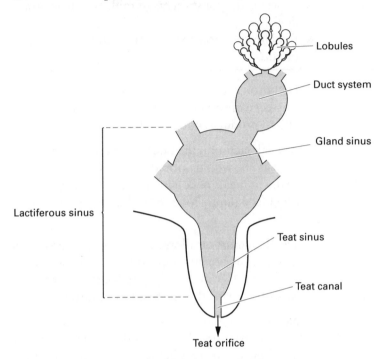

Figure 3.120   Diagram of the teat in the dog or cat.

- Mammary glands become developed and enlarged during oestrus in the non-pregnant animal, but regress during anoestrus.
- During pregnancy a number of hormones such as prolactin and glucocorticoids stimulate the production of milk (**lactogenesis**).
- Oxytocin stimulates special muscle cells within the mammary glands called **myoepithelial cells**. These squeeze milk out of the glandular tissue and stimulate milk let-down.
- Removal of milk by the offspring (suckling) is the main stimulus for the continued production of milk.
- As parturition approaches the glands become swollen and pendulous.

2.3.76   Lactation and neonatal care

What you need to learn

- You need to be able to explain the physiology of lactation and of the let-down of milk during feeding.

- Describe the care of the bitch and queen during lactation (nutritional needs and environment).
- Describe the care and management of a neonate until weaning.
- Describe the constituents of colostrum, its period of production and its functions in cats and dogs.
- Describe the constituents of milk and their proportions in cats and dogs.
- Explain common complications that may occur within the neonatal period.

Lactation causes a huge metabolic drain on the bitch. It is vital that she receives sufficient nutrients in her diet to sustain her own body and to produce enough milk to support and nourish her offspring.

At peak lactation the bitch or queen may need three times as much food as she would normally have. Often appetite is reduced so small, frequent meals of concentrated food may need to be fed. Breeders often feed puppy food to the bitch during peak lactation for this reason.

The dam must be allowed plenty of peace and quiet with her offspring to provide opportunities to suckle. Care must be taken to monitor the growth and vigour of the offspring. This is the simplest way of ensuring that each puppy or kitten is receiving sufficient milk.

Neonates should have sucked within 4 to 6 hours of birth. Most will suck almost immediately. As the offspring are born the dam should lick them clean. This helps to dry their coats and also encourages them to suck. This procedure is the first step in creating a bond between the dam and the litter. If the litter is very large or the mother is tired the pups or kittens may need towelling dry. Care should be taken to keep the litter warm. A lined box in a draught-free warm room is usually sufficient. Some breeders use heat lamps as an extra source of warmth.

Weaning is the process when the neonatal animal takes less milk from the dam and starts to lap liquid and eat solid food. It usually starts when kittens or pups are 3 to 4 weeks old and takes 2 to 3 weeks. The dam produces less milk in response to the decrease in demand and the mammary glands reduce in size.

The milk that is produced in the first 48–72 hours after birth differs in composition from the milk that is produced throughout the rest of lactation. This early milk is called **colostrum**. Colostrum has a number of functions:

- It provides a concentrated nutrient source. It is very rich in protein and glucose. New-born animals (**neonates**) are at risk from low blood glucose (**hypoglycaemia**) if they do not drink sufficient

colostrum. Colostrum also contains iron and the amino acid, proline which are used to make haemoglobin.

• The laxative effects of colostrum help the neonate to expel the foetal gut contents (**meconium**).

• It provides **immunoglobulins** (**antibodies**). These pass immunity from the dam to the offspring and provide some passive immunity against disease. The immunoglobulins are only absorbed through the neonatal gut for the first 24 hours of life. The maternal antibodies last for approximately 12 weeks. At this point the puppy or kitten has started to develop its own immunity to disease.

• It provides a warm drink for the neonate. Neonatal animals are wet and can chill very quickly.

After 48–72 hours the composition of the mammary secretion has changed into normal milk. Milk contains less protein and fat than colostrum. It contains carbohydrate in the form of **lactose**. It also contains minerals such as calcium, phosphorous, magnesium, sodium and chloride. These are vital for the development and growth of many tissues including bone and muscle. Vitamins A, E, K and B12 are also present in small quantities.

There are many problems which can arise during the neonatal period in the bitch or the queen, including:

• haemorrhage, uterine infection (**metritis**)
• mammary gland infection (**mastitis**)
• calcium deficiency (**hypocalcaemia**)
• lack of milk production, this is rare but there can be problems with milk let-down, injection of oxytocin usually stimulates release of the milk
• retention of placentas (rare).

Problems in neonates include:

• congenital abnormalities such as cleft palate, heart defects, deformities
• failure to suck – failure to suck colostrum will result in weak offspring which are vulnerable to disease
• rejection by mother – these animals often require hand-rearing
• disease numerous bacteria and viruses can infect neonatal animals worm infestations are common and can be very debilitating
• injury – there is a risk that the dam will lie on some of her offspring if there is too little room or a large litter.

2.3.77 Management of the orphaned newborn

What you need to learn

☙ You need to be able to explain how to nurse an orphaned neonate, including:
  ☙ environment
  ☙ nutrition
  ☙ excretion.
☙ Describe the methods of hand rearing, including:
  ☙ frequency of feeding.
  ☙ milk substitutes
  ☙ quantities.
☙ Explain the use of a foster mother.

Neonates can become orphaned for a number of reasons including illness or death of the mother; inability of the mother to cope with feeding the whole litter or simply being rejected by the mother.

Hand rearing orphans can be extremely difficult. A selection of commercial kitten and puppy milk substitutes are available. Examples are Welpi® and Cimicat®. Initially the orphans will need small amounts of concentrated milk substitute. As the animal grows a greater volume of more diluted milk can be provided. Special feeding bottles with small rubber teats are available for feeding orphans.

The orphan will need to be fed every 2 hours including through the night. The orphan will need to be encouraged to pass urine and faeces. The mother would do this by licking the perineum of the puppy or kitten. When hand rearing this can be simulated by wiping the perineum gently with a moist cotton bud. This should be done after every feed. Failure to perform this can result in the orphan's failure to thrive and even death.

It is sometimes possible to find a foster mother for the orphans. A foster mother can be a mother:

• who has lost her own litter but is still lactating
• who has plenty milk and only a small litter
• whose own offspring have been weaned but who still has plenty milk.

Care must be taken to ensure the orphans are not rejected by the foster mum as injury can result. Before introducing the orphans, attempts should be made to rub the smell of the bitch onto the pups or kittens. This can be done by allowing the orphans to sleep on a blanket belonging to the bitch.

Multiple choice questions

1. The cytoplasmic organelles which are closely involved with energy production are:
   - ☐ A lysosomes
   - ☐ B mitochondria
   - ☐ C ribosomes
   - ☐ D golgi apparatus

2. Simple ciliated columnar epithelia is found lining the:
   - ☐ A oesophagus
   - ☐ B trachea
   - ☐ C oviducts
   - ☐ D bladder

3. Nerve cells are known as:
   - ☐ A neurones
   - ☐ B nephrons
   - ☐ C neuroglia
   - ☐ D neutrophils

4. The haploid number is:
   - ☐ A the normal chromosome complement of a cell
   - ☐ B half the normal chromosome complement of a cell
   - ☐ C occurs during mitotic division
   - ☐ D found in dividing blood cells

5. The serous membrane which lines the abdominal cavity is the:
   - ☐ A parietal pleura
   - ☐ B visceral peritoneum
   - ☐ C visceral pleura
   - ☐ D parietal peritoneum

6. The pelvic bones are classified as:
   - ☐ A irregular bones
   - ☐ B flat bones
   - ☐ C long bones
   - ☐ D short bones

7. A dog breed which exhibits a dolicocephalic skull is a:
   - ☐ A saluki
   - ☐ B beagle
   - ☐ C pug
   - ☐ D boxer

8. The triceps brachii muscle inserts on the:
   - ☐ A   os calcis
   - ☐ B   olecranon
   - ☐ C   scapular tuberosity
   - ☐ D   tibial crest

9. The gastrocnemius muscle:
   - ☐ A   extends the hip and stifle
   - ☐ B   flexes the hock and extends the stifle
   - ☐ C   extends the hock and flexes the stifle
   - ☐ D   flexes the stifle and the hock

10. The outermost membrane covering the brain and spinal cord is the:
    - ☐ A   pia mater
    - ☐ B   arachnoid mater
    - ☐ C   dura mater
    - ☐ D   epidural mater

11. The inner layer of the eye is known as the:
    - ☐ A   limbus
    - ☐ B   sclera
    - ☐ C   choroid
    - ☐ D   retina

12. Mammalian erythrocytes are biconcave anuclear discs whose main function is:
    - ☐ A   antibody production
    - ☐ B   carriage of oxygen
    - ☐ C   clotting
    - ☐ D   phagocytosis

13. The commonest type of leucocyte in the dog is the:
    - ☐ A   eosinophil
    - ☐ B   basophil
    - ☐ C   monocyte
    - ☐ D   neutrophil

14. The mitral valve is also known as the:
    - ☐ A   right atrioventricular valve
    - ☐ B   left semilunar valve
    - ☐ C   tricuspid valve
    - ☐ D   bicuspid valve

15. The enzyme produced by the stomach which is involved in protein digestion is:
    - ☐ A   pepsinogen
    - ☐ B   trypsinogen
    - ☐ C   amylase
    - ☐ D   lipase

16. The hormone not produced by the anterior pituitary gland is:
    - ☐ A follicle stimulating hormone
    - ☐ B growth hormone
    - ☐ C oxytocin
    - ☐ D thyroid stimulating hormone

17. The lymph node located on the caudal aspect of the stifle is the:
    - ☐ A prescapular
    - ☐ B axillary
    - ☐ C popliteal
    - ☐ D inguinal

18. Vital capacity is defined as the:
    - ☐ A volume of gas inspired each breath during normal respiration
    - ☐ B maximal volume of gas that can be expired after a maximal inspiration
    - ☐ C reservoir of gas in the lungs after a normal expiration
    - ☐ D volume of gas left in the lungs after a maximal expiration

19. The thick muscular layer of the uterine wall is called the:
    - ☐ A endometrium
    - ☐ B myocardium
    - ☐ C myometrium
    - ☐ D mesometrium

20. The kidney is not responsible for the production of:
    - ☐ A erythropoietin
    - ☐ B urea
    - ☐ C renin
    - ☐ D hypertonic urine

Level 2: Unit 4

Principles of animal management and nursing

2.4.01   Legal and ethical aspects of practice

What you need to learn

* You need to be able to describe the legal accountability of the veterinary nurse:
  * criminal and civil law
  * employment.
* Professional regulation.
* Outline the provisions of the Veterinary Surgeons Act 1966 for the practice of veterinary nursing (Schedule 3 Amendment Order 2002).
* Outline the sphere of practice of student and qualified veterinary nurses:
  * interpreting schedule 3
  * supervision
  * direction
  * medical treatment
  * minor surgery.
* Explain what is meant by negligence:
  * duty of care
  * breach of duty
  * liability.
* Describe the role of the Royal College of Veterinary Surgeons (RCVS) in relation to veterinary and veterinary nursing practice
  * registration
  * listing
  * education
  * guidance
  * discipline.
* Outline the provisions of the RCVS Codes of Professional Conduct for veterinary surgeons and nurses.
* Explain the concept of ethics in veterinary practice (listed overleaf):

* morals
* balancing right and wrong
* common conflicts.
* Describe the protocols to be followed when dealing with a clinical referral to another veterinary surgeon (RCVS Guide to Professional Conduct).
* Outline current legislation and policies, both nationally and locally with regard to keeping and handling exotic species and wildlife. This covers:
* exotics
* birds
* reptiles
* amphibians
* fish.

Legal accountability

Legal accountability of the veterinary nurse is the responsibility of the employer. The veterinary nurse is subject to the criminal and civil law of the land like any other citizen. There is a contractual relationship between the veterinary nurse employee and the veterinary surgeon employer which is subject to relevant employment legislation.

Professional regulation

The Royal College of Veterinary Surgeons (RCVS) is the regulatory body in charge of veterinary nursing. The RCVS sets external examinations which a veterinary nurse must pass to enter the RCVS List of Veterinary Nurses.

The RCVS Veterinary Nursing Occupational Standards and Objective Syllabus set the level of practical competence and theoretical knowledge necessary to practice as a qualified veterinary nurse. The British Veterinary Nursing Association (BVNA) promotes the interest and standard of veterinary nursing.

Veterinary nursing bylaws

The Veterinary Surgeons Act 1966

Section 19 of this Act restricts the practice of veterinary surgery to registered members of the RCVS subject to a number of exceptions. Listed veterinary nurses are one of the exceptions.

Veterinary surgery includes:

• the diagnosis of diseases in, and injuries to, animals including tests performed on animals for diagnostic purposes

- the giving of advice based upon such diagnosis
- the medical or surgical treatment of animals
- the performance of surgical operations on animals.

Schedule 3 Amendment Order 2002

This is a correction made to the Veterinary Surgeons Act 1996 on October 2002. Veterinary nurses and student veterinary nurses may now perform the following:

- administer first aid and look after animals in ways which do not involve acts of veterinary surgery
- administer medical treatment or carry out minor surgery (not involving entry into a body cavity). This applies to all species (including exotics) kept as pets and does not include equine, wild or farm animals. If the person holds the equine veterinary nursing certificate (EVN) they are permitted to administer medical treatment or carry out minor surgery (not involving entry into a body cavity) on horses, donkeys and zebra.

Remember:

- A listed veterinary nurse may undertake such a procedure only if he/she is properly trained and competent to carry it out, understands the associated risks and has the necessary experience and good sense to react appropriately should any problems arise.
- A listed veterinary nurse may carry out these acts only under the direction of a veterinary surgeon. The animal must be under the veterinary surgeon's care and treatment must be carried out at his/her direction. The veterinary surgeon must be the employer of the veterinary nurse or acting on their behalf.
- The veterinary surgeon is accountable for what has been done by the veterinary nurse and should ensure that they are covered by professional indemnity insurance.
- Student nurses can carry out the procedures mentioned but under the direct, continuous and personal supervision of a veterinary surgeon or listed veterinary nurse.

Negligence

Negligence is carelessness, want of proper care and attention. Professional negligence is the failure to exercise the normal level of skill and judgement that would be expected of the average veterinary surgeon as a result of which damage has suffered. If a veterinary nurse is negligent the supervising veterinary surgeon is likely to be held liable.

Allegations of negligence are resolved directly between the veterinary surgeon and client or by the civil courts. The RCVS is involved only if negligence results in a complaint being made to the college or if it amounts to professional misconduct.

The practice can take disciplinary action to deal with a negligent veterinary nurse.

Duty of care

Nurses are personally responsible for their own professional standards and negligence and should act at all times in the best interest of the animal. Breach of duty is a lapse in the duty of care.

Liability

The employer of the veterinary nurse is legally held responsible (liable) for any work carried out by the veterinary nurse.

What is the role of the Royal College of Veterinary Surgeons?

The RCVS safeguards the health and welfare of animals committed to veterinary care through the regulation of educational, ethical and clinical standards of the veterinary profession, therefore protecting the interests of those dependent on animals and assuring public health.

The RCVS also acts as an impartial source of informed opinion on animal health and welfare issues and their interaction with human health.

Registration

A certificate of membership of the RCVS is legally required to practice veterinary surgery in the UK.

Listing

A veterinary nurse's name must be on the List of Veterinary Nurses maintained by the RCVS to perform Schedule 3 procedures.

Education

The RCVS supports training and continuing professional development of veterinary surgeons and support staff. Veterinary surgeons are expected to continue their professional development and that of their veterinary nurses and support staff by keeping up-to-date with developments, taking part in training and refresher courses and keeping records.

Guidance and discipline

Guidance to veterinary nurses is detailed in the Guide to Professional Conduct. Matters relating to veterinary nurse discipline are the responsibility of the veterinary surgeon employer and are subject to the disciplinary powers of the RCVS.

Provisions of RCVS Codes of Professional Conduct

Veterinary surgeons make a special declaration on admission to the RCVS in exchange for the right to practice veterinary surgery in the UK. They are then obliged to abide by a set of rules set out in the RCVS Guide to Professional Conduct to ensure that animal welfare is their most important consideration at all times.

Specific parts of the guide relate to veterinary nurses (bold text):

- The RCVS guide is divided into three parts. Part 1 lists the responsibilities of a veterinary surgeon.
- The Ten Guiding Principles summarise what clients expect a veterinary surgeon to do.
- The guide lists the responsibilities of a veterinary surgeon:
  - his/her parents
  - his/her clients
  - the general public
  - in relation to their professional colleagues
  - under the law – all relevant legislation
  - when things go wrong – Preliminary Investigation Committee, Disciplinary Committee.

Remember: The responsibilities of a veterinary surgeon in relation to the treatment of animals by non-veterinary surgeons – Section 19 of the Veterinary Surgeons Act 1996 restricts the practice of veterinary surgery to registered members of the RCVS subject to a number of exceptions – this applies to listed veterinary nurses.

Part 2 contains guidance on disclosure of information, fees and related matters, promoting the practice, maintaining practice standards and running the business.

Treatment of animals by non-veterinary surgeons – this applies to veterinary nurses.

Concept of ethics in veterinary practice

Morals

This is the distinction between right and wrong.

Right and wrong

A veterinary nurse must be able to differentiate between right and wrong in terms of actions and words.

Common conflicts

This is a clash between personal and professional interests eg matters regarding wages or hours.

Referrals

Also see 2.2.08.

Referrals are used when:

- a veterinary surgeon recognises that a case is outside their area of competence
- the client has requested a referral
- a case is referred to a referral practice for diagnosis and possible treatment after which the case is referred back to the original veterinary surgeon.

Other factors regarding referrals:

- The referring veterinary surgeon is responsible for ensuring that the client is fully aware of the level of expertise of the referral veterinary surgeon (specialist by experience, certificate holder, RCVS Recognised Specialist).
- The referral veterinary surgeon discusses the case with the client and reports back to the primary veterinary surgeon.
- The case history and reason for referral are supplied to the referral practice.
- Any further information requested should be supplied promptly.

2.4.02   Basic handling and restraint

What you need to learn

- You need to be able to recognise different behaviour traits and explain why these occur. These include:
  - causes of aggression
  - dominance

- ☙ possessiveness
- ☙ territorial or protective behaviour
- ☙ play
- ☙ predatory behaviour
- ☙ fear or pain-induced reactions
- ☙ maternal behaviour
- ☙ competitive aggression
- ☙ redirected and pathophysiological breeds (dogs).
- ☙ Knowledge of specific species behaviour, eg exotics and their normal habitat, coprophagia.
- ☙ Describe safe handling methods of common species including wildlife:
  - ☙ dogs
  - ☙ cats
  - ☙ exotics
  - ☙ birds
  - ☙ reptiles
  - ☙ amphibia
  - ☙ fish.
- ☙ Describe how to approach an animal according to its behaviour and know how to modify your approach accordingly (dogs and cats).
- ☙ Describe ways to handle animals appropriately. This includes
  - ☙ types of behaviour (normal, aggressive, hyperactive, timid, hypersexed.
  - ☙ equipment dog or cat crush cage
  - ☙ blanket or towel method
  - ☙ cat or dog catcher
  - ☙ net
  - ☙ gloves.
- ☙ Understand the principles of training and be aware of training techniques
  - ☙ reinforcement (negative or positive)
  - ☙ desensitisation and counter-conditioning
  - ☙ commands including come, down, sit, heel, stay.
- ☙ Describe basic training and be aware of factors influencing training:
  - ☙ check chain
  - ☙ slip lead
  - ☙ collar
  - ☙ dog alarm
  - ☙ flexi leads
  - ☙ halti
  - ☙ harness.
- ☙ Know safe handling methods for common species including wildlife.
- ☙ Describe the handling of birds, exotics and other animals commonly kept as pets.

Different behaviour traits

Causes of aggression include:
• dominance
• possessiveness
• territorial or protective behaviour
• play
• predatory – hunting behaviour
• fear or pain-induced reactions
• maternal behaviour – protecting litters
• competitive aggression – sibling rivalry
• redirected/pathophysiological breeds are more prone to aggression, eg American pit bull terrier, Rottweiler.

Safe handling of cats and dogs

• Always handle dogs and cats with an assistant.
• Dogs should wear a collar with a lead attached.
• Transport cats in a basket, never carry cats from room to room in your arms.
• Don't handle cats near dogs and vice versa.
• Always shut windows and doors.

How to approach cats and dogs

• Speak softly, move slowly and avoid startling them.
• Use a calm and pleasant manner.
• Approach dogs crouched on their level (only if safe to do so).
• Be confident, don't show fear (animals pick up on human body language).

Modified approach according to the animal's behaviour

• If the animal is behaving normally then approach it as already described.
• If the animal is aggressive put human safety first. Ask the owner to attach a collar and lead to the dog or transfer the cat from the basket to the cage themselves. Use firm tones and avoid eye contact.
• If the animal is hyperactive ask the owner to attach a collar and short lead, and be calm and firm.
• If the animal is timid stay calm and quiet and approach slowly.
• If the animal is a hypersexed male try and keep it away from females in season.

Principles of training

Training techniques

- Positive reinforcement is based on reward (treats, praise, attention) when the animal obeys a given command.
- Negative reinforcement is based on 'punishment' or an unpleasant experience eg shock and pain (ear pinching). It is used if the dog doesn't respond to positive reinforcement. Negative reinforcement should be used with great care. A short shock (eg loud noise or squirt from water pistol) can be useful but pain should never be used in training.
- Desensitisation is the gradual exposure of the animal to the source of the fear, eg for dogs that are afraid of fireworks the sound of a pre-recorded tape of fireworks is played quietly at home. Over a period of time the volume of the sound is increased until the dog is no longer concerned. Commercial tapes are available with noises such as fireworks and thunder storms.
- Counter-conditioning is correcting fear or anxiety by distracting the animal with treats or games but not attention. This can be used alongside desensitisation.

Use simple commands and always use the same word, eg

- no!
- come
- down
- sit
- heal
- stay
- wait
- fetch.

Factors influencing training

- Age – there is an optimal age when animals are most receptive to training (young vs old).
- Situation – choose a quiet area free from distractions.
- The trainer – the trainer's approach should always be pleasant.

Training aids

- Check chains should only be used by experienced people.
- Slip leads should only be used by experienced people.
- A dog should always wear a collar.
- Dog alarms are useful in vocal training, eg to prevent constant barking.

- Flexi leads are useful for teaching the retrieve command.
- Haltis are useful for dogs that pull but only work while the dog is wearing one. The halti won't teach the dog that it shouldn't pull on a normal collar and lead
- A harness is useful for a dog that pulls but is only suitable for small dogs as medium and large-sized dogs can throw their whole weight into the harness making the pulling action stronger.

Handling exotics

Birds

- All windows and doors must be closed, and fans switched off, before handling a bird in the examination room.
- Birds rely heavily on vision and so are more easily caught in subdued light. Birds see poorly in red or blue light, so the use of a red or blue filter over a torch in a completely dark room can aid in the capture of particularly difficult birds.
- Firm but gentle handling minimises stress. The bird should be handled for as short a period as possible.
- The neck of the bird should be steadied using the thumb and forefinger (or one hand in larger birds). The thumb can be placed beneath the lower beak to prevent biting.
- Care should be taken when holding a bird to avoid placing any pressure on the sternum as this can easily cause asphyxiation.
- Birds are often calmer if held on their backs.
- A towel should be used to protect the hands in all but the smallest birds. Larger birds such as the parrots and birds of prey can be handled with thick gloves if necessary to prevent injury to the handler.
- Birds may carry zoonotic diseases such as psittacosis so normal hygiene precautions must be taken.

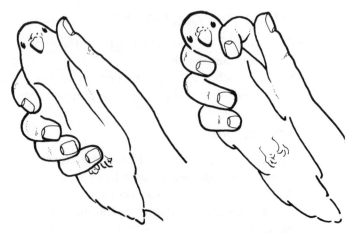

Figure 4.1 Diagram demonstrating the handling of a small bird.

Cage birds

• Toys should be removed from a birdcage before attempting to remove the bird.
• If possible it is better to remove a bird through the bottom of the cage than through a narrow door.
• Talking to a stressed cage bird and tickling the feathers on the back of the neck can help calm it.
• An owner of a sick or weak bird should be warned that the stress of examination can cause collapse.

Wild birds

• Care should be taken to avoid damaging any feathers as this will affect the bird's ability to fly. The wings should be held to the bird's sides to prevent injury from flapping.
• Larger birds can be very strong and care must be taken to avoid injury to the bird and handler. Special bags can be used to restrain and carry birds such as swans and geese.
• Some species will attempt to peck at the handler's eyes. Care must be taken to prevent this by wearing protective goggles when handling birds such as herons and gannets.
• Birds of prey have very sharp beaks and talons. Gloves or thick towels should be used for handling.

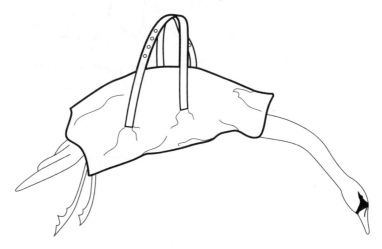

Figure 4.2   A bag for safe transportation of large birds.

Rodents and rabbits

• Friendly small rodents can be handled by gently holding the body over the shoulders or simply holding in cupped hands.
• Even small rodents can deliver a painful bite. Hamsters, for example, can be particularly aggressive if woken from sleep.

- Nervous rodents should be held firmly but gently by the scruff of the neck. If the grip is too tight the eyes will bulge and the animal could choke.
- The base of the tail can be used to steady the standing animal while the correct grip is achieved. Animals should never be held by the tail alone.
- Rabbits and heavier rodents such as guinea pigs should be restrained using both hands.
- When handling guinea pigs or chinchillas one hand should hold the shoulders and chest while the other hand supports the animal's weight at the hindquarters.
- Extra care should be taken with chinchillas as improper handling can result in patchy hair loss known as **fur slip**. Fur slip can also be caused by stressful experiences such as chasing the animal around a cage.
- Rabbits should be grasped with one hand under the chest or holding the scruff of the neck. The other hand is then used to support the abdomen and hind quarters.
- Wrapping the rabbit in a towel will aid in the restraint of fractious rabbits.
- Rabbits are at risk of spinal injury if they struggle during handling.

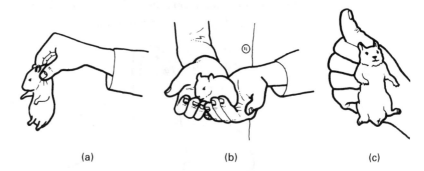

(a)   (b)   (c)

Figure 4.3 Diagram demonstrating the handling of a small rodent.

Reptiles

Careful attention should be paid to hygiene when handling reptiles as many carry potentially zoonotic diseases such as salmonella.

Chelonians

- Tortoises are very docile but can present a problem when handling by retracting the head and feet into the shell. Pushing the hindlimbs into the shell usually results in the head being extended. The head should be held gently between the finger and thumb.

- Terrapins and turtles can be more aggressive. They should be held by the caudal end of the carapace.

Lizards

- Lizards should never be held by the tail as they can shed it as a protective mechanism.
- Lizards can injure the handler with their teeth and claws. Some larger lizards such as the iguana can also inflict injury with their tails.
- Gloves or a towel can be used to protect the handler.
- Lizards should be held with one or both hands around the body, with the legs being held to the animal's side.

Snakes

- Care should be taken when handling snakes to avoid bruising the delicate flesh. Dropping a snake can cause potentially fatal injuries.
- If the species has not been identified the animal must be treated as potentially venomous.
- Non-venomous snakes can be handled with the thumb and finger of one hand behind the head while the weight is supported by the other hand.
- Large or aggressive snakes should be handled by more than one person to avoid injury.

Amphibians

- The skin of amphibians is covered with mucus which makes handling difficult.
- The hands should be cool and wet before attempting handling. Plastic gloves are useful.

Fish

- Handling fish out of water is difficult and poses a risk to the health of the fish.
- Anaesthesia is often required if a fish needs to be handled, eg for taking blood samples.

2.4.03   Animal accommodation

What you need to learn

- You need to be able to describe the requirements for animal accommodation within a veterinary practice (accommodation includes hospital, recovery and isolation wards).

☙ Explain the relevance of accommodation construction relative to its purpose:
  ☙ materials used are wood, stainless steel, metal, tiles, plastic, fibreglass, brick, glass, concrete
  ☙ equipment is heating, lighting, ventilation and power supply.
☙ Outline the advantages and disadvantages and suitability of bedding material according to species and condition of the animal, including:
  ☙ cats
  ☙ dogs
  ☙ exotics
  ☙ healthy, injured and special-care patients.
☙ Explain the optimum and acceptable environment and housing requirements of any individual species based upon knowledge of the animal's biology and basic requirements:
  ☙ birds
  ☙ rabbits and rodents
  ☙ reptiles
  ☙ amphibians
  ☙ fish.
☙ Outline the optimum environmental conditions for animal accommodation:
  ☙ noise
  ☙ temperature
  ☙ accessibility
  ☙ light
☙ Describe the feeding, housing and general husbandry of:
  ☙ exotics
  ☙ birds
  ☙ reptiles
  ☙ amphibia
  ☙ fish

Suitable accommodation

Suitable accommodation needs to be provided in the:

• hospital ward
• intensive care ward
• recovery ward
• isolation ward.

Construction of accommodation

The layout of the kennels can be:

• corridor type
• H-block type
• circular type.

Materials that can be used to construct the kennels include:

- wood – warmer than concrete, not very secure, could splinter
- stainless steel – easily cleaned
- metal – durable, easy to clean, cold
- acoustic tiles (soundproof) – deaden or reflect the sound, not easy to clean
- plastic – not as secure as stainless steel or fibreglass, warm, easy to clean
- fibreglass – easily cleaned, warmer than stainless steel
- brick – good for outside walls, cold, secure
- glass – may break
- concrete – good for outside areas, cold, secure.

Equipment that is needed in all kennel areas includes:

- heating with either central or local temperature control
- natural and artificial lighting
- active or passive ventilation
- power supply with sockets
- drafts prevention, eg self-shutting doors
- a sink with hot and cold water
- cupboards, shelves and worktops
- a general waste bin and clinical waste bin
- cleaning equipment, mops, brushes, hose pipe, disinfectant
- feeding equipment
- grooming equipment.

Bedding

See Table 4.1.

Housing requirements of exotics

Birds

- Pet birds are usually kept in cages.
- The cage should legally be at least big enough to allow the bird to stand and stretch its wings freely. Ideally a cage should be as large as possible, allowing the bird to fly and exhibit normal bird behaviour.
- Galvanised cages should be avoided as the zinc can cause toxicity in birds.
- Perches should be made of wood.
- If possible perches made from tree branches (fruit trees, willow and oak are suitable) are the best.
- Tree-branch perches have variable diameters which help keep the nails trim and provide exercise for the bird's feet.
- Branches also provide environmental enrichment for the bird as they enjoy stripping the bark.

Table 4.1

Type of bedding	Advantages	Disadvantages
Newspaper	Widely available Cheap Disposable Insulating layer Suitable for all patients	Can stain Not suitable as the only means of bedding
Shredded newspaper	As above but warmer	Can stain. Will entangle in patient's coat Not suitable for patients with wounds – use for healthy patients
Blankets	Warm Comfortable Re-useable Can use for all patients – use 2 or 3 for thin or recumbent patients	Expensive unless donated Patient may chew or tear them May aggravate dust allergies Laundry time and cost
Acrylic bedding, eg Vetbeds	Warm Provides more padding than blankets Less resistant to chewing Absorbs fluid away from the patient, eg urine Re-usable Can use for all patients – very good for thin, recumbent and incontinent patients	Expensive to purchase Laundry time and cost
Incontinence pads	Absorb urine and other fluids away from the patient Plastic backing prevents bedding underneath becoming soiled Disposable	May have to change regularly Not suitable as the only means of bedding

(**NB**: commercially available tropical hardwood perches should be avoided as the bark is too hard for the birds to strip, and they are often imported from non-sustainable rain forests.)
• Cages should be kept at a constant temperature and away from draughts. Room temperature is sufficiently warm for most species.
• Sand sheets are often used to line bird cages. These are usually unnecessary but are harmless.
• Toys should be provided to enrich the environment. These should

be indestructible, and should be rotated so that the bird has a new toy regularly.

- Birds are very intelligent and behaviour problems are common in the larger psittacines due to improper husbandry.
- Some birds are kept in aviaries. Care should be taken to provide protection against extremes of weather in this country.
- Aviary birds should be monitored closely for signs of contagious diseases which may spread to other birds.

Rabbits and rodents

- Numerous cages are available commercially for rabbits and rodents.
- Small rodents should be provided with escape-proof accommodation which cannot easily be damaged through gnawing.
- The cage should allow the animal as much room as possible.
- The environment should be enriched to allow the animal to express normal behaviour. This can be achieved by providing objects of interest to the animal. An example is providing a whole toilet roll which can be shredded by the animal to provide bedding.
- Exercise wheels can provide environmental enrichment but care should be taken that the wheel is solid rather than the ladder type which can cause tail and leg injuries.
- The best bedding material depends on the species:
  - wood shavings are good bedding materials for most rodents and rabbits. Wood shavings are very absorbent but can be dusty. Aromatic shavings should be avoided.
  - Gerbils prefer to burrow into their bedding. Suitable materials are peat-type soils mixed with sand. Shavings, shredded paper and straw can be incorporated into the burrow.
  - Tissue paper or cotton wadding should be provided as bedding for hamsters.
  - Guinea pigs are hardy rodents and can be kept outdoors providing the shelter and insulation is sufficient. Plenty of hay should be provided for food, bedding and environmental enrichment.
  - Chinchillas should be provided with dust baths for approximately 10 minutes each day, for grooming. Chinchillas prefer a cool environment and suffer from heat exhaustion very easily.
- Rabbits thrive when they are allowed some access to an outdoor run, although they can be kept completely indoors if care is taken to meet all their needs. Rabbit hutches should be as large as possible. If kept outdoors care should be taken to protect them from cold, draughts and predators. Rabbits can be litter trained.

- Rodents prefer different ambient temperatures although they will often tolerate a wide range of temperatures:
  - rats and mice 18–22 °C
  - gerbils 20–22 °C
  - hamsters 21–22 °C
  - guinea pigs 18–22 °C
  - chinchillas 10–16 °C.

Reptiles

The housing requirements vary between species.

- Land lizards and tortoises require a large floor space for wandering around.
- Terrapins and other semi-aquatic species need water for swimming and a dry land area for basking.
- Tree-climbing species require high enclosures to allow them to express their natural behaviour. Branches should be provided for climbing.
- Many species benefit from a hiding shelter within their accommodation.
- Snakes tend to require less space than other reptiles.
- The substrate should be easily cleaned. Newspaper or tissue paper usually suffices.
- The temperature of the accommodation depends on the species. Cold-blooded animals thrive better at their preferred body temperature. A hot spot for basking is appreciated. There should be a temperature gradient so that the animal can move away from the heat if it overheats.
- Correct lighting is vital for most reptiles (although some, such as geckos, are nocturnal). Broad spectrum 'natural' lighting which incorporates ultraviolet light is better for diurnal species. Many species require ultraviolet light for synthesis of vitamin D. Animals which are deprived of proper lighting do not grow well and fail to thrive.
- Humidity is important for some species. A dry atmosphere will interfere with a reptile's ability to shed its skin properly.

Amphibians

- Some amphibians are completely aquatic and are kept in a water-filled tank, eg the axolotl.
- Most amphibians require some land area as well as water.
- Water quality must be controlled carefully. Rotting food will quickly pollute the water and can cause disease in the animals. Water should be de-chlorinated.
- Amphibians are cold blooded. They should be kept at fairly low

temperatures and do not tolerate high temperatures well.
- Humidity must be carefully controlled as low humidity causes the animal to lose heat by evaporation while high humidity prevents the animal from dissipating heat.
- Correct lighting is vital for most amphibians. Broad spectrum 'natural' lighting which incorporates ultraviolet light is better for diurnal species. Many species require ultraviolet light for synthesis of Vitamin D. Animals which are deprived of proper lighting do not grow well and fail to thrive.

Fish

The husbandry of fish varies depending on the species and whether they are to be kept in an aquarium or a pond.

Aquarium fish

- Aquarium fish can be either fresh-water or sea-water and either cold-water or tropical. Tropical fish need a water heater.
- The aquarium should be sited away from direct sunlight and household heating appliances.
- Goldfish bowls should be avoided as they are prone to fluctuations in heat and oxygenation. They are also often overstocked and the water quality quickly deteriorates. Fish tanks are preferable.
- Fish tanks usually require a filtration system which maintain water quality and also aerate the water. Filters should be rinsed out regularly.
- Lighting is important to encourage healthy plant growth in an aquarium. Plants produce oxygen and are therefore important to the health of the aquarium.
- Partial water changes (replacing a quarter of the water with de-chlorinated fresh water) improves water quality.

Pond fish

- Most ponds contain cold-water fish.
- Ponds should be sited with some shade, and protection from the cold.
- Plants are usually used to improve the oxygenation of the water.
- Care should be taken not to overstock the pond.
- Ponds tend to have a more stable environment than aquaria and partial water changes may be unnecessary.

Prevention of the spread of infection

What you need to learn

☙ You need to be able to define the terms infection and contagion.
☙ Outline the major groups of infectious agents:
  ☙ viruses
  ☙ bacteria
  ☙ ectoparasites
  ☙ endoparasites
  ☙ fungi
  ☙ protozoa.
☙ Define terms associated with transmission of disease:
  ☙ direct contact
  ☙ indirect contact
  ☙ fomites
  ☙ vectors
  ☙ intermediate hosts
  ☙ airborne transmission
  ☙ faecal transmission
  ☙ oral and body fluids
  ☙ symptomatic
  ☙ asymptomatic.
☙ State the meaning of 'carrier animal' and define types of carriers.
☙ Briefly describe the various methods used in the prevention of transmission of disease:
  ☙ disinfectants
  ☙ isolation
  ☙ quarantine and treatment
  ☙ sterilisation.
☙ Describe the requirements of the pets passport scheme.
☙ State the diseases and parasites that are controlled by the pets passport scheme:
  ☙ rabies
  ☙ leishmaniasis
  ☙ tapeworm (*Echinococcus multilocularis*)
  ☙ ticks.

Infection

Infection is an invasion of the body by harmful micro-organisms that multiply during the incubation period before symptoms develop.

Contagious originally meant a disease spread by direct animal-to-animal contact, but it now also means any communicable disease.

Infectious agents

Infectious agents include:

- viruses, eg parvovirus
- bacteria, eg salmonella
- ectoparasites, such as fleas eg *Ctenocephalides felis*
- endoparasites, eg such as worms *Toxocara canis*
- fungi, eg aspergillus
- protozoa, eg *Toxoplasma gondii*

Transmission of disease

Disease is spread from one patient to another or others by several different methods:

- the direct method – animals with direct physical contact
- the indirect method – via the environment between animals that are not in physical contact
- by fomites – inanimate objects, eg feeding bowl, grooming brush
- by vectors – invertebrates, eg mites, ticks carrying infection or parasites from one vertebrate host to another
- by intermediate hosts – invertebrates or vertebrate animals that carry infection or parasites from one animal to another. If the parasite goes through part of the life cycle in the intermediate host
- by aerosols – suspension of particles of infection in the air (otherwise known as airborne transmission)
- by faeces
- by oral and body fluids
- by contaminated food and water.

Routes by which infectious agents leave a patient's body and increase the risk of causing infection in another patient are:

- urine and faeces
- vomit
- blood
- ocular, nasal and oral discharges
- body fluids, eg milk and semen
- parturition
- skin
- dead animals.

Symptomatic – a patient that is showing clinical signs of the infection.

Asymptomatic – a patient that is showing no clinical signs of the infection.

Carriers

A carrier is a patient who has come into contact with an infectious agent and may harbour that agent without showing any clinical signs.

A carrier may be a closed carrier, ie does not shed the agent into the environment or they may be an open carrier, ie they do shed the agent into the environment.

There are two types of carrier, both of which can be open or closed:

• A healthy carrier is a patient who has been exposed to the infectious agent but has never shown any clinical signs. They are usually immune to that particular agent.
• A convalescent carrier is a patient who has recovered from the infectious agent.

Prevention of transmission of disease

The following methods can be used to help prevent the transmission of infectious agents:

• disinfection – physical or chemical means of removing micro-organisms (not spores) from contaminated surfaces, eg kennels, equipment, floors, surfaces
• isolation – separate accommodation
• quarantine – a statutory isolation period usually longer than the incubation period of a disease for animals entering a country or region, eg rabies
• sterilisation – the process of destroying all micro-organisms and spores.

Pets passport scheme / Pets Travel Scheme (PETS)

Requirements for pets wanting to return to the UK

• The pet needs to be micro-chipped with an approved chip.
• Then the pet is vaccinated against rabies – a booster is required once a year.
• 30 days after the rabies vaccination the pet is blood tested to confirm there are sufficient antibodies present.
• A health certificate and vaccination certificated will be issued to the owner which must be taken with them.
• Worm treatment and examination of the pet by a veterinary surgeon should be carried out in the country they are visiting before returning to the UK.

The above information is correct at the time of writing, it is important to check the requirements of PETS regularly as they are changed and updated by DEFRA (Department for the Environment, Farming and Rural Affairs).

Diseases and parasites controlled by PETS

- Rabies
- Leishmaniasis
- *Echinococcus multilocularis* (tapeworm)
- *Ixodes* spp. (ticks).

2.4.05 Cleaning and maintaining clinical environments and accommodation

What you need to learn

- You need to be able to describe the principles of cleaning a clinical environment and appropriate cleaning systems:
  - examination rooms
  - preparation areas
  - minor treatment areas
  - disinfection systems
  - steam and pressure washing systems.
- Describe the principles of cleaning a kennel or cattery unit including:
  - hospitalisation
  - isolation
  - stray animals
  - long-stay animals
  - breeding kennels.
- Describe the principles of cleaning feeding bowls and equipment
  - mechanical and chemical methods
  - frequency.
- Define the terms disinfection, antisepsis and sterilisation.
- Explain the purpose of antiseptics, disinfectants and cleaning.
- Describe the common antiseptics and disinfectants and their safe usage. These include:
  - aldehydes
  - iodophores
  - iodine
  - quaternary ammonium compounds
  - oxidants
  - halogenated peroxide compounds
  - tertiary amines.
- Describe the susceptibility of a variety of microbes to disinfection:
  - viruses
  - bacteria

* fungi
* protozoa
* prions.
* Explain the disadvantages and dangers of disinfectants where appropriate and the risk of toxicity to patients and operators.

Protocol

All areas of the hospital need a high standard of hygiene to control micro-organisms and/or disease. A protocol should be drawn up for each of the following areas and adhered to:

- examination rooms
- preparation areas
- minor treatment areas
- waiting room
- theatre
- ward kennels
- recovery area and kennels
- isolation ward.

Cleaning equipment

- Disinfectants
- Steam cleaners and pressure washers
- Brushes
- Vacuum cleaners
- Mops and buckets
- Cloths or disposable tissue.

Daily cleaning of hospital kennels

For hospital patients (long and short stay):

- Clean and disinfect any used kennels and place in new bedding (in preparation for next patient).
- Ensure all equipment is stored away.
- Ensure all clinical waste is disposed of correctly.
- Clean and disinfect the walls and doors.
- Wipe down (with disinfectant) all surfaces, cupboards, fittings and any equipment present.
- Empty clinical waste bin and disinfect inside and out; replace with new clinical waste liner.
- Brush and/or vacuum the floor and disinfect, eg with a mop and bucket.

For isolation kennels instigate barrier nursing. For stray animals it is always better to place them in isolation until it is confirmed they are harbouring no infectious micro-organisms.

For breeding kennels:

- The whelping kennels should be treated as isolation kennels to prevent spread of infection to neonates.
- Check the whelping box is clean and has sufficient bedding.
- Check the kennel area is escape proof.

Cleaning feeding bowls and equipment

Mechanical methods

Physical scrubbing with brushes or cloths and detergent in warm water to remove dirt and debris.

Chemical methods

Use cold sterilisation fluids, stainless-steel bowls and equipment may be steam sterilised as well.

Frequency of cleaning

Clean the equipment each time it is used.

- **Disinfection** is the removal of micro-organisms but not always bacterial spores.
- **Antisepsis** is the agents which prevent sepsis by inhibiting or destroying micro-organisms.
- **Sterilisation** is the destruction of all micro-organisms including bacterial spores.
- **Disinfectant** is an agent that provides disinfection. Disinfectants are available as skin disinfectants or environmental disinfectants. The latter is for use on inanimate objects only.
- **Cleaning** is the mechanical removal of debris. It is important this process is carried out before using any antiseptics, disinfectants or sterilising methods, as debris will hinder their action.
  Protozoa: Unicellular parasitic organisms
  Prion: Minute particle smaller than viruses, of a protein-like nature, considered to be the infectious agents for Bovine Spongiform Encephalopathy (BSE), scrapie, new variant Creutzfeldt–Jakob Disease (CJD).

Table 4.2

Ingredient	Properties	Effect on micro-organisims	Safety precautions	Dangers
Aldehydes eg glutaraldehyde – Cidex®	Slow acting Not easily inactivated by organic material	Bacteria, spores and viruses	Wear gloves and mask as highly toxic to skin, eyes and respiratory tract	Not used routinely because of high toxicity, formaldehyde is even more irritant
Idophores, e.g. povidone iodine – Pevidine®	Inactivated by organic material Needs a 2-minute skin contact tine	Bacteria, fungi, viruses, some activity against spores	Leaves a yellow stain therefore primarily used on the skin and not the environment	Can be irritating
Quaternary ammonium compounds eg cetrimide – Cetavlon®	Environmental and skin use More resistant to inactivation by organic material	Bacteria, viruses, spores, fungi	Wear gloves as irritant at concentrate level	Low toxicity Low corrosion potential
Peroxides, eg peroxygen compound – Virkon®	Fast acting Not inactivated by organic material	Wide range of activity – bacteria, spores, viruses, fungi	Powder irritant until made into a solution Wear gloves	Causes metal corrosion
Tertiary amines, eg Trigene®	Non-corrosive Not easily inactivated by organic material	Wide range of activity – bacteria, spores, viruses, fungi	Wear gloves	Low toxicity
Alcohol, eg isopropyl alcohol 70% – surgical spirit	Inactivated by organic material	Bacteria (not spores), some viruses	Wear gloves as skin irritant	Highly inflammable Can increase hypothermia if overused on the skin
Phenols, eg black phenols – Jeyes fluid®	Inactivated by organic material	Bacteria, not very effective against viruses or spores	Wear gloves as skin irritant Leaves sticky residue	Toxic to cats Strong smelling
Halogen, eg hypochlorite – Domestos®	Inactivated by organic material	Wide range of activity – bacteria, spores, viruses, fungi	Wear gloves and apron as it will bleach clothing	Causes metal corrosion Will burn skin if undiluted Strong smelling

How much have you learnt?

1 Describe two techniques that can be used to train any of the eight commands.

2 What aids can be used with an aggressive dog?

3 What are the requirements for patients hospitalised in a kennel?

4 What is the difference between a carrier and an infection?

5 How are infections spread?

6 What is the difference between an antiseptic and a disinfectant?

7 How would you clean the kennel, bowls and other equipment that have been used by a cat with influenza?

8 Describe three commonly used disinfectants.

9 How does the current Schedule III amendment affect veterinary nurses?

10 Name three situations where confidentiality may be broken.

The answers can be found within this unit, up to page 256.

2.4.06 Observation and assessment of patients

What you need to learn

* You need to be able to describe the principles of a systematic patient assessment.
* Describe the factors assessed on initial observation:
    * behaviour
    * condition
    * demeanour
    * mobility.
* Describe the needs of an animal experiencing sensory loss:
    * sight
    * hearing
    * overcoming disorientation.

Systematic assessment

Patients who are hospitalised require systematic assessments on a daily basis. First, the veterinary nurse should inform the veterinary surgeon, plan nursing care and decide the need for treatment. The assessment needs to be methodical and performed in the same order each time. This provides continuity and prevents areas from being overlooked. Here is an example of the order of assessment:

* ears
* eyes
* nose
* mouth and teeth
* thorax
* abdomen
* perineum and tail
* limbs.

Factors assessed on initial observation

* Behaviour – ensure the patient is settled and not showing signs of pain, fear, anxiety or excessive vocalisation.
* Condition – check the coat is smooth and shiny, eyes are bright and the animal is not over or under weight.
* Demeanour – ensure the patient is responsive and not depressed.
* Mobility – ensure the patient can get up and move about their cage or kennel. Assistance may be needed to walk a patient if mobility is compromised.

Care of patients who have sensory loss

Blind patients

- Speak to the patient using their name before opening the cage or kennel door and approaching them. (A startled blind patient may bite or scratch.)
- Allow an opportunity for the patient to sniff and smell you before getting hold of them.
- Keep talking to them as they are being handled so they don't become frightened.
- Use physical contact such as stroking and petting.
- Keep the position of food bowls, blankets and litter trays constant so that the environment is familiar.
- Put food within easy reach so that they do not stumble over bedding or other items.
- Ask the owner for a favourite toy or an item of the owner's clothing for familiar smells.
- Keep the blind patient away from noisy animals.

Deaf patients

- Allow an opportunity for the patient to sniff and smell you before getting hold of them.
- Ensure the deaf patient can see you when approaching them and handling them.
- Create vibrations to alert the patient by knocking on the kennel or cage, or by tapping a foot.
- Separate dogs from cats, if they are within sight of each other it may cause distress.

Disorientation

- Talk to the patient on approach and while handling them.
- Use slow, gentle movements.
- Keep bedding and feeding bowls in the same place and fix to the cage or kennel.
- Try to use the same members of staff and a reduced number of staff when dealing with the patient to allow a bond to develop.

Loss of smell

- This is very common among cats suffering from cat flu. If cats can't smell they won't eat. Try the methods below to encourage eating.
- Ensure eyes, nose and mouth are free from crusts, saliva and any discharges.

- Use strong smelling foods – in the author's experience pilchards or sardines in tomato sauce work very well.
- Ask the owner what the pet would eat at home and what their favorite treats are.
- Warm the food to enhance its smell.
- Give steam baths by placing the animal in a basket, or tying it securely in a room full of steam. Never a leave a bowl of hot water where the patient can harm themselves and supervise all steam baths.
- Place a variety of foods within the kennel, eg cat or dog food, chicken, fish.

2.4.07   Assessing temperature, pulse and respiration

What you need to learn

- You need to be able to describe the safe use of a clinical thermometer:
  - digital
  - mercury
  - electronic
  - Celsius
  - Fahrenheit
- Describe methods used to measure the respiratory rate and character:
  - observation
  - auscultation.
- Describe common respiratory abnormalities
  - coughing
  - dyspnoea
  - apnoea
  - thoraco-abdominal and abdominal breathing
  - tachypnea
  - Cheyne–Stokes respiration
  - inspiratory.
- Describe methods used for assessing pulse rate and character:
  - palpation
  - auscultation
  - pulse oximeter.
- Outline the locations of palpable pulses:
  - femoral
  - carpal
  - sub-lingual
  - coccygeal
  - supra-orbital
  - carotid
  - brachial.

How to take a temperature using a mercury thermometer

- Wear gloves.
- The assistant should then restrain the patient.
- Shake the thermometer and ensure the mercury line is at the bulb.
- Place lubrication on the end of the thermometer and insert the thermometer into the rectum. This may be more difficult in the cat; it can help to twist the thermometer but never force it.
- Leave the thermometer in place while holding it for 1 minute.
- Remove the thermometer and wipe off excess faeces.
- Place the thermometer on the back of the hand with a tissue underneath and read off either the centigrade or farenheit scale – it may help to rotate the thermometer.
- Shake the thermometer, wipe with an antiseptic and place it back into the container.
- Record the reading – see Figure 4.4 for a centigrade and Fahrenheit scale.

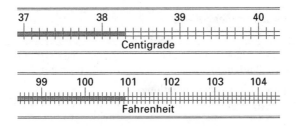

Figure 4.4   A Centigrade and Fahrenheit scale.

Digital thermometers are available, they can be placed in the patient's ear and are quicker to use. Electronic thermometers can be used in the rectum or in the oesophagus and provide a continuous reading.

Normal temperature readings are:

- dog: 38.3–38.7 °C/100.9–101.7 °F
- cat: 38.0–38.5 °C/100.4–101.6 °F.

Abnormal readings are:

- dog: below 38.3 °C/100.9 °F or above 38.7 °C/101.7 °F
- cat: below 38.0 °C/100.4 °F or above 38.5 °C/101.6 °F.

Assessing respiration rate and character

The character and the rate of respiration should be recorded. The character can be assessed by observing thoracic movements. Both of these parameters should be performed when the patient is at rest but not asleep.

How to measure the respiratory rate

To measure the respiratory rate by observation:

• An assistant is not required.
• Observe the patient and count either the inspirations or expirations.
• Count for 1 minute or for 30 seconds and multiply by two.
• Record the rate and pattern.

To measure the respiratory rate by auscultation use a stethoscope and place it over the lung fields.

Normal respiration rates are:

• dog: 10–30 breaths per minute
• cat: 15–30 breaths per minutes.

Inspiration: breathing in
Expiration: breathing out

Table 4.3

Respiratory abnormalities/ description	Causes
Coughing – harsh or dry, may produce fluid, blood, mucous	Congestive heart failure, kennel cough, bronchitis
Dyspnoea (difficulty in breathing) Inspiratory dyspnoea	Diseases or stenosis of the nasal cavities or upper respiratory tract
Expiratory dyspnoea	Collapsed trachea, bronchitis
Mixed dyspnoea (inspiratory and expiratory)	Pneumonia, pneumothorax
Apnoea (temporary cessation of breathing)	Anaesthesia
Thoraco-abdominal breathing	Ruptured diaphragm
Abdominal breathing	Asthma
Tachypnoea (increased respiratory rate)	Pain, hyperthermia, exercise, increased levels of carbon dioxide
Cheyne–Stokes respiration	Seen before death, demonstrated by an alternating pattern of deep, rapid breaths and shallow breaths

Assessing the pulse

How to take the pulse digitally (palpation)

• Restrain the patient using an assistant.
• Place two fingers on the selected artery.

- Count each pulse for 1 minute or for 30 seconds and multiply by two.
- Record the rate.

Auscultation of the heartbeat using a stethoscope can be performed as described in taking the pulse. The pulse and oxygenation can also be assessed by using a pulse oximeter (a machine that measures oxygenation concentration in the haemoglobin and digitally displays the pulse rate attached to the tongue, ear or in between the toes.

Normal pulse rates

- Dog: 60–180 beats per minutes
- Cat: 110–180 beats per minute

Table 4.4

Rate and character	Causes/effects
Increased pulse rate	Pain, pyrexia, exercise, shock, hypoxia, neonates
Decreased pulse rate	Effect of anaesthetic drugs, old age, unconsciousness
Weak pulse	Shock, dehydration, low blood pressure
Strong and jerky 'water hammer' pulse	Congenital heart defects, e.g. patent ductus arteriosis
Sinus arrhythmia	Increased rate on inspiration, decreased rate on expiration. This is a normal finding.
Pulse deficit	The pulse rate is lower than the heart rate. To assess this, take the pulse as outlined above and listen to the heart rate with a stethoscope at the same time. This is not a normal finding and can indicate dysrhythmias.

The pulse can be digitally assessed at the following areas:

- femoral – on the medial aspect of the femur
- carpal – on the palmer aspect on the carpus
- sub-lingual – underneath the tongue (reserve for anaesthetised patients)
- coccygeal – underneath the base of the tail
- supra-orbital
- carotid – on the sides of the neck
- brachial – on the medial aspect of the humerus.

2.4.08   Assessing appetite

What you need to learn

* You need to be able to describe the principles of assessing appetite and nutritional status and describe signs of weight loss and gain.
* Describe abnormalities in feeding pattern including:
    * vomiting
    * pica
    * capricious appetite
    * coprophagia.
* Describe the principles of assessing hydration:
    * dermal elasticity
    * capillary refill time.

Monitoring appetite

Appetite may be monitored by:

* observing the patient to see if they either refuse food or require more food
* recording the amount eaten and type of food eaten
* weighing the patient on a daily basis.

Signs of weight loss

* Reduced body weight, that continues to fall
* Poor coat
* Loss of muscle tone
* Bones such as the spine and ribs become visible
* Sunken eyes.

Signs of weight gain

* Increased body weight, that continues to increase
* Cannot tolerate exercise as well as before
* Coat may become scurfy in appearance
* Increased drinking
* Bones that were visible become covered with fat
* Arthritis may become more apparent.

How to assess adequate hydration

* Is dermal elasticity normal – to test this 'tent' the skin on the neck or on the top of the head. In a normal hydrated patient the skin should return to its normal position immediately. If it retains the tenting

Table 4.5

Abnormal feeding patterns	Causes/effects
Vomiting	Food is propelled from the stomach and out of the mouth
Pica	Eating non-food substances, eg stones
Voracious/capricious appetite	Eating large volumes of food, eg worms
Coprophagia	Eating faeces
Dysphagia	Difficulty in eating, eg caused by lacerated tongue
Selective eating	Animal picks certain foods, can be caused, eg, by pain due to dental disease
Dropping food from the mouth	Can indicate facial nerve damage
Anorexia	Absence of eating, eg caused by renal failure

position this is indicative of dehydration.
- Capillary refill time should be normal, ie less than 2 seconds.
- The eyes should be bright and not sunken.
- The mucous membranes should be moist.
- Record the patient's history.
- Packed cell volume and urine output should be normal.
- The patient should not be drinking more or less than usual.
- Measure the amount of water the patient is drinking to obtain an exact figure.

2.4.09 Assessing elimination

What you need to learn

- You need to be able to outline principles of assessing urinary output:
  - amount
  - appearance (presence of blood, clots or calculi)
  - frequency
  - odour
  - colour
  - quantity.
- Describe normal urinary deposits in various species:
  - birds
  - rodents
  - lagomorphs
  - reptiles.
- Outline the principles of assessing defecation:

☘ appearance
☘ amount
☘ consistency
☘ odour
☘ colour
☘ frequency.

☘ Describe the observations to be made of a vomiting animal:
  ☘ frequency
  ☘ force
  ☘ appearance (presence of blood or foreign material)
  ☘ odour
  ☘ quantity.

Urine

• Appearance – is the urine clear with no debris, blood or blood clots present?
• Frequency – does the animal urinate regularly throughout the day?
• Odour – is the smell of urine inoffensive?
• Colour – is the colour a medium yellow?
• Quantity – dogs and cats should pass 1–2 ml/kg/h.

Urinary sediments seen in exotic species:

• Birds and reptiles excrete the majority of their nitrogenous waste as uric acid and urates (compared with most mammals which excrete nitrogenous waste as urea). These urates form the normal white crystals which are seen in the urine of birds and reptiles.
• There is great variation in the colour of normal rabbit urine. The variation in colour is caused by a variety of pigments which come from plant material and can range from white through to dark red.
• Rabbits excrete excess calcium via the urine as calcium carbonate. This results in creamy urine.
• Struvite crystals can also be found in small amounts in normal rabbit urine.
• Other herbivorous rodents such as guinea pigs can show a similar range of colour for normal urine.

Faeces

Defecation is the act of passing faeces:

• Appearance – the faeces should be sausage shaped.
• Amount – two to three 'sausages' should be passed.
• Consistency – the faeces should be formed, not hard or watery.
• Odour – there should be a typical faecal smell.
• Colour – faeces are normally medium brown in colour.
• Frequency – faeces are normally passed once or twice a day.

Vomit

Vomiting or emesis is defined as the forceful emission of the stomach contents via the mouth. Any vomiting should be recorded with the following details:

• frequency
• force and type of vomit
• appearance – any blood, bile or foreign material present (some blood can look like coffee granules)
• odour
• quantity.

2.4.10   Assessing activity and behaviour

What you need to learn

❧ You need to be able to explain reasons of unusual restlessness:
  ❧ anxiety
  ❧ pain
  ❧ need to defecate
  ❧ urinary retention
  ❧ hunger.

Restlessness

If a patient is becoming restless (pacing the kennel, unable to settle or sleep) it may be due to one of the following reasons:

• They may be feeling nervous or anxious – plenty of tender loving care should help.
• They may be in pain – inform a veterinary surgeon if you suspect this.
• They may need to urinate or defecate – take them out for a walk or clean soiled litter trays.
• They may have urinary retention making them uncomfortable – inform a veterinary surgeon.
• They may be hungry or thirsty – offer food or water if appropriate.
• They may have an abnormal temperature.
• Dressings or bandages may be overtight and uncomfortable.

2.4.11   Providing essential patient care

What you need to learn

❧ You need to be able to describe common signs of pain:
  ❧ panting

- ❀ whining
- ❀ cowering
- ❀ aggression
- ❀ hiding
- ❀ immobility
- ❀ elevated temperature
- ❀ prayer position.
- ❀ Recognise signs of pain or distress exhibited by the various species and outline pain assessments based on subjectivity, clinical indications and responses:
  - ❀ exotics
  - ❀ birds
  - ❀ reptiles.
- ❀ Describe general care necessary for all inpatients:
  - ❀ environment
  - ❀ monitoring
  - ❀ nutrition
  - ❀ physical and mental support.
- ❀ Outline the needs for critically ill patients and neonates:
  - ❀ environment
  - ❀ monitoring
  - ❀ nutrition
  - ❀ body temperature control
  - ❀ urination
  - ❀ defecation.
- ❀ Describe methods of transporting animals of all sizes when unconscious or anaesthetised:
  - ❀ stretchers
  - ❀ baskets
  - ❀ trolleys
  - ❀ blankets.

Common signs of pain

If the patient is in pain they may exhibit one or more of the following signs:

- they may show increased panting, whining, barking or crying
- they may be more subdued than normal, or may cower away from people
- they may show more aggression than usual
- they may hide under blankets
- they may refuse or limit movement
- they may have increased temperature, pulse and respiratory rate
- they may adopt the prayer position
- they may refuse to eat or drink.

Signs of pain in exotics

Many exotic species and wild animals are prey animals so avoid showing signs of pain, as any weakness could be detected by a predator. This often results in illness being overlooked by the owner until it is advanced and can no longer be disguised by the animal.

- Care must be taken to observe an animal for subtle changes in behaviour which could suggest the animal is unwell or in pain.
- A report from an owner that an exotic animal is 'not himself' should therefore always be taken seriously and investigated.
- Sick rabbits and rodents will be less mobile and often have a hunched stance.
- Teeth grinding (bruxism) is often a sign of pain.
- A sick animal or an animal in pain may show signs of aggression.
- Refusal to eat and weight loss is usually a sign of ill health in exotics.
- Sick birds often have a hunched stance with ruffled feathers.
- The skin of brightly coloured reptiles may become dull when the animal is unwell.

Daily care of all inpatients

Environment

- Provide separate housing areas for dogs and cats.
- Maintain temperature between 21–23 °C with adequate ventilation.
- Clean kennels daily including the door.
- Supply fresh bedding if it is soiled.

Monitoring the patient

All the following parameters should be taken and recorded twice daily. Any abnormalities (including those such as pain and vomiting) should be noted and must be reported to the veterinary surgeon:

- temperature
- pulse
- respiratory rate
- mucous membrane colour
- capillary refill time (CRT)
- notes on urination and defecation – walk dogs frequently
- notes on eating and drinking
- notes on medication.

Nutrition

- If appropriate, patients can be fed two to three times daily; ask the owner what the animal likes to eat at home.
- Hand/syringe/spoon feed to help tempt a patient to eat.
- Patients may require specially formulated diets, eg those made specifically for kidney disease or urinary calculi.
- If nursing a diabetic patient always check with the veterinary surgeon what the feeding regime is. It is important to strictly adhere to this so food and insulin can work in harmony and not cause complications.
- Fresh water should always be available unless contraindicated. Avoid giving milk as this can cause diarrhea.

Physical support

- Give plenty of tender loving care.
- Take the patient outside for walks.
- Clean soiled litter trays and kennels.
- Administer any medication.

Mental support

- Groom the patient.
- Clean the patient's face and paws.
- Give plenty of tender loving care.
- Place their favourite blanket or toy in the kennel.
- Provide a variety of toys.

Needs of critically ill patients and neonates

Care of the critically ill patient

The critically ill patient will require more frequent checks – every 10 minutes in some cases. As well as the daily care described earlier the following must also be considered.

Environment

- Maintain the temperature between 21–23 °C with adequate ventilation.
- Clean kennels daily including the door.
- Supply fresh bedding if soiled.

Monitoring the patient

- Temperature
- Pulse
- Respiratory rate

- Mucous membrane colour
- CRT
- Notes on urination and defecation
- Notes on eating and drinking
- Notes on medication
- Signs of pain or anxiety.

Is nutrition correct?

- Are they eating?
- Do they need a special diet?
- Fluid therapy – Is hydration correct?

If they are receiving intravenous fluids – see monitoring
the patient receiving intravenous fluid therapy (see p. 291).

Temperature control

Many critically ill patients cannot regulate their own body
temperature. Take the temperature at regular intervals. If they
become hypothermic then warm with blankets, space blankets,
bubble wrap, heat lamps and heat pads may be used but with care as
they may not be able to move away from them. Ensure fluids and
diets (if tube fed) are at body temperature. If suffering from
hyperthermia then cool with wet towels, ice packs, cold
baths/showers.

Are they incontinent or unable to urinate/defecate? See elements
2.4.17, 2.4.18 and 2.4.19.

Transporting unconscious or anaesthetised patients

Patients should, wherever possible, be transported by the following
methods to avoid injury to yourself and the patient:

- stretchers
- baskets
- trolleys
- blankets – use as a makeshift stretcher
- mobile tables.

2.4.12   Wound management, dressings and bandages

What you need to learn

- ☙ You need to be able to outline the process of wound healing.
- ☙ Explain how the local application of moisture, heat or cold may
  affect the process of healing.

- Explain how local therapeutic applications may affect the process of healing:
  - ultrasound
  - laser light.
- Describe the functions of a wound dressing:
  - protection
  - absorption
  - pressure
  - therapeutic effect.
- Describe groups of dressing materials in common use:
  - dry (cotton/cellulose)
  - non-adherent
  - interactive (hydrogel, hydrocolloid, foam, alginate, film).
- Explain the use of interactive dressings in wound management.
- Describe the functions of a bandage:
  - support
  - compression
  - protection.
- Describe materials in common use for bandaging:
  - conforming
  - non-conforming
  - adhesive
  - non- and self-adhesives.
- Outline materials in common use for casting:
  - plastic polymers
  - plaster of Paris
  - fibreglass.
- Describe the health and safety precautions to be taken when handling casting materials:
  - wearing gloves
  - protective clothing.
- Describe the observations to be made following application of the bandage or cast:
  - protection
  - exercise
  - observation.
- Describe special types of bandages:
  - Ehmer sling
  - Velpeau sling
  - Robert Jones bandage
  - pressure bandage
  - Spica bandage
  - head bandages (eye and ear).
- Explain measures to be taken to prevent the animal interfering with bandages:

* Elizabethan collar
* bitter sprays or paints
* distraction.

Stages of wound healing

- Haemostasis – all wounds have varying degrees of haemorrhage which need to be controlled. Blood clots inhibit wound healing by increasing the amount of devitilised cellular debris (removed by the inflammatory process), enlarge dead space and provide media for bacterial growth.
- Inflammatory process – this is the activation of inflammatory mediators.
- Proliferation – this stage occurs 24–36 hours after the wound has occurred and the tissue that was destroyed begins to regenerate.
- Maturation and remodelling – begins 15 days after the wound occurred and can continue for many months. Tissue continuity and strength is restored. The strength of the scar depends on this stage.
- Contraction – this is reduction of the wound by movement of normal tissue migrating towards the centre of the wound. Starts after the wound occurred and continues for 2–3 weeks.
- Epithelialisation – begins 10 days after the wound occurred and is the regeneration of tissue over the wound.

Local applications

Moisture

A wound that has a moist environment will heal more rapidly. The moisture can be provided by wound dressings, eg hydrogels, or it can be provided by swabs soaked in saline or Hartmann's solution.

Heat

Applications of heat, eg swabs soaked in hot water, aid wound healing by causing vasodilatation, this in turn increases blood supply to the wound and also helps to drain fluid from the area.

Cold

Applications of cold, eg swabs soaked in cold water, can be used in wound care to reduce heat and blood loss by causing vasoconstriction.

Therapeutic applications

Ultrasound and lasers

Can also help wound healing by reducing inflammation.

Wound dressings

Wound dressings provide protection from outside sources, provide an area of absorption for exudates, can apply pressure and also provide a comforting therapeutic effect. Dressing materials commonly used:

- Dry – cotton/cellulose pad with semi-permeable film on one side, these can stick to the wound, they are useful for covering surgical incisions, eg Melolin® (Smith and Nephew)
- Non-adhesive – these dressings don't stick to the wound, they have good absorptive properties (foam type) and maintain a moist environment, eg foam-type Allevyn® (Smith and Nephew)
- Impregnated gauze-type dressings (Inidine®, Johnson and Johnson)
- Semi-permeable adhesive film – suitable for use with small or no exudates, the film maintains moisture but doesn't adhere to normal skin well, eg Opsite® (Smith and Nephew). Bioclusive® (Johnson and Johnson)
- Hydrogels – also known as interactive dressings. Amorphous hydrogel is applied directly to the wound and covered with a non-adhesive dressing, eg Intrasite® (Smith and Nephew), Nu-Gel® (Johnson and Johnson)
- Hydrocolloids – also known as interactive dressings. A self-adhesive gel containing the hydrocolloid is held in place by a thin layer of plastic, eg Tegasorb® (3M), Granuflex®, (ConvaTec)
- Calcium alginate – also known as interactive dressings. Derived from seaweed woven into pads. They exchange sodium ions for calcium ions to aid wound healing and also help to stop haemorrhage, however they are not intended for intraoperative use, eg Kaltostat® (ConvaTec), Tegagel® (3M).

All of these dressings can be used in both open and closed wound management.

Interactive wound dressings

Interactive wound dressings maintain a moist environment, encourage epithelisation and are not painful to remove.

Bandaging

Functions of a bandage

- To provide support, eg post-surgery, fractures
- To provide pressure or compression, eg haemorrhage, anticipated dead space
- To provide protection, eg wounds

- To prevent patient interference, eg bandaging paws to prevent scratching
- To provide absorption, eg exudation from wounds
- To limit mobility, eg fractures, comfort.

Materials

Materials used for the primary layer (to provide padding, absorption and hold the wound dressing in place):

- cotton wool
- commercially prepared padding layers, eg Soft Ban® (Smith and Nephew).

Materials used for the secondary later (to provide support and hold the primary layer in place):

- conforming bandage, eg Knit-fix® (Millpledge)
- crepe bandage.

Materials used for the tertiary layer (to provide protection from the environment):

- non-adhesive (self-conforming) eg Co-Plus® (Smith and Nephew)
- adhesive, eg Elastoplast®.

Materials used for casting:

- thermoplastic (plastic polymers) – dry within minutes, lightweight
- plaster of Paris – takes several hours to dry, heavy
- resin-impregnated (fibreglass) materials – dry within minutes, lightweight.

Precautions to take when handling casting materials:

- wear gloves
- wear a disposable apron
- wear a mask – especially on removal of a cast
- wear goggles or a visor – especially on removal of a cast
- cover the table in newspaper or some form of disposable covering

Observation of the bandage or cast

The following need to be monitored regularly when the patient has a bandage or cast applied.

- Check there are no smells – an offensive smell indicates infection.
- Check it is not too tight – you should be able to insert three fingers.
- Check it is not too loose or it will slip down or come off.
- Check there is no swelling above or below the bandage or cast – swelling indicates it is too tight.

- Check there are no pressure sores – red, sore and ulcerated areas indicate too much pressure. Some sores are seen at the top or bottom of the bandage or cast, others will only be visible on removal. Check for these at each re-dress. Use extra padding in bony and thin-skinned areas.
- Check the toes are not cold – this indicates poor circulation and an over-tight bandage.
- Check there is no weeping of the tissues or exudate around and under the bandage or cast – this indicates infection.
- Check there is no redness or heat around the surrounding areas – these indicate inflammation and infection.
- Check for signs of pain or anxiety in the patient.
- Ensure the bandage is dry at all times – a wet bandage will be cold and will induce sore skin. Change wet bandages or casts immediately. A plastic bag or an old drip bag can be placed over the bandage or cast and secured with an elastic band.
- Ensure the patient can walk and rest correctly.
- Check with the veterinary surgeon if there are limits on the amount of exercise or movement and adhere to this.

Care of the cast or bandage

- Protection – keep the cast or bandage dry by covering it with a plastic bag.
- Exercise – limit the patient to lead exercise only.
- Observation – monitor the cast or bandage as described above.

Special types of bandages

Ehmer sling

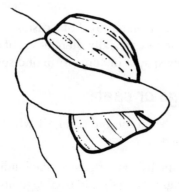

Figure 4.5

To support the hind limb eg after hip dislocation.

Velpeau sling

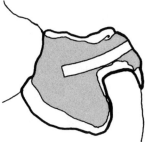

Figure 4.6

To support the shoulder, eg after shoulder dislocation.

Robert Jones bandage

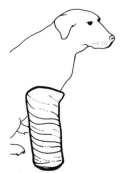

Figure 4.7

To aid support, should be three times the diameter of the limb and on flicking it should sound like flicking a water melon.

Pressure bandage

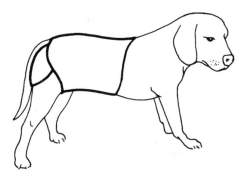

Figure 4.8

A tightly applied bandage to aid haemostasis – do not leave on for more than 10 minutes.

Spica bandage

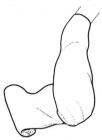

Figure 4.9

Wind the bandage around repeatedly in a figure of eight pattern so a series of V marks appear on the outside surface of the bandage.

Head bandage

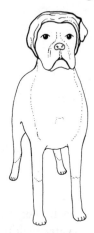

Figure 4.10

Can be adapted to include the ears or eyes. Use Elastoplast for the tertiary layer as a self-conforming bandage can tighten and may obstruct the neck, causing breathing difficulties.

Body bandage

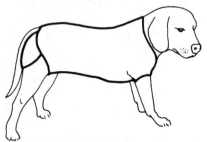

Figure 4.11

Can be used on the thorax or abdomen to aid decompression of air, fluid or blood. Use Elastoplast for the tertiary layer as self-conforming bandage can tighten and may obstruct breathing.

Preventing patient interference

The following methods can be used alone or together to help prevent the patient licking or biting at a wound, or trying to remove the bandage or cast.

- Use an Elizabethan collar.
- Bitter-tasting substances can be placed onto the area (if appropriate) to help prevent licking and biting, eg mustard.
- Bandage the paws to help prevent scratching.
- Use devices such as neck braces to stop the animal from reaching the affected area.
- Use a good surgical technique, eg no clipper rash, sutures are not too tight.
- Ensure adequate analgesia is given; sedation may also be used.

2.4.13 Care of hospitalised and recumbent patients

What you need to learn

- You need to be able to explain the meaning of recumbency
- Outline the conditions that may result in recumbency:
  - debilitating disease
  - neurological disease
  - trauma
  - old age.
- Outline the psychological needs of the recumbent animal:
  - contact
  - mental stimulation.

Care of the recumbent patient

Recumbency – a recumbent animal is unable to stand.

Table 4.6

Causes	Resulting conditions	Treatment and prevention
Debilitating disease, eg severe gastroenteritis	Hypostatic pneumonia Hypothermia	Turn every 2 hours, perform coupage and position to aid postural drainage
Neurological disease, eg coma	Decubitus ulcers Muscle wastage	Take temperature regularly, use heat pads (carefully as the patient can't move away from them), keep room warm and use bubble or space blankets
Trauma, eg fractures to the pelvis	Incontinence or soiling of bedding	
Old age	Constipation or impaction	
	Inability to eat or drink, spillage	See Care of the patient with loss of mobility
	Dyspnoea	See Care of the patient with loss of mobility
	Depression	See Care on nursing the incontinent patient
		Administer faecal softeners. Care with opiate analgesia. Perform an enema
		Hand/syringe/spoon feed, can feed via a tube. Use non-slip bowls within easy reach and keep bedding clean and dry
		Support in sternal recumbency for 30–40 minutes at regular periods. Use foam wedges to aid positioning and respiration. Supply oxygen if necessary
		Lots of TLC and mental stimulation, eg grooming and toys

Psychological needs include tender loving care (TLC), personal contact and mental stimulation.

2.4.14 Mobility

What you need to learn

* Explain how reduced mobility may affect muscles, joints and skin:
    * muscle spasms
    * muscle wasting
    * pressure sores.
* Describe how physiotherapy may be used to maintain joint flexibility and muscle tone. This includes:
    * passive physiotherapy

- exercise (active physiotherapy)
- flexion
- rotation
- assisted exercise
- hydrotherapy
- massage.

Describe how positioning may be used to maintain normal limb function and muscle tone. This includes:
- bedding
- manipulation
- foam wedges
- air or fluid-filled support.

Explain the underlying causes of pressure sores (decubitus ulcers):
- pressure
- shearing forces.

Describe measures which may be used to prevent the development of pressure sores (decubitus ulcers):
- repositioning
- observation of pressure areas
- hygiene
- pressure-relieving equipment (bedding, positioning aids).

Outline the management of an established pressure sore or decubitus ulcer:
- pressure relief
- hygiene
- wound care
- nutrition.

Describe the principles of moving and handling immobile animals:
- manual lifting
- transferring
- slings
- hoisting systems

Care of the patient with mobility loss

Patients with loss of mobility include **paraplegics,** and those with fractured limbs and **paresis.** Loss of use of one or more limbs can lead to:

- muscle spasms – paraplegic – loss of use of hindlimbs
- muscle wastage – tetraplegic – loss of use of all four limbs
- urinary scalding – paraparesis – weakness of hindlimbs
- pressure sores – tetraparesis – weakness of all four limbs
- joints becoming stiff.

Physiotherapy

This helps to maintain supple flexible joints and muscle tone, and improves circulation:

- passive physiotherapy: efflurage (smooth hand movements in the direction of the heart)
- active physiotherapy: flexion, extension and rotation of joints
- assisted walking and exercises
- hydrotherapy
- acupuncture and massage.

Bedding, foam wedges and airbags can all be used to aid limb positioning and function. Reposition the patient at regular intervals. Feeding a high protein diet can also help towards preventing muscle wastage.

Decubitus ulcers

These are also known as pressure sores or bedsores. They are a particular problem in thin, bony dogs, eg greyhounds, and occur over bony prominences. Because of the decreased amount of subcutaneous tissue and the constant pressure exerted, blood supply and oxygen to the area is diminished causing a decubitus ulcer.

Table 4.7

Areas	Prevention	Treatment
Olecranon	Turn the patient every 2 hours	Clip area
Hock		Clean area regularly with antiseptic and keep dry
Wings of ilium	Use double or triple thickness bedding – blankets, vetbeds, bubble wrap	Apply barrier cream
Shoulder		Inspect regularly
Greater trochanter of femur	Place pressure ring bandages or padding over problem areas	
	Place foam wedges under problem areas	

Moving and handling immobile animals

Always think of your own safety first. The following methods can be used:

- manual lifting – use two people
- transferring
- slings
- hoisting systems.

2.4.15   Respiration

What you need to learn

❧ You need to be able to explain how respiration may be compromised in the recumbent animal:
  ❧ hypostatic pneumonia
  ❧ dyspnoea.
❧ Describe how an animal may be positioned to facilitate the respiratory function:
  ❧ sternal recumbency
  ❧ rotation of position
  ❧ positioning aids.
❧ Describe physiotherapy techniques used to aid the respiratory function:
  ❧ postural drainage
  ❧ coupage (percussion).

How respiration may be compromised

Respiration may become comprised in the recumbent patient due to there only being one dependent lung. The following may then follow:

• Hypostatic pneumonia – the non-dependent lung becomes fluid filled and therefore compromises breathing.
• Dyspnoea – this will occur as there is only one functioning lung; pre-existing disease may also cause this.

The following methods will help to facilitate respiration in these cases:

• sternal recumbency – sitting the patient on their brisket
• rotation of the patient every 2 hours – helps to prevent hypostatic pneumonia
• the use of positioning aids such as foam wedges aids sternal recumbency.

Physiotherapy can also aid respiration and the following techniques may be used:

• postural drainage – sitting the patient in sternal recumbency to aid drainage of any fluid
• coupage (percussion) – external slapping of the thorax with cupped hands.

2.4.16 Food and fluid intake

What you need to learn

☙ You need to be able to explain how hospitalisation and recumbency affect nutritional requirements:
- ☙ balance of nutrients
- ☙ energy requirement.

☙ Outline the physical difficulties associated with feeding and drinking for a hospitalised or recumbent animal:
- ☙ access to food and water
- ☙ spillage.

☙ Outline the conditions which may lead to a requirement for assisted feeding:
- ☙ psychological condition
- ☙ trauma
- ☙ alimentary surgery
- ☙ illness
- ☙ medication.

☙ Describe methods used for assisted feeding. These include:
- ☙ handfeeding
- ☙ syringe feeding
- ☙ spoon feeding
- ☙ pharyngostomy
- ☙ naso-oesophageal tube
- ☙ gastrostomy tube.

☙ Describe the use of assisted feeding and oral therapy in exotic species and the correct methods of placing an orogastric tube:
- ☙ exotics
- ☙ birds
- ☙ reptiles.

☙ Describe the nursing care of a patient requiring tube feeding:
- ☙ placement and patency of tube
- ☙ feeding frequency
- ☙ stoma care.

☙ Outline methods of calculating nutritional requirements for tube feeding:
- ☙ basal energy requirements
- ☙ fluid requirements.

☙ Explain the causes of vomiting and regurgitation:
- ☙ bolting food
- ☙ gastrointestinal tract disorders
- ☙ metabolic disease
- ☙ medication
- ☙ poisoning
- ☙ obstruction
- ☙ toxaemia.

☙ Describe the observations to be made of a vomiting patient. This includes:
   ☙ nature of vomiting
   ☙ content
   ☙ frequency and volume of vomitus (sick).
☙ Outline methods of assessing the degree of hydration:
   ☙ tenting
   ☙ dry mucous membranes
   ☙ observe sunken eyes
   ☙ packed cell volume.
☙ Describe the principles of re-introducing oral food and fluids to a recovering animal. This covers:
   ☙ gradual re-introduction
   ☙ observation
   ☙ possible complications.
☙ Describe the care of a hospitalised patient with an intravenous infusion and the required equipment checks:
   ☙ protection and observation of infusion site
   ☙ drip rate
   ☙ pulse and respiration
   ☙ urine output.
☙ Describe how to change an infusion bag.

Nutrition

Both hospitalisation and recumbency affect the nutritional requirements of patients as they may refuse to eat or have difficulty in eating. Disease, injury and surgery can increase the amount of calories needed each day.

Feed a highly digestible diet that includes a highly digestible high biological value protein, eg chicken; highly digestible carbohydrate, eg rice; and reduced fibre. Adjust the amount required to compensate for illness, cage rest and stress.

Patients may find it difficult to reach their food and water if they are recumbent. If so, you can hand feed, syringe feed or spoon feed, or you can feed via a tube (see Table 4.8). Use non-slip bowls within easy reach and keep bedding clean and dry.

Conditions that lead to the need for assisted feeding include:

• a psychological condition, eg depression from being recumbent
• trauma, eg road traffic accident causing a fractured mandibular symphysis
• alimentary surgery, eg recovery from intestinal surgery
• systemic illness, eg renal failure

- medication, eg some animals may require assisted feeding to medicate them
- oral surgery, eg if oral surgery has been performed the animal may be physically unable to eat.

Assisted feeding

- Hand feeding – offer food to the patient on clean hands or fingers.
- Syringe feeding – use liquefied diets and feed into the side of the mouth. Ensure the patient can swallow and that their head is in a natural position to avoid **aspiration pneumonia.**
- Spoon feeding – feed diets into the mouth from a spoon.
- Tube feeding – see Table 4.8.

Table 4.8

Tube type	Naso-oesophageal	Pharyngostomy	Gastrostomy	Jejunostomy	Parental feeding
Placement	In the oesophagus via the ventral meatus	In the oesophagus via the pharynx. Incision made on the left side of the neck.	In the stomach by laparotomy incision or by endoscopy – percutaneous endoscopically placed gastrostomy tube	In the jejunum passed by percutaneous gastrostomy tube	Intravenous
Indications	Burns/lacerations to the mouth Fractures/trauma to the head Inappetance	Facial disease or surgery	Anorexia, the upper gastro-intestinal tract can be used	Following major surgery on the stomach, gastric or oesophageal dysfunction	A non-functioning gastro intestinal tract, pancreatitis?
Anaesthesia required	No – can be placed with the animal conscious or under sedation	Yes	Yes	Yes	No
Lubrication	Yes	No	No	No	No
Prevention of patient interference	Elizabethan collar, bandage paws	A bandage around the neck, can bandage the paws	Abdominal bandage, bandage paws, Elizabethan collar	Elizabethan collar, bandage paws	Bandages
Contra-indications	Unconscious patients, disease of the oesophagus/pharynx/larynx and stomach	Persistent vomiting, Pharyngeal disease	Persistent vomiting, a non-functioning gastro-intestinal tract	Non-functioning gastro-intestinal tract	Non-skilled staff. Availability of equipment

Exotics

Anorexia is a major symptom of ill health in exotics so the provision of nutrition is often vital in restoring the health of the patient.

Birds

- If a bird is unable or unwilling to eat, or if its food intake is insufficient, supplementary food can be given by **crop-tube feeding**.
- Special crop tubes are available but a blunt-ended needle such as a Spreull's needle is suitable. The tube is lubricated and inserted into the side of the mouth and directed over the top of the opening to the trachea and down the oesophagus as far as the crop.
- Small amounts of liquefied food can be given in this way at each session.
- The procedure can be repeated every few hours.
- Great care should be taken to clean the equipment thoroughly.

Rabbits and rodents

- Oral feeding (**gavage**) can only be performed if the animal is strong enough to hold its head up and swallow.
- Small amounts of liquefied food can be passed from a syringe through a soft tube into the back of the animal's mouth.
- Care should be taken to allow the patient to swallow each mouthful so that food is not aspirated into the lungs.
- Naso-oesophageal tubes can be used for feeding rabbits. A feeding tube is lubricated and fed gently for a measured distance into the nostril after the application of a local anaesthetic.
- A radiograph should be taken to check that the tube is not resting in the trachea.
- The tube is then glued or sutured in position and a collar fitted to prevent the rabbit from removing the tube.
- Liquefied food can be passed down the tube, which should be flushed with sterile water or saline before and after use.
- Caecotrophs can be liquidised and fed in this way to aid in digestion and provide gut flora for the rabbit.

Reptiles

- Stomach tubing is used with care in anorexic reptiles. Care should be taken to avoid damaging the animal's mouth while holding it open.
- Sedation or anaesthesia may be necessary to restrain an unco-operative or belligerent reptile.
- **Chelonians**: the mouth is held open by an assistant while the

lubricated tube is passed a measured distance down the oesophagus
to the stomach (Figure 4.12).

- **Snakes:** the stomach tube must pass into the stomach as snakes can
easily regurgitate. The stomach is approximately one third of the
way along the snake. The snake's glottis is often firmly closed so
there is little chance of passing the tube into the trachea. The mouth
may need to be held open with a speculum but care must be taken
not to damage the teeth.

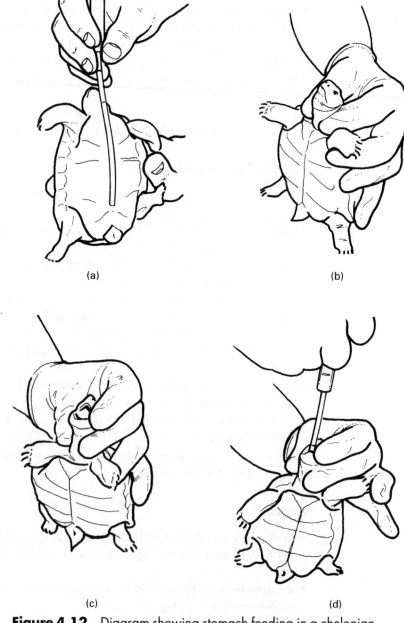

(a)

(b)

(c)

(d)

Figure 4.12 Diagram showing stomach feeding in a chelonian.

• **Lizards:** lizards will often open their mouths fairly easily with gentle tension on the lower jaw. A speculum can be inserted and the lubricated tube advanced into the oesophagus.

Feeding via a tube

The tube should be flushed with 5–10 ml water before and after each feed to avoid blockages. If a blockage does occur then Coca Cola can be used to dislodge it. Replace the cap each time it is removed.

• On the first day one third of the total amount is given.
• On the second day two thirds of the total amount is given.
• On the third day the total amount is given.
• If using a percutaneous endoscopically placed gastrostomy tube withhold food for the first 24 hours.
• The amounts given should be divided between four to six meals a day.

This same process should be repeated in reverse when the tube is to be removed to avoid **hypoglycemia**.

Warm the food to body temperature and give slowly to avoid overload, vomiting and diarrhoea.

Stoma care

The skin and area around the exiting tube should be bathed daily, kept clean and dry. Any soiled or wet bandages should be changed.

Nutritional requirements

Calculations for the basal energy requirements (BER) for animals over 5 kg are:

BER = 30 × bodyweight + 70

and for animals under 5 kg are:

BER = 60 × bodyweight

If disease, injury or surgery is present a disease factor needs to be added to the calculation as follows:

BER × disease factor = daily calorie requirement

Disease factors are:

• cage rest 1.2
• surgery or trauma 1.3
• multiple surgery 1.5
• sepsis or cancer 1.7
• burns 2.0

Fluids should be maintained at 40–50 ml/kg/d to replace inevitable and urinary losses. If the patient is vomiting or has diarrhoea 4 ml/kg/episode should be added.

Complications of tube feeding

Complications of tube feeding include:

- occlusion of the tube
- vomiting and/or diarrhoea
- oedema and/or haemorrhage
- aspiration of food
- hypoglycemia
- peritonitis.

Vomiting

Types of vomiting
Table 4.9

Type of vomit	Description	Causes
Projectile vomit	Forceful ejection of stomach contents	Gastritis, foreign bodies, ingestion of poisons
Bilious vomit	Vomit containing bile	Pancreatitis, intestinal foreign bodies
Haematemesis vomit	Vomit containing blood	Gastric ulcer
Stercoraceous vomit	Vomit containing faeces	Severe constipation
Cyclic vomiting	Repeated acts of vomiting	Inflammatory intestinal disease
Retching	Failure in attempts to vomit, 'heaving'	Gastric dilatation/volvulus (GDV)
Regurgitation	Undigested food ejected from the oesophagus (sausage-shaped)	Reflux oesophagitis

Vomiting or emesis is defined as the forceful emission of the stomach contents via the mouth. Any incidents of vomiting should be recorded with the following details:

- the nature of vomiting
- contents:
  - any blood within the vomit (some forms of blood can look like coffee granules)
  - any mucus within the vomit
  - any foreign material within the vomit
  - any bile within the vomit
- frequency

- volume
- general appearance of the vomit.

Assessing the degree of dehydration

- Dermal elasticity (tenting) – in the dehydrated patient this will be increased.
- Mucous membranes will be dry or tacky.
- Eyes will look sunken.
- Packed cell volume will be increased.
- Serum total protein can be increased.
- Urine output is reduced.
- Lethargy is increased.
- Coma and death at the most severe level.

Causes of dehydration

- Decreased water intake, eg reduced access to water and inability to drink.
- Increased water loss, eg diarrhoea/vomiting; chronic renal failure; burns; excessive panting.

There are often electrolyte imbalances in the dehydrated patient.

Re-introducing oral fluids and food

The process described for gradual introduction of fluids and food should be repeated in reverse when discontinuing tube feeding to avoid hypoglycemia.

Complications of tube feeding include the same as those mentioned under the Feeding via a tube section.

Monitoring the patient receiving intravenous fluids

The following parameters should be monitored along with the daily care described earlier:

- Protection – change the dressing on the leg (protecting the catheter and attached giving set) if it becomes soiled or wet.
- Observation – if the catheter is not in the vein, the following will be seen:
  - a wet bandage and leg swelling above the catheter site
  - the catheter may be visible if the patient has pulled it out completely.
- Check the drip is running and not occluded by kinks in the giving set or by the patient pulling their leg back.
- Check the patient's pulse and respiration rate.
- Urine output – this can only be measured accurately if collected into

a collection bag. Alternatively the urine could be collected in a kidney dish and measured. Urine output should be 1–2 ml/kg/h.
• Check mucous membrane colour and capillary refill time.
• Record any signs of noisy breathing or coughing.

How to change a drip (infusion) bag

• Close off the giving set.
• Remove the tag from the new bag by twisting it.
• Take the giving set out of the old bag.
• Place the giving set into the new bag with a rotating movement; be careful not to twist it in as this will twist the giving set tubing.
• Open the giving set to the appropriate level.
• Place the old bag in the clinical waste bin.

Standard giving set = 20 drops/ml
Paediatric giving set = 60 drops/ml

Fluids should be maintained at 40–50 ml/kg/d to replace inevitable and urinary losses. If the patient is vomiting or has diarrhoea 4 ml/kg/episode should be added. For example, to calculate the maintenance fluid requirement of a 5 kg cat using a standard giving set:

Maintenance fluid requirement = 50 ml/kg/d = 50 ml × 5 kg
= 250 ml per 24 h
Requirement per hour = 250 ml/24 h = 10 ml
Requirement per minute = 10 ml/60 min = 0.16 ml
Giving set drop rate = 20 × 0.16 ml = 3.2 drops per min
Drip rate = 60 seconds/3.2 drops = 1 drop every 18 sec

2.4.17 Urination

What you need to learn

☙ You need to be able to describe the urinary problems that may affect recumbent patients:
  ☙ retention
  ☙ incontinence
  ☙ urine scald
  ☙ urinary tract infection (UTI).
☙ Describe methods of assisting urination in the recumbent animal:
  ☙ position
  ☙ support
  ☙ manual expression
  ☙ catheterisation
  ☙ cystocentesis.

- Outline the methods for manually expressing the bladder.
- Outline the indications for urinary catheterisation. These include:
    - retention of urine
    - incontinence
    - diagnostic procedures
    - monitoring urine output
    - abdominal surgery, eg male dog.
- Explain the principles of urinary catheterisation for cats and dogs, both male and female.
- Describe the different types of urinary catheter available for use with cats and dogs:
    - self-retaining catheter
    - Foley catheter
    - Tiemann's catheter
    - nylon disposable catheter
    - Jackson cat catheter.
- Describe the equipment needed for undertaking catheterisation, including:
    - gloves
    - vaginal speculum
    - stylet
    - sterile water
    - syringe
    - antiseptic solution
    - lubricant
    - catheters of appropriate size and type
    - collection bag.

Urinary problems affecting recumbent patients

These include:

- urinary retention – holding urine
- urinary incontinence – leaking urine
- urine scald – skin damage due to urine soaking
- urinary tract infections (UTI).

Assisting urination in the recumbent patient

- Position the patient, eg in their litter tray.
- Support the patient, eg towel-assisted walking.
- Manual expression of the bladder, repeat this throughout the day.
- Use catheterisation to drain urine from the bladder via a catheter (repeated catheterisation or an **indwelling** catheter can be used).
- Use cystocentesis to drain the bladder via a sterile needle and sterile syringe.

Manual expression of the bladder

A patient's bladder can be expressed manually when they are
conscious, sedated or under general anaesthesia:
• restrain the patient in the standing position
• lift the tail and gently squeeze the caudal abdomen
• collect urine in a kidney dish, universal container or boric acid
container.

Indications for placing a urinary catheter

These include:
• urinary retention
• urinary incontinence
• diagnostic procedures, eg to introduce radiographic contrast media
• to monitor urine output
• before and during abdominal surgery – to prevent contamination of
the surgical field
• following surgery – when the patient can't move or it is unadvisable
for the patient to move
• urinary calculi and obstruction
• to prevent urinary scalding
• to obtain a less contaminated urine sample.

Principles of urinary catheterisation

Male dog

• General anaesthesia may be needed.
• Restrain the patient in lateral recumbency or in the standing
positioning.
• Cut the top off the plastic wrapper of the catheter.
• Extrude the penis.
• Gently insert the catheter by feeding from the remaining plastic
wrapper.
• Stop advancing the catheter when urine is seen in the catheter.

Female dog

Catheterisation can be done with the patient either in the standing
position or in dorsal recumbency and requires two people. The
technique which follows is used in dorsal recumbency using a Foley
catheter.

• General anaesthesia is usually needed.
• Restrain the patient in dorsal recumbency.
• Draw the patient's hind legs in a cranial direction.

- Lubricate the speculum and insert it into the vagina.
- Insert the catheter and on advancement of the catheter slowly release the hind legs caudally.
- Inflate the balloon – resistance will be felt if the catheter is not in the bladder.
- Remove the stylet and urine will be seen.

Male cat

- General anaesthesia is needed.
- Restrain the patient in right lateral recumbency.
- Extrude the penis.
- Insert the catheter using slight rotation.
- Advance the catheter until urine is seen.
- Suture the catheter in place if it is being used as indwelling catheter.

Female cat

- General anaesthesia is needed.
- Restrain the patient in right lateral recumbency.
- Cut the top off the plastic wrapper.
- Insert and advance the catheter along the floor of the vagina.
- Stop advancing the catheter when urine is seen.

Types of urinary catheter

- Metal bitch catheter
- Foley catheter
- Tiemann's catheter
- Portex dog catheter (nylon disposable)
- Jackson cat catheters
- Dowse catheter
- Conventional cat catheters.

Equipment needed

The equipment needed to catheterise a patient includes:

- gloves (sterile or non-sterile depending on procedure)
- vaginal speculum
- stylet
- sterile water
- syringe
- swabs and antiseptic solution
- lubricating jelly
- catheter
- urine collection bag, universal container, boric acid container
- kidney dish

- clippers
- contrast media (if needed).

For a Foley catheter

As already described, plus:

- spigot or adapter
- sterile water for inflating the balloon – the amount needed is specified on the catheter
- stylet
- Elizabethan collar.

For Jackson cat catheters

As already described, plus:

- Elizabethan collar
- needle and suture material, eg nylon
- needle holders and rat tooth forceps.

2.4.18   Defecation

What you need to learn

🐾 You need to be able to explain how bowel movements may be affected in the recumbent animal:
  - 🐾 constipation
  - 🐾 impaction
  - 🐾 soiling.
🐾 Describe how constipation may be prevented:
  - 🐾 mobility
  - 🐾 diet
  - 🐾 management
  - 🐾 hydration
  - 🐾 laxatives and bulking agents
  - 🐾 enemas.
🐾 Describe the principles of administering enemas. This includes:
  - 🐾 introduction per rectum of fluid
  - 🐾 suitable volume of fluid
  - 🐾 monitoring effects.
🐾 Outline the types of enemas used:
  - 🐾 phosphate
  - 🐾 micro-enemas
  - 🐾 oil-based enemas
  - 🐾 warm water.

Recumbency often results in slow intestinal movements which in turn can cause constipation and impaction. A recumbent patient may become soiled.

- Constipation – faeces are retained in the rectum and large intestine.
- Impaction – faeces cannot be passed.
- Soiling – faecal material sticks to the coat, on the tail and on the hindlegs, there is faecal material on the bed and floor.

Preventing constipation

Measures to prevent constipation include:

- increasing mobility (exercise)
- feeding a high-fibre diet
- adding fibre to the food
- general management (taking the patient out for regular exercise and cleaning litter trays frequently)
- increasing hydration by offering more water or moist food
- using laxatives to increase intestinal mobility
- using bulking agents to increase the faecal amount
- performing enemas.

Principles of administering an enema

Equipment

- Two bowls – one with solution in and one empty.
- Apron and gloves.
- Newspaper.
- Higginson's syringe or lamb feeder and attached syringe with lubrication.
- Contrast media if needed.

Method

- General anaesthesia is needed apart from the ready-to-use brands.
- Prepare all the above equipment using warm water to heat it to body temperature.
- Restrain the patient in lateral recumbency.
- Lubricate the tip of the chosen applicator.
- Insert the nozzle of the applicator into the anus, rotate and advance into the rectum.
- Introduce the chosen solution. The recommended amount for olive oil, glycerin and water is 5–10 ml/kg, and for liquid paraffin is 3 ml/kg.
- Digitally remove the faeces; it can help to palpate the faeces in the abdomen and propel them forward.

- Once all the faeces are removed, shampoo and rinse the caudal quarters – pre-warn the owners that their pet's fur may look greasy, especially if liquid paraffin is used.
- When appropriate supply litter trays and take the patient outside for exercise, monitor the amount of faeces passed, the consistency of the faeces and note if it contains blood or mucus.

Types of enemas used

Solutions used as enemas include:

- phosphate enemas
- micro-enemas, eg ready-to-use types
- oil based enemas – liquid paraffin or glycerin
- warm water.

2.4.19   Hygiene

What you need to learn

☙ You need to be able to explain the principles of maintaining hygiene in the recumbent animal:
  ☙ skin
  ☙ bathing
  ☙ grooming.
☙ Describe the nursing management of an incontinent animal:
  ☙ skin care
  ☙ bedding.

Maintaining hygiene

It is important to maintain hygiene in the recumbent patient to prevent urine scalds, soiled and stained fur and bacterial infections. This is achieved by protecting the skin, bathing the patient and grooming the patient at regular intervals throughout the day.

Nursing management of an incontinent animal

- Apply barrier cream to the skin around the vulva or prepuce to prevent urine scalds, eg vaseline, sudocrem.
- Bath and groom the patient once daily or more often if needed.
- Clip fur from around the vulva or prepuce – this prevents staining and it is easier to keep the skin clean and dry.
- Ensure bedding is kept clean and dry at all times.
- Place an indwelling catheter if appropriate.

2.4.20 Advising clients on the care of animals, essential grooming and hygiene

What you need to learn

❧ You need to be able to explain the principles of grooming a hospitalised animal.

❧ Outline areas requiring particular attention. These include:
  ❧ ears
  ❧ eyes
  ❧ orifices
  ❧ feet.

❧ Describe correct use of grooming equipment:
  ❧ electric clippers
  ❧ scissors
  ❧ comb
  ❧ brush.

❧ Explain the reasons an animal may require bathing:
  ❧ skin conditions
  ❧ parasites
  ❧ hygiene
  ❧ wounds.

❧ Describe the principles of bathing an animal. These include:
  ❧ equipment
  ❧ methodology
  ❧ safety.

❧ Describe the principles of how to clip claws and beaks:
  ❧ equipment
  ❧ methodology
  ❧ safety.

Principles of grooming a hospitalised animal

Patients are groomed within the hospital to keep them free from debris and to provide mental stimulation and comfort.

Areas needing particular attention

The following areas should be bathed twice daily with warm water and then dried (if appropriate):

• eyes
• ears
• orifices, eg nose
• feet.

Use of grooming equipment

The following equipment may be used on a daily basis. One or all of these items can be used during the grooming routine.

- Electric clippers – use these with the blade parallel to the skin to prevent clipper rash and nicks in the skin. Keep cool by spraying regularly with the clipper spray. For use on heavily matted areas.
- Scissors are useful for cutting out knots, use scissors that have blunt blades, use with caution near the skin as it is very easy to cut the skin as well as the fur.
- Combs – various sized tooth combs or dematting combs are used for grooming once all the matts and knots are removed. Comb from root to tip every day to prevent matts and knots from forming.
- Brushes – soft/hard/wire/double-sided/slicker/hound glove brushes can all be used to groom the patient once all matts and knots have been removed. Brush from root to tip every day to prevent matts and knots from forming.

Reasons why a patient may require bathing

A patient may require bathing for:
- treatment of skin conditions, eg scurfy dry skin, greasy skin
- treatment of external parasites, eg sarcoptes
- treatment of hygiene, eg urinary or faecal incontinent patients, long-haired patients
- treatment of wounds, eg some wounds may require daily bathing.

How to bath a patient

- Wear an apron and gloves, especially if using medicated products.
- If using a bath, run warm (not hot) water so it is a quarter full. Test the temperature of the water. Place the patient in the bath and use a second assistant to restrain them. Use jugs or containers to carry out the procedure. Refill with fresh water if a rinse is required.
- If using a shower, stand the patient in the area near the shower. Use a second assistant to restrain the patient. Adjust the temperature of the shower so it is warm. Carry out the procedure.
- After bathing ensure the patient is dried. If using a hairdryer, use the lowest heat setting, hold well away from the patient and keep the dryer moving at all times.

How to clip claws and beaks

- Use a second assistant to restrain the patient.
- Use sharp nail clippers of an appropriate size depending on the size of the patient.
- Hold the foot and expose the claw.
- Cut the claw above the level of the quick; this is easily seen in white claws. In black claws take repeated small bites.
- For beaks follow steps one and two. Hold the head and clip off the point. The beak also has a quick so take small bites to avoid bleeding.

2.4.21 Advising clients on the care of animals, basic nutrition and feeding

What you need to learn

- You need to be able to define nutrition.
- Explain the components of a healthy diet:
  - protein
  - fat
  - carbohydrate
  - vitamins
  - trace elements.
- Describe the differences in dietary requirements for animals commonly kept as pets:
  - dogs
  - cats
  - exotics.
- Outline the advantages and disadvantages of foodstuffs available for animals commonly kept as pets:
  - cats
  - dogs
  - exotics
  - fresh prepared foods
  - type of animal, cost, convenience, preference.
- Describe how to prepare and present complete foods:
  - young and elderly patients
  - in-patients
  - convalescing patients.
- Explain the importance of a balanced and complete diet at each life stage
  - young and elderly patients
  - inpatients
  - convalescing patients.

☙ State and understand the dangers of deficiencies and excesses in the diet:

☙ taurine
☙ B vitamins
☙ vitamin C
☙ vitamin A
☙ calcium
☙ phosphorus.

Nutrition

Nutrition is a solid or liquid that is capable of nourishing a living being, allowing normal function of cells and promoting life.

Components of a healthy diet

A complete diet should contain the following nutrients.

Protein

Chains of amino acids are linked by peptide bonds. Amino acids are divided into non-essential amino acids of which there are 12 and essential amino acids of which there are 11. Each protein has its own combination of amino acids. The biological value (BV) of the protein refers to the quality of that protein; the higher the BV the less is needed in the diet as it is utilised well. Protein is needed for tissue growth and repair, energy production and transportation of oxygen. In commercially prepared food protein levels are approximately 70%–85%.

Fat (also known as lipids)

Fat is formed from fatty acids and glycerol. Fatty acids are either saturated (no double bonds) or unsaturated (one or more double bonds). Unsaturated fats containing more than one double bond are then referred to as polyunsaturated. There are three essential fatty acids (EFA):

• linoleic
• alpha-linolenic
• arachidonic acid.

Fat provides energy, is a carrier for fat-soluble vitamins, it increases palatability and provides the above essential fatty acids.

Carbohydrates

The main source of carbohydrates is plants. There are four groups of carbohydrate:

- monosaccharides – single molecule sugars which are the main carbohydrates used by animals, eg glucose and fructose
- disaccharides – two sugar molecules linked by an alpha bond, eg lactose and sucrose
- oligosaccharides – a chain of 3–10 monosaccharides (can be all the same or a mixture)
- polysaccharides – thousands of monosaccharides.

Carbohydrates provide 40%–50% energy in dogs and 30% energy in cats. In commercially prepared food, carbohydrates are present at approximately 85% in dog food and 75% in cat food.

Other nutrients

- Vitamins – with water-soluble vitamins (vitamins B and C) any excess is excreted in the urine. With fat-soluble vitamins (vitamins A, D, E and K) any excess is stored within the body.
- Micro-minerals (also known as trace elements), eg iron, zinc, selenium, maintain metabolic processes.
- Water – a daily intake is required to replace obligate water loss from the body. Intake can be derived from drinking water and from food (70% water content in moist food, 10% water content in dry food). Water is needed to maintain normal electrolyte balance and is essential in thermoregulation and lubrication of body tissues.

Dietary requirements

A complete diet containing all the above components is required by both dogs and cats. Cats have two extra requirements that are added into feline diets. These are:

- taurine – an essential amino acid
- arachidonic acid – an essential fatty acid derived from animal origin.

Cats also require lower levels of carbohydrates as they are unable to metabolise large amounts. They derive most of their energy from proteins and fats.

Advantages and disadvantages of types of foodstuff

Table 4.10

Food type	Advantages	Disadvantages
Dry	Convenient Cheap Complete diet Aids dental care Diets are available for both dog and cat	Some dogs and cats may not find them palatable Storage May drink more
Mixers	Convenient Cheap Diets are available for both dog and cat Aids dental care	Some dogs and cats may not find them palatable Storage Not a complete diet May drink more
Semi-moist	Available as a complete diet and as treats or snacks Diets are available for both dog and cat More palatable than dry food	More expensive than dry food Not as convenient as dry food Does not aid dental care
Moist	Diets are available for both dog and cat Very palatable Available in cans, trays and pouches, promotes easy storage Complete diet	Expensive Does not aid dental care Not as convenient as dry food

- Cats and dogs may be fed fresh or preparatory food (ready made food in tins or dry formula). Dry food is cheaper and more convenient to feed than moist or semi-moist foods.
- Most cats and dogs will have a preference for moist, semi-moist or dry food.

Preparing and presenting complete foods

All diets should be prepared on clean work surfaces with clean bowls and utensils. Any unused canned food should have a cover placed over the top and put in the fridge. Dry food should be stored in a sealed container.

- Shallow, wide bowls or saucers should be used for puppies and kittens.
- Shallow, wide, non-slip bowls should be used for elderly patients or bowls they are used to feeding from.
- Feed inpatients from a suitable sized bowl, eg don't give a narrow bowl to a large dog; if infection is suspected, feed from stainless steel bowls as these can be sterilised.
- Convalescing patients may prefer to be fed from a bowl they would

use at home, or use easy-to-reach shallow bowls.
• Cats prefer to eat from shallow, wide bowls; metal bowls are preferable as the plastic type can give off a certain smell which cats do not like.

Life-stage diets

There are various stages to an animal's life. Each one requires different amounts of nutrients and supplementation is not required if a complete diet is fed for that particular life stage.

• Puppies and kittens require increased protein, energy and minerals; this diet is also suitable for pregnant and lactating bitches or queens.
• Large-breed puppies require a diet with a reduced energy and fat content, and reduced calcium and phosphorus.
• Senior animals need reduced energy and protein; calcium and phosphorus are also reduced to avoid excessive intake.
• Hospitalised patients should be fed an adult maintenance diet if they are not suffering from disease or injury. These diets contain maintenance levels of carbohydrates, protein, fat, vitamins and minerals. Maintenance diets with reduced levels of energy and fat are available to control weight or maintain weight loss.
• Convalescing patients – these patients may need a specific diet relative to their disease or injury, eg a high-quality protein diet for renal failure patients.

Vitamins
Table 4.11

Vitamins and elements	Excess	Deficiency
Taurine	Non-toxic	Central retinal degeneration, dilated cardiomyopathy, reduced growth rate
Vitamin B	None reported	Anorexia, skin disorders, neurological disorders
Vitamin C	Non-toxic	Scurvy
Vitamin A	Liver damage, ankylosis of joints especially the cervical vertebrae	Seborrhoeic coat conditions, night blindness, crusting lesions of the external nares and nasal discharge
Calcium and phosphorous	Hip dysplasia, oestochondrosis syndrome	Nutritional secondary hyperparathyroidism

Feeding exotics

All animals must be provided with fresh water daily. The water should be provided in a suitable receptacle with which the animal is familiar.

Birds

- Diet varies greatly depending upon the species encountered.
- Anyone considering owning a bird should obtain as much information on the diet and husbandry of the species as possible.
- All birds need to eat fragments of grit and other abrasive materials. These fragments pass into the gizzard where they help to grind food.

Caged birds are often divided into **hardbills** and **softbills**.

Hardbills (most of the parrot-like birds and finches) remove the outer husk to reach the nutritious kernel from seeds and nuts. Their beaks are specially adapted for this purpose.

Softbills eat food such as fleshy fruit, invertebrates (eg many garden birds including blackbirds and tits), or pollen and nectar (eg hummingbirds and lorikeets).

The distinction between softbills and hardbills is not always clear-cut. Psittacines will eat fruit and some softbills will eat seed as a supplement to their diet.

Water fowl, including ducks, geese and swans, will often eat bread, mixed corn and water plants. Birds such as swans often prefer the food to be fed in a bowl of clean water.

Some water birds such as seabirds and herons are fish eaters. Care should be taken when feeding birds on white fish as it contains an enzyme which causes thiamine deficiency. Captive fish-eating birds should therefore be provided with a vitamin B supplement.

Birds of prey such as eagles, hawks, falcons and owls require a carnivorous diet. Whole animals should be fed to provide a balanced diet. Day-old chicks, or dark mice (as wild birds will often not recognise white mice as food) fed with a vitamin and mineral supplement will usually suffice. Larger birds can be fed on pigeons and rabbits.

NB It is illegal to offer live vertebrate food.

Rodents

- Omnivores such as rats, mice and hamsters can be fed with well-balanced, commercially available diets.
- Food should be stored in a cool dry place to prevent spoiling.
- Treats such as raw fruit and vegetables can be offered.
- Chocolate and sweet treats should be fed only very occasionally as they can cause obesity.
- Gerbils can be fed on well-balanced, commercially available diets but these should be supplemented with seeds, fruits and leafy vegetables.
- Guinea-pigs are naturally herbivorous. They can be fed with well-balanced, commercially available diets which have been **specifically** designed for guinea-pigs.
- Guinea-pigs, like humans, are unable to synthesise vitamin C and therefore obtain it from the diet. Many commercial rodent foods lack sufficient vitamin C and contain too much vitamin D for guinea-pigs.
- The diet of a guinea-pig should be supplemented with good quality hay and grass, along with a variety of fruit and vegetables.
- Chinchillas may be fed with a well-balanced, commercially available diet.
- Pelleted food can be supplemented with a small amount of fresh or dried fruit and vegetables. Fresh good quality hay should be available.

Rabbits

- Rabbits are grazing animals. Their natural diet is grass and hay. The digestive system of rabbits is designed to digest this high-fibre, low-protein diet.
- Commercial diets are usually too low in fibre and too high in protein which results in digestive and dental disorders.
- Many rabbits will eat their commercial diets selectively so that much of the fibre is ignored in favour of the grains and pulses. This leads to obesity and, because of the low calcium content, problems with the teeth and bones.
- An ideal diet for a rabbit consists of good quality grass and hay.
- A small amount of a good quality commercial diet should be fed only as a supplement. A suitable commercial diet would be one which consists of just one type of pellet therefore avoiding selective feeding.

Reptiles

- A balanced diet is essential in keeping a healthy reptile. Most of the disorders encountered in reptiles are a direct result of improper feeding and husbandry.
- Reptiles are cold blooded and will eat more when they are warm.
- Obesity and anorexia are both common problems in reptiles. The weight of an animal should be monitored if the animal is not feeding properly.
- Great care should be taken to ensure that the diet contains sufficient calcium and phosphorous in the correct proportions to prevent metabolic bone disease.
- The actual diet fed depends upon the species. Anyone considering owning a reptile should obtain as much information regarding the diet and husbandry of the species as possible.

Chelonians

Tortoises are mainly herbivorous although there are some species which occasionally eat meat or insects. A variety of fruit and vegetables should be offered.

NB It should be noted that lettuce contains very little in the way of nutrients and should be avoided because it is often eaten preferentially by tortoises.

Lizards

- Some lizards, such as geckos, are insectivorous and should be fed on locusts, crickets and occasional mealworms. The feed should be dusted with a vitamin and mineral supplement. It is important to also feed the locusts well as an undernourished locust will provide little nourishment for the lizard.
- Larger lizards such as iguanas are predominantly herbivorous and should be fed a wide variety of fruit and vegetables.
- Water dragons are insectivorous when very young but become omnivorous as they age.
- Carnivorous lizards can be fed on mice. The whole animal, rather than pieces of meat, should be fed to provide a balanced diet.
- Chameleons are difficult animals to feed as they are very fastidious, preferring a variety of winged insects, caterpillars and crickets.

Snakes

- All snakes are carnivorous although the kind of meat they eat varies between species.
- Most species will eat small mammals. The whole animal, rather

than pieces of meat, should be fed to provide a balanced diet.
- **Pinkies** are bald baby mice and can be fed to small snakes.
- **Fuzzies** or **furries** are young mice with a fine coat.
- Adult mice and rats can also be fed.
- The size of the snake determines the size of food which should be provided. A small snake will refuse food which is too big to swallow whole. A large snake will often refuse prey which is too small, or lose weight because it will often only eat one animal at each feeding time.
- Some snakes are fish eaters (eg garter snakes). Fish should be fed whole to provide a balanced diet. Care should be taken when feeding snakes on white fish as it contains an enzyme which causes thiamine deficiency.
- Some snakes are cannibalistic or eat prey such as lizards. Owners should be advised to obtain all the necessary information before deciding to take on these species.

Amphibians

- Almost all adult amphibians are carnivorous.
- Anyone considering owning an amphibian should obtain as much information on the diet and husbandry of the species as possible.
- Aquatic species can usually be fed on mealworms or earthworms.
- **Terrestrial** (land-living) species can usually be fed on maggots, crickets or small mice.
- **Arboreal** (tree-living) species can be fed on flies such as fruit flies.

Fish

- Fish can be herbivorous, carnivorous or omnivorous.
- Most commonly kept fish can be fed with a well-balanced, commercially available diet. These are usually in the form of pellets or flakes.
- Live foods such as daphnia and bloodworms are available but care should be taken when feeding these as they can introduce parasites to the pond or aquarium.
- Care must be taken not to overfeed fish as the tank can become polluted with rotting surplus food.
- If an owner is considering keeping fish such as Koi carp or discus on a larger scale they should be advised to obtain as much information on the diet and husbandry of the species as possible.

How much have you learnt?

1 In what order would you perform an examination on a patient?

2 What are the normal temperature, respiratory and pulse rates?

3 Describe the signs of pain.

4 Describe four wound dressings.

5 What equipment is needed to a remove a plaster of Paris cast?

6 Explain how you would nurse a recumbent patient.

7 How could you increase a patient's mobility?

8 List the indications for placing an indwelling urinary catheter.

9 Describe the different methods of assisted feeding.

10 Describe the contents of a complete balanced diet.

The answers can be found within this unit, up to page 309.

2.4.22 Medicines and their management

What you need to learn

☙ Outline the provisions of legislation relating to medicines and therapeutic agents:
  ☙ Misuse of Drugs Act 1971
  ☙ Misuse of Drugs Regulations 1985
  ☙ Medicines Act 1968
  ☙ Health and Safety legislation (COSHH) 1995.
☙ Describe the requirements for the safe storage of medicines and therapeutic agents:
  ☙ legal requirements
  ☙ temperature
  ☙ humidity
  ☙ light
  ☙ shelf life.
☙ Outline the principles of pharmacy stock management:
  ☙ ordering
  ☙ rotation
  ☙ seasonal goods
  ☙ stock lists
  ☙ auditing.
☙ Describe the legal requirements for record keeping of pharmacy stock
☙ Describe the legislation affecting the use of controlled goods (CD) and explain associated drug schedules (Misuse of Drugs Regulations 2001).
☙ Outline the categories in use governing the sale and supply of medicines:
  ☙ general sales list (GSL)
  ☙ pharmacy list (P)
  ☙ prescribing merchants list (PML)
  ☙ prescription-only medicines (POM).
☙ Explain the difference between proprietary and generic names for medications.
☙ Describe the principles of safe and effective dispensing.
☙ Describe the weights and measures used in the prescription of medicines:
  ☙ standard units: ml, l, mg, g, kg
  ☙ international units: IU
☙ State the recommended containers for different medicines. These include:
  ☙ colour
  ☙ fluted bottles
  ☙ plain glass bottles

* wide-mouthed jars
* paper board cartons/wallets
* air-tight glass
* plastic/metal containers.
* Describe the formulae used to calculate required dosages and quantities for dispensing:
  * reduction
  * conversion of fractions.
* Explain the precautions to be taken when handling medicines. These include:
  * sensitivity reactions
  * ingestion/inhalation by dispenser
  * contamination
  * absorption
  * accidental ingestion by child or animal.
* Outline common abbreviations in prescribing use
  * SID
  * BID
  * TID
  * QID
  * BD
  * EOD
  * OD.
* Explain the risks involved in the use of prescribing abbreviations.

Legislation

The use of drugs in veterinary medicine is covered by a number of laws:

* **The Misuse of Drugs Act (1971)** details the legal aspects of misuse of drugs; this includes import, export and use of controlled drugs. It also covers production and supply and possession of controlled drugs. Controlled drugs are classified as:
  * Class A (examples of Class A drugs used in veterinary medicine include fentanyl, morphine, diamorphine and pethidine)
  * Class B (examples of Class B drugs used in veterinary medicine include codeine and dexamphetamine)
  * Class C (no Class C drugs are used in veterinary medicine on a regular basis).
* **The Misuse of Drugs Regulations (1985).**
* **The Medicines Act (1968)** covers the legal aspects of the licensing of drugs used for medical purposes. It also covers pharmacy use of drugs; packaging and containers; identification of drugs; and the legal sale and promotion of drugs.
* **Health and Safety legislation COSHH (1995).** This covers the

Control of Substances Hazardous to Health. This provides guidelines on the use of substances (including disinfectants, medicines, anaesthetics and radiation) which are potentially hazardous. It details the legal responsibilities of the company to protect its workers against such hazards, and the action which should be taken if an accident occurs.

Various amendments have been made to all these laws since their creation.

Safe storage of medicines

Proper storage of drugs and medication is important in maintaining sterility and preventing damage to the product. Consideration must be given to:

- **Temperature:** most drugs can be stored at room temperature although some products require refrigeration (eg insulin, most vaccines) to maintain their efficacy. High temperatures will cause degradation of most medications. Gaseous substances such as anaesthetic gases can become dangerous if subjected to high temperatures.
- **Humidity:** medications should be stored in a dry environment. Increased humidity can cause the medicine to degrade.
- **Light:** some substances can be degraded by exposure to light. Products should be kept in a dark environment if they are to be stored for a prolonged period. Contrast media, such as those used to provide contrast during radiography, will become degraded if exposed to light. These products must be kept in the dark at all times.
- **Shelf life:** all products are marked with an expiry date. After this date has passed these drugs should be carefully disposed of as their efficacy and safety can no longer be guaranteed.

Pharmacy stock management

Pharmacy stock management is extremely important in the smooth running of the practice. Running out of a particular product is inconvenient, and at worst it can threaten the health of a patient.

Most practices receive regular deliveries from a pharmaceutical wholesaler. These can be daily or weekly. The pharmacy should carry enough stock of the regularly used products to last until the next order arrives. The pharmacy should also stock any products which could be needed in an emergency (eg soluble insulin, adrenaline, etc).

There is a variation in demand for certain products at different times of year. Examples are flea treatments which are in greater demand from spring to autumn, and antihistamines are more likely to be required through the summer months. Stocking of the pharmacy should reflect these seasonal variations.

It is useful to carry a list of the stock in the pharmacy. This should be regularly updated so that the amount of stock being carried can be assessed quickly and easily when auditing or stock-taking is performed.

Record keeping

Special legislation exists regarding the use of controlled drugs:

- Controlled Drugs (CDs) must be recorded in the controlled drugs register.
- This register must be a bound book which is only used for recording CD use.
- Separate pages are provided for different classes of drugs.
- Entries should be indelible and written in chronological order. Alterations may not be made. Any corrections can be recorded at the foot of the page.
- The register should be kept for 2 years after the last entry.
- Details of drugs supplied to the practice are recorded (date, supplier, amount and form of the drug).
- Details of the drug used are recorded (date, name and address, amount and form of the drug).
- The CD register is covered by the **Misuse of Drugs Regulations 2001.**

Categories

Medicines are divided into categories which relate to how they may be supplied to the public:

- **General sales list (GSL):** these products can be sold without veterinary supervision. These can often be found in pet shops and supermarkets. Examples are some wormers (anthelmintics), parasiticide shampoos, laxatives and nutritional products. Most disinfectants are GSL.
- **Pharmacy medicines (P):** these products can be sold over the counter. There should be veterinary supervision but the animal does not have to be under the care of the veterinary surgeon.
- **Prescribing merchants list (PML):** these products can only be sold if an animal is under the care of the veterinary surgeon. The product does not have to be dispensed by the vet.
- **Prescription only medicines (POM):** these can only be supplied if an animal is under the care of the veterinary surgeon. The veterinary

surgeon must prescribe these medications and supervise the dispensing. Prescribing the medicine involves stipulating which medication is to be given, the strength, the dosage and the length of the course.

The name of the active ingredient in each medication is called its generic name. When a drug is packaged into a product by a drug company it will often be given a different name. This is the proprietary (brand or trade) name of the product. This name differentiates between similar products from various companies.

For example: Clavulanate-potentiated amoxycillin is the generic name of the drug. It has various proprietary names such as Synulox® (Pfizer) or Clavulox®.

Safe and effective dispensing

Dispensing of medication must be performed very carefully as mistakes can be easily made and have potentially serious consequences. Each label must include:

• name and address of the veterinary practice
• name and address of the client
• name of the animal
• date the product was dispensed
• name and strength of the product
• quantity of product dispensed
• the phrases 'For animal treatment only' and 'keep out of reach of children'.
• precautions such as 'for external treatment only', or 'wear gloves when handling this medication'.

Care must be taken to ensure that the labelling is correct. The correct quantity and strength of medication should be given and the expiry date of the product should be checked.

It is advisable to explain to the client about what medication is being dispensed and how it should be used. If there are any queries on medication the supervising vet should be consulted.

Any unlabelled products should be disposed of carefully. Packaging should be intact and, where possible, childproof.

Weights and measures

A variety of weights and measurements are used in dispensing. The metric system (kilograms, litres) should be used rather than the more old-fashioned imperial system (pounds, ounces, fluid ounces).

• Mass is measured in kilograms (kg).

- One kilogram contains 1000 grams (g).
- One gram contains 1000 milligrams (mg).
- One milligram contains 1000 micrograms (µg).
- Volume is measured in litres (l).
- One litre contains 1000 millilitres (ml).
- Dosages can also be described in International Units (IU). For example, insulin is administered in terms of international units. One international unit of insulin is equivalent to 0.1 ml.

Recommended containers

Various types of containers are available for packaging medications. The most appropriate container should be selected so that the medication retains its efficacy and sterility for as long as possible.

Liquids

These are dispensed in bottles.

- Bottles can be made from glass or plastic.
- Fluted bottles contain medicines for external applications.
- Wide mouth jars contain creams and powders.
- Plain bottles contain oral medication.
- They are often brown in colour which prevents damage from sunlight.
- Glass containers must be handled with care because of the risk of breakage.
- Bottles should be airtight to prevent evaporation and contamination with bacteria.
- Tamper-proof lids should be used routinely although some clients may request normal screw caps.

Tablets

These are dispensed in bottles or packets.

- Packets can be paper envelopes or cardboard boxes.
- Many tablets are provided in foil or paper blister packs which protect the tablets from moisture and provide a sealed environment.
- Other containers used include plastic and metal containers.

Useful calculations

Fractions and percentages

It is important to understand the relationship between fractions and percentages. For example:

- The whole (1) of an object is 100%

• Half (1/2) of the whole is 50%
• One quarter (1/4) of the whole is 25%
• One tenth (1/10) of an object is 10%.

So fractions and percentages are two different ways of describing a part of the whole.

Fractions should be reduced to the smallest way they can be expressed:

For example four out of twenty could be expressed as $\dfrac{4}{20}$

But four and twenty can both be divided by two and four. This fraction can therefore also be expressed as $\dfrac{2}{10}$ or $\dfrac{1}{5}$

To calculate a percentage from a fraction the following formula can be used:

$$\frac{\text{Part of the whole amount}}{\text{Whole amount}} \times 100 = \text{percentage}$$

Example 1: What percentage of dogs have been affected by kennel cough if four dogs have been affected in a kennel full of twenty dogs?

$$\frac{4}{20} \times 100 = 20\%$$

Example 2: If 25% of the remaining healthy dogs were previously vaccinated, how many of the healthy dogs were vaccinated?

Number of remaining healthy dogs = 20 – 4 = 16

$$\frac{\text{Number of vaccinated dogs}}{16} \times 100 = 25\%$$

Rearranging the equation gives:

$$\text{Number of vaccinated dogs} = \frac{25 \times 16}{100}$$

Number of vaccinated dogs = 4

Calculation of doses is important in ensuring that the animal receives the therapeutic (effective) dose of medication.

Solutions

• A solution which contains 1 kg of drug in 1 litre is a 100% solution.
• A solution which contains 1 g (1000 mg) in 1 ml is a 100% solution.
• A solution which contains 10 mg in 1 ml (10 mg/ml) is a 1% solution.

• In the same way a solution containing 25 mg/ml is a 2.5% solution.

A formula for performing this calculation is:

$$\frac{\text{Mass of drug (in g)}}{\text{Volume of liquid (in ml)}} \times 100 = \% \text{ solution}$$

Example: What weight of drug x should be dissolved in 50 ml to create a 10% solution?

$$\frac{\text{Mass of drug (in g)}}{50 \text{ ml}} \times 100 = 10\% \text{ solution}$$

Rearranging the equation gives:

$$\text{Mass of drug (in g)} = \frac{10 \times 50}{100}$$

Mass of drug x = 5 g

Handling medication

Care should be taken when handling medication. Gloves should be worn whenever medication could come into contact with skin. The reasons for this are:

• to avoid possible sensitivity reactions (many people are allergic to penicillins for example)
• to avoid absorption of medication through the skin (ointments containing steroids can be absorbed through the skin)
• to prevent contamination of the medication by bacteria from the skin of the dispenser
• to avoid ingestion of the medication if material is left on the hands after handling a drug.

If gloves are not worn the hands should be washed thoroughly before and after handling. Care should be taken to avoid inhaling medication in the form of aerosols (including flea sprays and anaesthetics), or dust from medication. The dispensary should be well ventilated.

Medication should be properly labelled, and stored out of the reach of children and animals to prevent accidental ingestion. Medical attention should be sought if there is accidental ingestion of medication, hypersensitivity reaction, splashing of medication in the eyes, or inhalation of medication.

Abbreviations

Abbreviations are often used for prescribing. Great care should be taken with these as they can be misread or misunderstood. Everyone who is involved with dispensing should understand all the abbreviations used. Examples are:

- SID: once daily dose (sometimes OD)
- BID: twice daily dose (sometimes BD)
- TID: three times daily dose
- QID: four times daily dose
- PRN: when required
- EOD: every other day
- PO: (per os) by mouth.

2.4.23 Elementary pharmacology

What you need to learn

- You need to be able to explain the meaning of terms used in pharmacology:
  - therapeutic effect
  - absorption
  - half-life
  - side effect
  - reaction
  - interaction.
- Outline the pharmacology of medicines in common veterinary use:
  - action
  - uses
  - nursing implications
  - common side effects
  - handling precautions
  - contra-indications of use of medicines.
- Describe the routes by which medicines may be administered:
  - oral
  - parenteral
  - rectal
  - topical
  - inhaled.
- Explain the reasons for use of different routes for administration:
  - absorption
  - speed of effect
  - duration of effect.
- Describe the advantages and disadvantages of various routes of administration.
- Explain the reasons for availability of different pharmaceutical presentations of a medication. This includes:
  - speed of absorption
  - duration of action
  - unpalatability.
- Outline types of complementary or alternative therapy available in the field of veterinary medicines and understand their application:

* homeopathy
* acupuncture
* herbal remedies
* aromatherapy.

Terms used in pharmacology

* Therapeutic effect is the intended effect which the medication has on the patient either in the management of disease or the manipulation of physiological function.
* Absorption is when the drug is taken from the outside of the body (including the gut) into the body. It can occur across a surface such as skin, gut lining or mucous membrane.
* The half-life of a drug describes the length of time before half of the drug is removed from the body. Drugs are often altered by the liver then excreted through the kidney or gut.
* Side effects are unintended effects of the drug on the body. They are usually inconvenient but can occasionally be harmful. Examples of side effects are diarrhoea when animals are treated with antibiotics, or polydipsia and polyuria as a result of treatment with corticosteroids.
* Drug reactions are adverse reactions to drugs which compromise the health of the patient. They suggest that the animal is particularly sensitive to a drug. Reactions are often severe side effects. An example is skin reaction in animals that are sensitive to penicillin.
* Interaction describes the situation involving two or more drugs where one drug is altering or modifying the effects of the other. Interactions often involve one drug affecting the uptake of another, or one drug potentiating (enhancing) the effect of another. Drug interactions can be useful, for example clavulanic acid enhances the ability of the antibiotic amoxycillin to kill bacteria. Drug interactions can often be harmful, for example glucocorticoids and non-steroidal anti-inflammatory drugs used together greatly increase the risk of gastric ulceration.

Pharmacology of commonly used veterinary drugs

Analgesics (painkillers)

Opioid analgesics

* These relieve pain by acting on receptors in the brain.
* They can have a sedative effect.
* High doses can cause respiratory depression and changes in gut motility.
* Opioids are controlled drugs.

- Examples are morphine, buprenorphine, codeine, pethidine, fentanyl.
- They are usually given by injection, but slow-release patches are occasionally used.

Non-steroidal anti-inflammatory drugs (NSAIDs)

- These relieve pain by blocking the release of substances which cause inflammation.
- They also reduce the temperature of pyrexic animals.
- Examples are carprofen, meloxicam, ketoprofen and phenylbutazone.
- NSAIDs can contribute to ulceration of the gastrointestinal tract so should always be given with food.
- Vomiting is an occasional side effect.
- NSAIDs can contribute to chronic renal failure if used for long periods or at high doses.

Local anaesthetics

- These relieve pain by reversibly blocking nerve impulses in the area surrounding the application site.
- They are occasionally used during orthopaedic surgery to numb the surgical area in the early post-operative period (examples are lignocaine and bupivicaine).
- They can be applied topically to reduce sensation of the skin.

Anti-convulsant drugs

- These are used in the treatment of seizures, particularly in epileptic animals.
- They act centrally (ie on the brain) to suppress seizures.
- They include phenobarbitone, diazepam, and potassium bromide.
- The side effects can include lethargy and sedation.
- Long-term treatment with phenobarbitone can have adverse effects on the liver.

Antihistamines

- These prevent the release of inflammatory substances (histamine) during hypersensitivity reactions.
- They are used for allergies and in the treatment of bites and stings.
- An example is chlorpheniramine.
- Lethargy is an occasional side effect.

Anti-neoplastic drugs

- These are drugs which selectively target rapidly dividing cells (such

as tumour cells) and are used to treat tumours.
- They must be handled carefully because they damage cells (cytotoxic).
- Examples are doxirubicin, chlorambucil and cyclophosphamide.
- They have a number of side-effects because they affect rapidly dividing normal body cells including the cells of the gastrointestinal tract and the immune system. As a result immune suppression and vomiting and diarrhoea are frequent side effects.

Antimicrobial agents

Antibiotics

- Antibiotics are drugs which selectively kill bacteria (bactericidal) or prevent them from growing and dividing (bacteriostatic).
- They vary greatly as to which organisms they can affect. They can be broad spectrum or narrow spectrum. They can affect gram positive or gram negative bacteria, or both. They can affect aerobic bacteria or anaerobic bacteria or both. Different classes of antibiotic have different modes of action.
- The most common side-effect is diarrhoea due to alteration of the normal gut micro-organisms (flora). Hypersensitivity reactions are occasionally seen. Some antibiotics should be avoided in young animals (enrofloxacin, tetracyclines).

Antifungal drugs

- These are drugs which kill (fungicidal) or retard the growth (fungistatic) of fungi.
- They can be given orally (griseofulvin) for the treatment of dermatophytoses such as ringworm; but are more commonly used in mixed topical preparations for use in treating yeast infections in the ears or on the skin (clotrimazole, miconazole).
- Care must be taken in handling griseofulvin as it can cause deformities in foetuses (teratogenic).

Antiprotozoal drugs

- These drugs are used to treat protozoal infections.
- Examples include clindamycin (used to treat toxoplasmosis).
  NB Clindamycin is more commonly used for its antibiotic effects.

Antiviral drugs

- These drugs prevent multiplication of viruses.
- They are used infrequently and tend to be expensive.
- Examples are idoxuridine (used topically to treat feline herpes virus).

Cardiovascular drugs

Drugs acting on the heart

- Drugs which stimulate the heart to beat more strongly are called positive inotropes. An example is digoxin.
- Drugs which are used to treat alterations in the rhythm of the heart are called antidysrhythmics. Diltiazem, propranolol and lignocaine are examples of these. Propranolol and diltiazem are negative inotropes in that they reduce the strength of the heart beats.
- Drugs which are used to increase the rate and strength of the heart beat. An example is adrenaline. These drugs are called sympathomimetics because they mimic the effects of the sympathetic nervous system.
- Drugs which are used to treat slow heart rates and heart blocks. An example is atropine, these drugs are called parasympatholytics because they banish the effects of the parasympathetic nervous system.

Drugs acting on the blood vessels

- Drugs which cause blood vessel dilation thereby reducing peripheral resistance are called vasodilators. They have the effect of reducing the amount of work that the heart needs to do to pump blood around the body.
- The biggest group of these is the ACE Inhibitors (angiotensin converting enzyme inhibitors). Examples are enalapril, ramipril, and benazepril.
- A drug which dilates the veins is called a venodilator. An example is glyceryl trinitrate (GTN). This is applied to the skin (usually inside ear flaps).
- If given at a high dose these drugs can cause hypotension (low blood pressure).
- Gloves must be worn when applying GTN as it is absorbed across the skin and can cause fainting.

Drugs acting on the blood clotting system

- Drugs which prevent blood clotting are called anti-coagulants. They work by blocking part of the clotting cascade.
- They can be used to treat blood clots.
- Examples are heparin and warfarin. They must be used with extreme caution as high doses can cause potentially fatal bleeding.
- Cases of warfarin poisoning are commonly seen because warfarin is used commercially as rat poison
- Drugs which are used to cause coagulation include adrenaline and ferric chloride. They are applied topically, eg to a bleeding nail.

Corticosteroids

- These are very potent anti-inflammatory drugs. They prevent the release of substances which cause inflammation.
- Examples are prednisolone, cortisone, dexamethasone and betamethasone.
- They also suppress the immune system when used at high doses.
- They have many uses including treatment of hypersensitivity reactions, immune-mediated diseases, pain caused by inflammation, and in some cases tumours. Steroids are used at high doses to treat shock.
- Side effects are common and range from polydipsia, polyuria, polyphagia, weight gain, lethargy and restlessness, to muscle weakness, skin problems (calcinosis cutis) and immune suppression. The effects are reversible if the steroid treatment is withdrawn.
- Steroids must be handled carefully as they can cause abortion.
- At the end of a course of steroids the dose must be lowered stepwise over a period of time. This is because negative feedback effects cause the animal's own steroid production (adrenal cortical function) to be greatly reduced. Sudden withdrawal of steroids can cause hypoadrenocorticism (Addison's disease).

Diuretics

- These increase the amount of fluid excreted from the body at the kidneys.
- They are usually used in the treatment of heart failure, to treat pulmonary oedema and reduce the circulating blood volume.
- There are a number of types of diuretic:
  - loop diuretics act at the Loop of Henlé (eg Frusemide)
  - thiazide diuretics include hydrochlorothiazide.
  - potassium-sparing diuretics include spironalactone.
- Side effects of diuretics can include dehydration and electrolyte imbalances. If a diuretic is being used which does not spare potassium there is a risk of hypokalaemia (low potassium). Oral potassium supplements should be used in this case.

Ectoparasiticides (drugs that kill external parasites)

- Fleas, ticks and lice are usually treated with topical sprays and spot-on treatments.
- Examples of ectoparasiticides are fipronil, selamectin and the synthetic pyrethroids such as permethrin.
- Mites, such as ear mites, are usually treated with topical preparations.

- Organophosphate preparations (such as dichlorvos) are sometimes used to treat burrowing mites such as sarcoptes scabei and demodex. Injectable preparations such as ivermectin can be used against most parasites. Selamectin is effective against sarcoptes mites.
- Toxicity is often seen with the use of synthetic pyrethroids in cats.
- Organophosphates can cause toxicity in humans and can cause major environmental damage if released into waterways. For this reason organophosphates are avoided where possible.
- Ivermectin can be very toxic in some collie-type breeds and therefore is usually avoided in dogs.

Endoparasiticides (drugs that kill internal parasites)

Anthelmintics

- Anthelmintics are drugs which kill helminth parasites (worms).
- Helminths include nematodes (roundworms), cestodes (tapeworms) and cestodes (flukes).
- Examples of these drugs are praziquantel (Drontal®) and fenbendazole (Panacur®).
- Occasionally vomiting is encountered as a side effect.

Sedatives and anaesthetics

Sedatives

- These drugs act on the brain to produce drowsiness and sedation.
- They are often used as anaesthetic premedicants.
- They often have depressive effects on the cardiovascular and respiratory system.
- Examples of sedatives are acepromazine, xylazine and medetomidine.
- The effects of medetomidine can be reversed by the antidote atipamezole.
- Medetomidine and xylazine usually cause vomiting.
- Sedated animals must be monitored closely for signs of inhalation of vomit or loss of consciousness.

General anaesthetics

- General anaesthetics induce and maintain a state of unconsciousness.
- They allow procedures to be performed which would be too painful or distressing in the conscious patient.
- Anaesthesia involves the anaesthetic triangle:
  - loss of consciousness
  - pain relief

- relaxation of muscles.
- Induction agents are injected, usually into a vein. Examples are thiopentone, propofol and alphaxolon/alphadolone.
- Agents which maintain anaesthesia are usually inhaled through a mask or endotracheal tube. Examples are halothane, isofluorane, sevofluorane and desfluorane.
- Nitrous oxide is often used alongside inhalational anaesthetics. This is because nitrous oxide provides very effective pain relief for the anaesthetised animal.
- Sometimes atropine is used during anaesthetics to counteract bradycardia (slow heart rate) and to reduce the production of salivary and bronchial secretions while the animal is asleep.
- Muscle relaxants are occasionally used during general anaesthesia. These block control of skeletal muscle (including respiratory muscles). An example is atracurium.
- Ventilation is required for animals which have been treated with muscle relaxants.

Vaccines

Vaccines are used to induce immunity against a range of diseases. Usually a primary course is provided followed by regular injections (usually annual or 6 monthly).

Dog vaccines are available to provide immunity against:

- parvovirus
- distemper
- leptospirosis
- parainfluenza
- infectious canine hepatitis
- rabies
- *Bordetella bronchiseptica*
- coronavirus.

Cat vaccines are available to provide immunity against:

- feline panleucopaenia
- feline herpes virus
- feline calicivirus
- feline leukaemia virus
- chlamydia.

Occasional vaccine reactions are seen. These usually manifest as pyrexia, lethargy and stiff joints. The effects are usually short lived. Vaccine breakdown can occur rarely.

Miscellaneous drugs

- Drugs used to treat urinary incontinence, eg phenylpropanolamine.
- Drugs used to treat endocrine disorders, eg:
  - insulin for the treatment of diabetes mellitus
  - trilostane for the treatment of hyperadrenocorticism
  - thyroxine for the treatment of hypothyroidism
  - methimazole or carbimazole for the treatment of hyperthyroidism
  - sex steroids such as testosterone and oestrogen used for reproductive disorders.
- Central nervous system stimulants, eg doxapram, which is used as a respiratory stimulant.
- Drugs used to treat gastrointestinal disorders eg
  - adsorbents which line the gastrointestinal tract to protect the mucosa, eg sucralfate
  - drugs which reduce the amount of gastric acid, eg cimetidine and ranitidine, they are used to prevent or treat gastrointestinal ulceration
  - laxatives are used to treat constipation, eg lactulose (taken orally)
  - drugs used to stimulate gut motility, eg metoclopramide (metoclopramide is also used as an anti-emetic to prevent vomiting)
  - anti-diarrhoeal drugs, eg loperamide or kaolin
  - pancreatic enzyme supplements which are used to treat deficiencies.
- Drugs used to treat the respiratory system, eg:
  - mucolytics are used to reduce the viscosity of mucus in the airways, bromhexine
  - bronchodilators such as theophylline and terbutaline widen the airways to ease respiration
  - anti-tussives suppress the cough reflex, eg butorphanol (care must be taken with this because coughing is a protective mechanism)
  - steroids and antihistamines are often used to reduce inflammation in the respiratory tract
  - essential fatty acids are used as dietary supplements in the treatment of skin and joint conditions.

NB This list is a summary of the commonly used medications. It is by no means exhaustive.

Routes of administration of medication

Medicines can be administered by a number of routes. The choice of route depends on a number of factors:

- speed of action
- compatibility of drug and route, eg some drugs are digested when

given orally, while a number of drugs cause reactions when injected under the skin
- area to be treated – administering medication straight onto the site is often used if a whole body effect is to be avoided
- availability of preparation
- amount of drug to be administered.

Table 4.12

Route	Advantages	Disadvantages	Examples
Oral	Painless No preparation required Owners can treat the animal at home Can give long-term therapy Available in slow-release forms to prolong duration of action	Slow onset of action Absorption depends on food in the gut, solubility of drug, gastrointestinal tract motility, etc Difficulty medicating some animals Not absorbed if animal vomits Can be unpalatable	Tablets, capsules, liquid medication, soluble powder, pastes (sugar-coated and sweet-tasting medication is used to improve palatability)
Parenteral (avoiding the gastrointestinal tract – used to describe injected medication)	Very quick action Large volumes can be given Direct effect Can be given over time (eg drip infusion) Accurate dosing possible Can give depot injections (slow release over prolonged period)	Aseptic preparation required Assistance and specialised skill may be required May be painful Difficult in fractious animals Possible allergic reactions	Injectable suspensions and solutions Intravenous, subcutaneous, intramuscular, intra-peritoneal, etc
Rectal	Painless Local effect	Often slow onset Messy Limited absorption	Suppositories, enemas
Topical	Direct action, little systemic effect Usually easy to apply. Can be used at home	Can be licked off Sometimes resented by animal (eg ear medication) Can cause irritation Messy Requires careful handling	Ointment, cream, shampoos, solutions, emollients
Inhalational	Direct action Rapid uptake due to large surface area and blood supply	Skill required to administer May be resented by patient	Anaesthetic gases, nebulised medication, some vaccines (*Bordatella* sp.)

Complementary and alternative medicine

Alternative medicine is used as an alternative to conventional medicine. Complementary medicine is used alongside conventional medicine as an aid to treatment. A variety of alternatives to conventional medicine are available:

- **Homeopathy**: this involves treatment of symptoms with an extremely diluted solution of a substance which is capable of causing the same symptoms. Treatments are usually given as liquid or sweetened tablets.
- **Herbalism**: this involves the use of herbal remedies. It should be noted that many modern medicines are derived from plant sources, eg digoxin which comes from *digitalis* (Foxglove), and atropine which comes from *belladona* (Deadly Nightshade).
- **Acupuncture**: this involves the use of very fine needles inserted at key points on the body. It can be used to treat a wide range of disorders but is most commonly used to treat pain, eg arthritic pain. When performed properly acupuncture should be painless.
- **Aromatherapy**: this involves the use of inhaled substances (usually herbal) to treat a range of disorders.

As the law currently stands homeopathy, herbal medicine and acupuncture can only be performed by veterinary surgeons who are trained in those disciplines. It may not be performed by non-vets.

Other forms of complementary treatments are used such as Reike healing, crystal healing, magnetic therapy and swimming. When used carefully complementary therapies can be a useful adjunct to conventional therapy. They are usually used alongside conventional medicine and can help in reducing the dose of medication required.

It is important that only skilled practitioners are employed to perform complementary therapy.

2.4.24   Administration of medicines prescribed by a veterinary surgeon

What you need to learn

- You need to be able to describe the principles of interpreting a prescription. These include:
  - legibility
  - written in indelible ink
  - drug name not abbreviated
  - dose expressed clearly
  - route of administration clear

* prescription signed in full and dated
* intended patient clearly identified.
* State the legal requirements for POM prescriptions:
  * written in indelible ink
  * veterinary surgeon's name, address and signature
  * owner's name and address.
* State name, dose, strength and directions prescribed of dispensed medicine
  * date.
* Outline the principles of administering oral medication:
  * temperament of animal
  * suitable and minimal restraint
  * use of oral syringe or tablet administrator
  * placing of medication
  * assisted swallowing.
* Explain the principles of administering medications by injection subcutaneously, intramuscularly and intravenously:
  * suitable sites
  * underlying anatomy
  * volume accommodated
  * technique
  * hygiene.
* Identify the intramuscular, subcutaneous and intravenous sites commonly used for exotic species:
  * rabbits
  * rodents
  * birds
  * reptiles
  * reptiles.
* Describe the equipment required for the administration of an injection:
  * syringes
  * needles
  * intravenous catheters (sizes and gauges).
* Describe the requirements for the safe handling and disposal of syringes, needles and ampoules.
* Explain the requirements for nursing observation following the administration of medication:
  * monitor therapeutic effect
  * report adverse reactions and side effects.

Interpreting a prescription

A prescription is a set of instructions directing a dispenser to provide medication for a patient. Prescriptions must be carefully interpreted as mistakes can be very serious. To interpret a prescription properly it must be:

• legible
• written in indelible ink
• the identity of the patient should be made clear
• the drug name should be spelled correctly and not abbreviated
• the dose and route of administration should be clearly stated
• the length of the course should be stated
• the full amount of product to be dispensed should be stated
• the prescription should be fully signed and dated.

Prescriptions for prescription-only medicines

In addition to these details a prescription for a POM drug is legally required to have:

• the veterinary surgeon's full name and practice address
• the name and address of the patient's owner.

Oral medication

Before giving oral medication the temperament of the patient should be assessed. Oral medication should not be attempted in aggressive animals because of the risk of injury. PO = per OS (by mouth).

The degree of restraint required for the technique to be performed will vary with the temperament of the animal. Restraint should be the minimum with which the procedure can be performed safely.

The animal's mouth should be held open with the head tipped back while the medication is placed as far back on the tongue as possible.

The use of a tablet administrator (pill giver) aids in the placement of the medication as far back as possible without putting fingers in the animal's mouth.

Liquid medication is usually given by syringe. Care should be taken to avoid giving too large a volume. There is a risk of choking if a large volume of liquid is placed in the mouth. Once the medication is inside, the mouth should be held closed. Swallowing can be encouraged by stroking the throat.

Injection techniques

There are numerous injection techniques. When preparing a syringe full of medication it is important that the solution is thoroughly mixed and all air bubbles are removed.

Subcutaneous injection SC (injection under the skin)

- The most commonly used site is the scruff of the neck but anywhere where there is plenty loose skin can be used.
- If the injection is not a vaccine the site can be swabbed prior to injection. (swabbing can inactivate vaccines).
- The skin is lifted with one hand.
- The needle is pushed through the skin into the subcutaneous layer.
- The plunger is pulled back to check that the needle is not within a blood vessel.
- The plunger is depressed and the medication deposited.
- The injection site should be gently massaged to disperse the medication.

Intramuscular injection IM (injection into the muscle)

- The most commonly used sites are the quadriceps muscles at the front of the thigh, the lumbar muscles, and the muscles of the scapula.
- The injection site can be swabbed before injection.
- The muscle to be used is palpated. The injection should be placed in the widest part of the muscle.
- The needle should be inserted at an angle of 90° to the skin.
- The plunger is pulled back to check that the needle is not within a blood vessel.
- The plunger is depressed and the medication deposited.
- The injection site should be gently massaged to disperse the medication.

Intravenous injection IV (injection into a vein)

- The most commonly used veins are the cephalic vein in the foreleg, the saphenous vein in the hindleg and occasionally the jugular vein in the neck.
- Hair at the injection site should be clipped and the skin prepared aseptically.
- An assistant restrains the patient and occludes the proximal part of the vein. This causes the vein to fill with blood and appear more prominent.
- The needle is inserted at a shallow angle.
- The plunger is pulled back to check that the needle is within the blood vessel.
- The assistant releases the pressure on the proximal vein.
- The plunger is depressed and the medication deposited.
- The rate of administration depends on the medication.
- The needle is withdrawn. The assistant puts pressure on the

injection site to prevent bleeding from the punctured vein. After a minute or two a clot will form over the puncture site within the vein so the pressure can be released.

Table 4.13 summarises the uses for these techniques.

Table 4.13

Route	Volume	Irritant effect	Prolonged administration	Rate of absorption
Subcutaneous	Fairly large volumes can be given although they may need to be split over several sites	Fairly frequent	Fluid absorbed over a few hours	Fairly slow
Intramuscular	Small volumes only	Frequent	Usually only short duration although depot injections can be used	Fairly swift
Intravenous	Very large volumes can be given over time (e.g. through a drip)	Fairly infrequent Drip fluids are isotonic and therefore non-irritant	Drip infusions can be given over very long periods providing the vein remains healthy	Very swift

Other injection techniques used are:

• intraperitoneal (injection into the peritoneal cavity)
• intracardiac (injection into the heart – painful and damaging, used occasionally for euthanasia)
• intra-articular (injection into the joint cavity)
• intrathecal (injection within the meninges of the spinal cord)
• epidural (injection into the epidural space)
• sub-conjunctival (injection into the conjunctiva of the eye).

Equipment required for injections

• Syringe (these vary in size from 0.5 ml to 50 ml). The smallest syringe possible should be used.
• Needle (some syringes have needles attached). Needles vary in length (5/8", 1" and $1\frac{1}{2}$") and in gauge (bore diameter).
• Needle gauges are colour coded:
  • 25 g (smallest needle) are orange
  • 23 g are blue
  • 21 g are green
  • 20 g are yellow
  • 19 g are brown
  • 18 g are pink

- 16 g are white
- 14 g are dark green.
- Larger gauge needles tend to be reserved for use in farm animals and horses.
- Smaller bore needles are less painful on insertion but injection takes longer.
- Catheters (flexible plastic tubes which are placed in a vein for up to 3 days) are also available in various lengths and gauges. The colour coding is different from the colour coding of needles.

Table 4.14 Injection techniques in exotic species

Species	Subcutaneous	Intramuscular		Intravenous
Rabbits	As for dogs and cats	As for cats and dogs		As for dogs and cats but also marginal ear vein
Small rodents	As for dogs and cats	As for cats and dogs		Usually jugular, may require anaesthesia
Birds	Skin over the neck or over the breast	Pectoral (breast) muscles or thigh muscles	Jugular vein, ulnar vein (medial elbow), saphenous vein, tarsal vein (larger birds) May require anaesthesia	
Reptiles	Skin of the neck and trunk	Forelimb muscles (avoid hind limb muscles because of renal toxicity caused by altered renal blood circulation in reptiles)		Jugular vein,coccygeal vein (underside of tail), intracardiac (not tortoises)

Disposal of materials

Disposal of injection materials is covered by the COSHH regulations as improper disposal poses a threat to health. Needles and stylets from catheters are classed as 'sharps'. They must be disposed of in a special sharps container. These are usually yellow plastic containers.

Used ampoules (glass injection vials) must also be disposed of in sharps containers. Used syringes (without needles) are not sharps but must be disposed of in a clinical waste bin. They are then sent for incineration.

Monitoring the patient

After an injection has been given the patient should be monitored closely. Treatments should be recorded on a file (or on a hospital chart for in-patients). Patients should be monitored for therapeutic effect (improvement in clinical signs) and for adverse effects (allergic reaction or side effects).

Adverse effects should be recorded and reported to the supervising veterinary surgeon immediately. Unexpected adverse reactions should also be reported to the drug company.

2.4.25 Providing first-aid and emergency treatment – aims and limitations

What you need to learn

* You need to be able to outline the aims of first-aid treatment. These include:
  * preservation of life
  * prevention of further suffering
  * prevention of the deterioration of the patient's condition
  * relief of acute conditions.
* Outline the legal position of the lay person and the veterinary nurse in providing first aid to animals:
  * Veterinary Surgeons Act 1966 and animals under the veterinary surgeon's care.

Aims and limitations

The aims of first-aid treatment are to:

• preserve life
• alleviate pain and make the patient as comfortable as possible therefore preventing further suffering
• prevent deterioration, ensuring no further damage occurs and avoiding damage becoming permanent
• relief of acute conditions.

The veterinary surgeon is legally obliged to provide 24-hour emergency cover. Emergency cover in this instance means first aid and pain relief (Veterinary Surgeons Act 1966).

The nurse is often responsible for obtaining information from the client about the condition of the animal. This information is often received over the phone. The nurse should be able to differentiate between life-threatening emergencies, immediate emergencies and minor emergencies.

As the law stands at the moment, anyone who is involved in a road traffic accident where a dog is injured must report the incident to the police. At this stage the veterinary surgeon is usually contacted.

The same law does not apply to cats or wildlife although drivers have a moral obligation to organise emergency treatment for an animal. Often the RSPCA become involved if the injured animal is a stray.

2.4.26   Principles of first aid

What you need to learn

- You need to be able to describe the four basic rules of first aid:
  - safety of personnel
  - airway
  - breathing
  - circulation
  - also contact the veterinary surgeon as soon as possible.
- Describe situations requiring first aid:
  - unconsciousness
  - convulsive states
  - scalds and burns
  - serious haemorrhage
  - penetrating wounds
  - possible poisoning
  - shock.
- Describe the essential observations to be made during first-aid treatment:
  - airway
  - respiration
  - colour of mucous membranes
  - level of consciousness
  - haemorrhage
  - distress.
- Explain the principles of managing a patient requiring first aid:
  - life-threatening and non-life-threatening situations
  - minor emergencies.
- Explain the principles of nursing an animal requiring first aid treatment:
  - warmth
  - quiet
  - comfort
  - monitoring.
- Identify special requirements of caring and nursing wild animals normally presented as casualties.

❧ Describe the principles of managing a telephone report of a
veterinary emergency:
  ❧ ascertain the animal's condition
  ❧ advise emergency treatment
  ❧ restraint and transport the animal.

Four basic rules

When there is an emergency you should follow four basic rules:

- **Safety:** great care must be taken to avoid injury to anyone, including
  veterinary staff and lay-people. Injured animals are frightened and
  will often bite. Wild animals can often be dangerous. If the
  emergency is away from the surgery no risk to human health should
  be taken (for example after a road traffic accident the animal must
  be carefully moved away from the road before medical attention
  can be given).
- **Airway:** the airway must be clear. The head and neck should be
  extended. Collars should be removed if they are restrictive. The
  throat should be checked for foreign bodies.
- **Breathing:** oxygen should be provided through a mask, tent, or
  endotracheal tube if necessary. If the airway is obstructed an
  emergency tracheotomy may be performed by the veterinary
  surgeon.
- **Circulation:** the animal should be checked for a pulse. If circulation
  has ceased (cardiac arrest) resuscitation can be attempted. The
  quality of circulation can also be assessed, eg in cases of shock or
  haemorrhage.

In any emergency situation a veterinary surgeon must be contacted
as soon as possible.

Situations requiring first aid

First aid should be provided in any of the following situations:

- respiratory difficulty or respiratory arrest
- unconsciousness
- convulsions (seizures, fits)
- severe haemorrhage or wounding
- shock
- scalds and burns
- possible poisonings.

During the initial assessment of the patient the nurse needs to check:

- airway

- breathing
- circulation (colour of mucus membranes, capillary refill time, pulse quality)
- level of consciousness
- degree and site of haemorrhage
- pain and distress.

Life-threatening situations require the most urgent management. These include:

- cardiac arrest
- complete obstruction of the airway (foreign body, injury, disease)
- unconsciousness
- status epilepticus (severe persistent fitting).

Non-life-threatening emergencies require urgent attention although life is not in immediate danger. These include:

- road traffic accident
- poisoning
- extreme pain
- dystocia (difficulty with parturition)
- severe haemorrhage
- circulatory abnormalities (dysrhythmias, fainting, pallor of mucous membranes, etc)
- inability to urinate
- burns
- fractures
- shock
- prolapses
- gastric torsion.

Minor emergencies warrant prompt attention although the animal's health is not severely compromised. These include:

- minor haemorrhage
- worsening of an existing medical problem
- hypo/hyperthermia
- most flesh wounds
- pain.

When an animal is being given first aid it is important that it is made as comfortable as possible. Warmth and bedding should be provided. Most animals will relax better in a calm, quiet and darkened environment.

Careful monitoring of the patient is vital as deterioration in the condition must be addressed as soon as possible. Improvements in the animal's condition should also be noted as some treatments may be discontinued.

Wild animals

Wild animal casualties are common. Important principles to note include the following:

• Safety is the most important consideration. Badgers and foxes can be very strong and very aggressive and should be suitably restrained. Birds will often peck at the eyes of a handler. Protective goggles must be worn with some species (herons, gannets, etc).
• Wildlife casualties will be extremely traumatised. A quiet, dark environment must be provided.
• Nursing wildlife casualties is often extremely difficult and specialist advice and assistance should be sought.
• Wild animals carry a number of diseases which can be transmitted to humans, eg sarcoptic mange, leptospirosis, ornithesis, also known as psittacosis chlamyolosis. Suitable hygiene precautions should be taken.
• Myiasis (fly-strike) is common in injured wildlife. This is also life threatening and must be addressed when providing first aid.
• Remember that the aim of treating wildlife casualties is to return them to the wild. Few species (with the exception of hedgehogs, rabbits and some bird species such as crows) will adapt to living in captivity. If an animal is too badly injured euthanasia should be considered.
• It is illegal to release non-indigenous (non-native) species into the wild in the UK. Non-indigenous species include grey squirrels, rabbits and some species of deer (muntjac, Chinese water deer).

Managing the telephone report

The veterinary nurse is often responsible for obtaining information from the client about the condition of the animal. This information is often received over the phone. During the phone conversation important details which should be obtained include:

• age, sex and breed of the animal
• owner's name and address
• information about the nature and extent of the condition.

The nurse will then be able to classify the emergency and advice can be provided for the owner on how to proceed with treatment, restraint and transport of the animal to the surgery.

The owner of an injured animal will often be distressed and need reassurance.

2.4.27 Restraining an injured animal

What you need to learn

☙ You need to be able to describe suitable methods of restraint and transport for animals. These include spinal injuries, fractures and abdominal or thoracic injuries. Consider:
  ☙ use of blankets
  ☙ padded clothing
  ☙ stretchers
  ☙ boards
  ☙ travelling boxes
  ☙ muzzles.

☙ Outline acceptable methods of transporting wild animals and exotic species:
  ☙ wild animals
  ☙ birds
  ☙ reptiles
  ☙ amphibia
  ☙ fish.

☙ Describe the value of using subdued light with diurnal birds and mammals.

Restraint

- Injured animals are frightened and will often bite. Great care must be taken to avoid injury to any person, including veterinary staff and lay-people. Wild animals can often be dangerous.
- Advice on restraint of the animal should be given over the phone.
- If treating an emergency away from the surgery it is important not to chase the animal away. The animal should be approached slowly and spoken to in a quiet reassuring voice.
- Do not risk being bitten. Blankets or towels can be thrown over an aggressive cat. Graspers can be used to restrain an aggressive dog until a muzzle can be placed on it.
- If the animal has a lead this should be caught underfoot, then carefully lifted.
- If possible, obtain a hold of the animal on the scruff of the neck. It is more difficult for the animal to bite in this position.
- Dogs, foxes and badgers should be muzzled. Injured animals are unpredictable.
- If a spinal injury is suspected the animal should be supported (using one or more assistants) and slid carefully onto a hard board. This will prevent unnecessary movement during the journey to the surgery.
- A stretcher can be made from a solid board or a blanket.

- Cats should be placed in a closable box, basket or bag.
- Fractures are extremely painful when moved. If a broken bone has been identified care should be taken to avoid moving the fracture during transport.
- Thoracic injuries can result in breathing difficulties. The animal should not be turned over if it is managing to breathe. This is because it is possible to cause respiratory difficulty or failure by, for example, laying an animal on its only inflated lung.
- Abdominal injuries are likely to result in haemorrhage and intense pain. The abdomen should be supported during the journey. If there are penetrating wounds these should be covered to limit damage to abdominal contents.

Wild animals and exotic species

Similar principles apply when restraining wildlife casualties:

- Injured birds can cause themselves further injury by flapping their wings in panic. The wings should be held to the animal's side. This can be achieved by wrapping the bird lightly in material. Do not obstruct the bird's airway. Special carrying bags are available for the safe transport of large birds such as geese and swans.
- Large exotic birds such as parrots have strong beaks which can easily remove a human finger.
- Birds of prey have extremely sharp, strong beaks and claws.
- If an animal is caught in netting or has fishing line in its beak the excess material should be cut away but do not try to remove material which is wrapped tightly unless respiration is being obstructed. This material should be removed under control at the surgery.
- Fish should obviously be transported in water. If possible they should be transported in the water in which they were living rather than tap water.
- Amphibians should be transported in a moist container (eg plastic container lined with moist kitchen paper. They should not normally be transported in water because of the risk of drowning if they are very weak.
- Potentially dangerous exotic animals such as snakes and spiders should not be handled directly. A blanket can be thrown over them, and the animal moved with the blanket into a container. Snakes can be carried in a cloth bag.
- **NEVER** handle bats without wearing gloves. Bats can transmit a virus which is similar to rabies.
- Wild animals panic less if they are transported in the dark. Throw a blanket over the carrying box. Deer should have a blindfold placed gently over the eyes to prevent panic.

2.4.28 Collapse, unconsciousness and death

What you need to learn

* You need to be able to describe the vital signs of life:
  * pulse
  * respiration
  * eye position
  * movement.
* Describe the signs of death and differentiate between collapse and unconsciousness:
  * collapse
  * unconsciousness
  * death.
* Outline conditions which may result in collapse and/or loss of consciousness
  * major injury
  * heart failure
  * poisoning
  * stroke
  * metabolic disease
  * toxicity
  * electrocution.
* Describe the principles of managing an unconscious animal (clearing and maintaining the airway).
* Explain the principles of emergency rescusitation:
  * clearing and maintaining the airway
  * intubation
  * ventilation
  * cardiac compression.

Vital signs of life

When the animal arrives at the surgery it should be checked for signs of life. Signs of life are known as vital signs. These can be assessed by checking:

• a pulse (ie cardiac output)
• respiration (or attempts at respiration)
• eye position, corneal reflex and pupil size
• movement (conscious movement, seizures)

Signs of death

The signs of death are:

• absence of a pulse (ie no cardiac output) for more than 3 minutes

- breathing has ceased
- there is no corneal reflex, the pupils are fixed and dilated
- there is no movement (gasps and muscular twitches often occur just after death but will cease after a few minutes)
- the mucous membranes are pale (beware – a normal capillary refill time can persist for some minutes after death)
- the temperature of the body starts to fall and eventually the body starts to stiffen (rigor mortis).

Collapse and loss of consciousness

Loss of consciousness is manifested by the following signs:

- collapse with flaccid muscles (although muscular spasm and movement occur during seizures)
- the animal is unaware of its surroundings
- loss of continence is common (urination and defecation)
- the reflexes are usually still intact
- pulse and respiration are present although they may be altered.

Collapse without loss of consciousness (locomotor collapse) can occur as a result of:

- weakness due to pain, eg arthritic old dogs that are unable to stand
- neurological disorders.

Collapse with or without unconsciousness can occur due to:

- weakness from circulatory compromise (heart failure, anaemia, haemorrhage)
- severe disease such as metabolic or endocrine disorders (uncontrolled diabetes mellitus, Addison's disease, etc)
- toxicity or poisoning
- electric shock
- shock.

Principles of emergency resuscitation

Basic first-aid principles should be applied to the unconscious patient:

- a clear airway should be obtained and maintained
- the animal should be kept warm and treated for any pain
- treatment of the underlying condition should start (control haemorrhage, give fluid therapy, etc).

If respiration and heartbeat cease resuscitation can be attempted. This is often called **cardiopulmonary resuscitation (CPR)** or **cardiopulmonary–cerebral resuscitation (CPCR)**.

All staff should be aware of CPR procedures as prompt treatment is vital:

- The **airway** is cleared and intubation is performed (the tube should be cuffed to prevent inhalation of foreign material). Tracheotomy may be performed where necessary.
- **Breathing**: ventilation should begin as soon as possible to provide oxygen.
- **Circulation**: compression of the chest wall should be performed. The aim is to push blood through the heart and therefore provide cardiac output.

In cats and small dogs the chest wall can be compressed from side to side. In larger dogs the chest is compressed from one side with the animal in lateral recumbency.

Drugs (such as adrenaline, atropine or lignocaine) may be administered once airway, breathing and circulation have been established.

CPR should only be performed if the animal has a disease which is treatable.

If possible the owner's consent should have previously been sought. CPR should not be attempted if the:

- animal is in the terminal stages of disease such as kidney or liver failure
- animal has severe head injuries which make recovery of mental function unlikely
- owner has asked that CPR should not be attempted.

2.4.29   Shock

What you need to learn

- You need to explain what is meant by shock:
  - hypovolaemic
  - cardiogenic
  - anaphylactic
  - endotoxic.
- Describe the principles of managing shock:
  - fluid replacement
  - warmth
  - quiet.

What is shock?

Shock is a group of symptoms resulting from a severe deterioration in the animal's clinical signs. It occurs when there is inadequate perfusion of all the body tissues with blood resulting in widespread cell damage.

Shock manifests as circulatory compromise (reduced capillary refill time, pallor of mucous membranes, tachycardia, weak or irregular pulses, cold extremities) and alteration in the level of consciousness.

There are different types of shock:

- **Hypovolaemic shock:** loss of circulating blood volume causes the change in perfusion of the tissues. Hypovolaemic shock can be caused by blood loss or severe dehydration. After trauma extensive tissue damage and severe pain can further exacerbate the compromise to tissue perfusion.
- **Cardiogenic shock:** failure of the heart to pump blood causes a decrease in tissue perfusion.
- **Anaphylactic shock:** this is the immediate response of the body to the entry of an antigen to which the animal is sensitised (allergic). Large amounts of antibodies are produced which have wide-ranging effects. Hypovolaemia is caused by the loss of plasma into the tissues from leaking blood vessels.
- **Endotoxic shock:** this is caused by an inflammatory response to severe infection. It is usually caused by bacteria.

How to manage shock

Treatment of shock involves supportive therapy and the treatment of the underlying problem. Fluid therapy is vital in restoring circulating blood volume, and improving tissue perfusion (although care should be taken with fluid therapy in animals with heart failure). Shocked animals must be kept warm and a quiet, comfortable environment aids in recovery.

2.4.30 Abdominal injuries

What you need to learn

- You need to be able to describe the management of closed and open abdominal injuries:
  - non-penetrating wounds
  - penetrating wounds
  - herniation

    ❧ haemorrhage
    ❧ lacerations.

Managing closed and open injuries

- Abdominal injuries can be described as open (where there is penetration of the abdominal wall) or closed (no penetration of the abdominal wall).
- The patient should be assessed following the first-aid rules. Once the animal is stable investigation of the trauma can begin.
- Abdominal wounds and lacerations should be assessed to determine whether penetration of the body wall has occurred.
- Radiography and ultrasound are useful tools in the assessment of abdominal injuries.

Non-penetrating wounds

These should be cleaned and flushed. Haemorrhage should be controlled and then repair can be attempted under general anaesthesia. Blunt trauma to the abdominal contents is possible with non-penetrating wounds.

Penetrating wounds

- Thorough examination of the abdominal contents is needed.
- If the penetrating object is still in the animal it should be left in place until the situation has been fully assessed. The foreign body may be occluding a damaged blood vessel so removal would cause haemorrhage.
- Under general anaesthesia damage to abdominal organs is assessed and repair performed where needed. Foreign material must be flushed out of the abdomen.
- There is high risk of peritonitis (infection and inflammation of the peritoneal cavity) with penetrating abdominal wounds. Thorough lavage of the peritoneal cavity and antimicrobial treatment is necessary.

Herniation

- There is a risk of herniation of gut contents through the damaged abdominal wall. There is often severe compromise of any herniated organ as the blood supply is occluded. Hernias must be reduced (organs must be returned to the abdomen) as soon as possible. Once reduced, the viability of the tissue is assessed and repair performed where necessary.
- Herniation can still occur if the wound is non-penetrating. In these cases the body wall is damaged although the skin remains intact.

• Once the abdominal cavity and organs have been treated the wound itself can be addressed. The wound must be thoroughly cleaned and any devitalised tissue removed. The wound is then sutured.

Haemorrhage

• Haemorrhage into the abdomen occurs when a blood vessel or organ is damaged.
• Haemorrhage can occur in closed and open injuries.
• The liver and spleen are susceptible to injury through blunt trauma. The spleen stores blood, so injury results in severe haemorrhage. If the damage is severe the spleen may need to be removed.
• In closed abdominal injuries haemorrhage manifests as hypovolaemic shock coupled with a distended, fluid-filled abdomen.
• When free abdominal fluid is present the fluid should be sampled. This procedure is called paracentesis. An area of skin on the ventral abdomen is clipped and aseptically prepared. A needle is inserted into the abdominal cavity and fluid is collected. With abdominal haemorrhage whole blood will be detected.
• Bladder damage is not uncommon in abdominal injuries. The bladder should be palpated and urine output monitored following abdominal trauma.

2.4.31   Thoracic injuries

What you need to learn

☙ You need to be able to describe the management of open and closed wounds including:
  ☙ non-penetrating wounds
  ☙ penetrating wounds
  ☙ pneumothorax
  ☙ haemothorax.

Open and closed wounds

• Thoracic injuries can be described as open (where there is penetration of the chest wall) or closed (no penetration of the chest wall).
• The patient should be assessed following the first-aid rules. Once the animal is stable investigation of the trauma can begin.
• Chest wounds and lacerations should be assessed to determine whether penetration of the chest wall has occurred.
• Radiography and ultrasound are useful tools in the assessment of thoracic injuries.

Non-penetrating wounds

These should be cleaned and flushed. Haemorrhage should be controlled and then repair can be attempted under general anaesthesia. Blunt trauma to the thoracic contents is possible with non-penetrating wounds.

Penetrating wounds

These are likely to cause pneumothorax. If the penetrating object is still in the animal it should be left in place until the situation has been fully assessed. The foreign body may be occluding a damaged blood vessel so that removal would cause haemorrhage.

Pneumothorax

- Damage to the lung tissue can result in air leaking into the pleural cavity. This is called pneumothorax. It is a common result of blunt trauma to the chest.
- As air builds up in the pleural cavity the pressure causes the lungs to collapse, resulting in respiratory distress.
- If a small volume of air has escaped and the animal is not in respiratory distress it is not necessary to drain the air.
- If a large volume of air is leaking the air must be drained from the chest using a needle (thoracocentesis). The damaged lung will often seal itself so that repeated thoracocentesis is not necessary. However, if the pneumothorax is recurring a chest drain may need to be placed to allow continuous removal of air.
- Pneumothorax can also occur as a result of injuries which penetrate the thoracic wall. In this case the air in the chest comes from the outside of the body, through the wound and into the pleural cavity. In these cases the wound must be repaired and air drained as described.

Haemothorax

- Bleeding into the thoracic cavity is known as haemothorax. As blood builds up the lungs collapse under the pressure as with a pneumothorax.
- Thoracocentesis is only performed if the animal is in severe respiratory compromise. This is because clots could be dislodged and the condition exacerbated. Once bleeding has stopped the animal will reabsorb the blood over time.
- Fractured ribs are fairly common and very painful.
- If only one or two ribs are damaged treatment is rest and pain relief only.

- If a series of ribs are broken the loose segments can move freely as the animal breathes. This is called flail chest and may require surgical stabilisation.
- Tears in the diaphragm are common following abdominal or thoracic injury and can result in diaphragmatic hernia.
- Diaphragmatic hernia usually involves the movement of abdominal organs through the tear into the thorax.
- Animals usually present in severe respiratory distress due to the pressure of the organs on the lungs. Damage to the herniated organs can also occur.
- Diaphragmatic hernia requires surgical repair.

2.4.32 Burns, scalds and cold injury

What you need to learn

- You need to be able to describe the first-aid management of burns, scald and cold injury:
  - electrical burns
  - dry heat
  - scalds
  - corrosive chemicals
  - cold injury.

Causes

Burns usually result from the application of heat (thermal burns). Thermal burns can be caused by:

- dry heat: fire, hot household appliances, heat pads, hairdryers and contact with hot parts of a car (exhaust-pipe burns are common following a road traffic accident).
- scalds: heated liquids including water and oils.

Other types of burn include:

- electrical burns: following electric shock or lightning strike
- chemical burns: caustic materials or acids
- radiation: microwaves, radiation therapy of tumours
- cold injury: prolonged contact with ice, liquid nitrogen burns.

Assessment and first-aid treatment

- Thermal burns should be cooled using cold water or ice.
- Any remaining liquid should be washed out of the coat in cases of scalding.
- In severe burning there is substantial loss of fluid. Patients are likely

to be suffering from shock. Burns are very susceptible to infection. Fluid therapy, pain relief and antibiotics should be provided.

• Splinting the injury can prevent movement of the burn site.

• Moist dressings can be applied. These prevent infection, keep the wound moist to aid healing and provide some relief from the pain of a burn.

• The depth and extent of the burn should be assessed. Burns are described in terms of depth (superficial partial thickness, deep partial thickness and full thickness) and in terms of what proportion of the body surface area has been affected (expressed as a percentage).

• The full extent of a burn is not always immediately clear. Lesions may take up to 48 hours to become visible.

2.4.33   Fractures and spinal injuries

What you need to learn

☙ You need to be able to describe the principles of transporting an animal with suspected fractures or spinal injury. This includes:
  ☙ maintaining spinal alignment
  ☙ use of stretcher
  ☙ box
  ☙ board
  ☙ restraining ties
  ☙ enveloping blanket.

Fractures

Fractures are rarely life threatening and are usually not dealt with until the animal's condition is stable.

• Fractures which are potentially life threatening include cranial fractures and spinal fractures.

• If the broken end of the bone is penetrating the skin the fracture is described as open. Compound open fractures should be treated as soon as possible as there is an increased risk of infection. If there are lots of pieces, the fracture is comminuted.

• Other fractures which require prompt treatment are fractures which involve a growth plate or a joint surface.

• Other fractures should be treated within 4 to 5 days of the injury.

• Symptoms of a fracture are usually very clear. There is marked pain, swelling and bruising over the fracture site; there is often deformity and instability of the affected area and crepitus can usually be palpated (crunching sensation on palpation due to the edges of the fracture scraping together).

• Sprains and dislocations can be mistaken for fractures.

- Radiography is required to identify bony injury.
- First-aid management of fractures includes providing pain relief and limiting further damage to the fracture site.
- Movement of a fracture causes intense pain. For this reason animals with suspected fractures should be moved with great care. If possible the fracture should be stabilised with a splint or bandage.

NB During first aid no attempt should be made to straighten a broken bone. The splint should conform to the shape of the fracture.

If the fracture is open care must be taken to avoid dislodging blood clots or touching the ends of the bones. Major blood loss can occur with long bone fractures. Fluid therapy may be required.

Spinal injuries

- If a spinal fracture is suspected immediate veterinary attention is required as prompt treatment can limit damage to the spinal cord.
- It is vital that there is no movement of the fracture site during transportation.
- A number of assistants may be required to move the patient taking care to maintain the alignment of the spine.
- The animal should be moved onto a stretcher or board. Cats can be placed in a rigid box.
- Blankets can be used to envelop the patient and restrict movement.
- If the animal is amenable it is possible to further restrict movement with the use of restraining ties.

2.4.34   Gastric dilatation and volvulus (GDV)

What you need to learn

- You need to be able to describe the signs of GDV in relation to the bloat-prone breeds. These are:
  - restlessness
  - discomfort
  - abdominal swelling
  - respiratory distress
  - collapse.
- Explain the emergency treatment of GDV:
  - passage of stomach tube
  - gastrocentesis.

Dilatation of the stomach

Dilatation of the stomach with or without a volvulus (torsion or twist) is a life-threatening condition which requires emergency treatment. The stomach becomes distended with food and gas. This affects blood flow by pressing on the vena cava. The dilated stomach can twist so that the outflow is occluded. More gas is produced. The animal very quickly becomes shocked and will die if the condition is not corrected surgically.

Symptoms include:

• unproductive retching (animal tries to vomit but is unable to because of the volvulus)
• bloated abdomen, (often feels like a balloon on palpation).
• restlessness and discomfort
• respiratory distress
• shock
• death.

Breeds which have a deep chest are most commonly affected because the stomach has more room to move (and therefore becomes twisted). Examples of commonly affected breeds are great Danes, wolfhounds, greyhounds, Dobermans, Weimaraners.

However, GDV can occur in any breed and does occur occasionally in cats.

Overfeeding followed by exercise is a common cause of GDV.

Emergency treatment

• First-aid treatment is aimed at reducing the pressure in the gas-filled stomach, and treating shock.
• Attempts should be made to pass a tube through the mouth into the stomach. If the stomach is not fully twisted the stomach tube will pass into the stomach and release some of the gas.
• If passage of a stomach tube is not possible the gas can be released by passing a wide-bore needle through the body wall into the distended stomach (gastrocentesis).
• Fluid therapy should begin as soon as possible. The animal will usually be in shock.
• Surgery to correct the disorder should then be performed as appropriate.

2.4.35 Emergencies occurring in elderly animals

What you need to learn

❧ You need to be able to describe disorders in the elderly that can give rise to an emergency situation requiring basic first aid:
❧ cardiac failure

* fits
* metabolic failure
* cerebrovascular accident (CVA).

Elderly animals are more prone to ill-health. First aid may be required in the following circumstances.

Cardiac failure

This is often but not always a chronic condition. First aid may involve CPR or providing comfort for the animal while medical treatment is administered.

Seizures

Seizures in elderly animals can be due to metabolic disorders, organ failure and neoplasia. First-aid treatment is as for seizures in younger animals.

Metabolic failure

Older animals are more likely to develop organ failure such as liver or kidney failure. First-aid treatment is usually the provision of supportive treatment while the investigation of the problem proceeds. The animal should be kept warm and quiet. Fluid therapy will usually be urgently required particularly if there is vomiting and diarrhoea.

Cerebrovascular accident (CVA, stroke)

A true stroke (rupture of a blood vessel in the brain) is an uncommon condition in the dog. The symptoms of vestibular syndrome are often described as a stroke by the owners.

Vestibular syndrome

This is often mistaken for a stroke. It occurs commonly in elderly animals. The condition results in disruption of the balancing mechanisms. Symptoms vary in severity and include head tilt, circling, ataxia, nystagmus (flicking of the eyes from side to side), and often nausea and vomiting.

The cause is often unknown (idiopathic) but can be related to inner-ear infection.

First-aid treatment involves settling the animal in a comfortable kennel so that injury due to falling is prevented. Owners are often extremely distressed. Reassurance should be given as the condition is not painful and animals usually recover without treatment.

2.4.36	**Haemorrhage**

What you need to learn

* You need to be able to differentiate between venous and arterial bleeding.
* Describe the basic methods of controlling haemorrhage and outline the risks associated with the use of tourniquets:
    * digital pressure
    * pressure pads and bandages
    * tourniquets.
* Describe sites of commonly used pressure points:
    * medial elbow (brachial artery)
    * inside thigh (femoral artery)
    * tail (coccygeal artery).

Blood loss

Haemorrhage (blood loss) can be caused by trauma, surgery, neoplasia and parasites. Blood loss from the gut (ulceration, neoplasia) or urogenital system (parturition, trauma) is not uncommon. Blood can be lost:

* **externally**: blood leaves the body through a wound or through the gut, urogenital tract or other body orifices)
* **internally**: blood is lost into body tissues and cavities, internal bleeding includes bruising, organ damage, and erosion of blood vessels by a tumour.

Blood can be lost from the following vessels.

Arteries (arterial bleeding)

This is the most serious and spectacular bleeding. Arterial blood is oxygenated (except in the pulmonary artery) and is pinker than venous blood. Arterial blood is often lost under pressure in a pulsatile fashion (blood spurts from the wound).

Bleeding from a major artery will rapidly cause hypovolaemic shock and death.

Veins (venous bleeding)

This is less serious than arterial bleeding as blood loss tends to be slower. Venous blood is deoxygenated (except in the pulmonary vein) and appears dark red in colour. Venous blood loss is rarely pulsatile. Blood loss from a large vein can cause hypovolemic shock and death.

Capillaries

This occurs in all wounds. Capillary blood oozes from numerous pinpoint sites in the wound. Capillary blood is rarely dangerous unless a clotting disorder is present. Blood loss usually comes from a mixture of arteries, veins and capillaries.

How to control haemorrhage

Digital pressure

Pressure is applied directly to the site of haemorrhage using clean fingers. This occludes the bleeding vessel and prevents further loss. This method is fast, easy and effective during first aid. It is only a temporary measure and is not used for longer term control of haemorrhage. Applying pressure for 5 minutes will give enough time for a clot to form in small damaged blood vessels.

Pressure pads or bandages

Absorbent padding is applied to the wound. This is then bandaged firmly in place. If blood seeps through, another bandage can be placed over the top (do not remove the padding). The whole limb will need to be bandaged if the haemorrhage is proximal. This is to prevent swelling of the distal limb. Pressure dressings can be used to control haemorrhage for longer than digital pressure.

Tourniquets

A tourniquet is a bandage or cuff tightly applied proximal to a wound. This occludes blood vessels and stops haemorrhage. Tourniquets should be used with great care because they can cause permanent damage to the nerves and blood vessels of the limb. A tourniquet should not be left in place for more than 3 or 4 minutes. Tourniquets are usually only used in limbs which are to be amputated, or distal to the carpus or tarsus (where there are fewer motor nerves).

Pressure points

Pressure points are sometimes used to reduce haemorrhage. A pressure point is the point where an artery courses over a bone and pressure can be applied to occlude the vessel. Pressing on a pressure point will prevent arterial bleeding distal to the pressure point.

Examples of pressure points are:

• brachial artery (medial elbow)
• femoral artery (medial (inside) thigh)
• coccygeal artery (underside of tail).

Minor haemorrhages can be stopped using coagulant agents. An example is the use of ferric chloride to treat a bleeding nail. Adrenaline causes constriction of blood vessels and so can be applied with care directly to a bleeding vessel. This aids in control of the haemorrhage. It should not be used in distal limbs as it can affect blood flow, causing necrosis.

2.4.37   Insect stings

What you need to learn

❧ You need to be able to describe the first-aid management of insect stings (wasps, bees).
❧ Explain what is meant by anaphylaxis and outline the management of this condition:
  ❧ adrenaline
  ❧ corticosteroids
  ❧ resuscitation.

First-aid treatment

Stings from wasps and bees are common in the summer months. Stings are rarely dangerous and can often be treated by the owner at home. Wasp stings are alkaline, so can be treated by applying a weakly acidic substance such as vinegar. Bee stings are acidic so can be treated by applying a weakly alkaline substance such as bicarbonate of soda.

Mild allergic reactions can be seen following a sting. Symptoms include swelling of the affected area (usually the face), prorates (itching) and raised skin lesions (urticaria). These cases resolve quickly on treatment with antihistamines or steroids. Severe allergic reaction occurs occasionally. This is called anaphylaxis and can be life threatening.

Symptoms include:

• severe swelling along with laryngeal swelling
• tachycardia
• respiratory distress
• shock.

First aid treatment can involve:

- oxygen supplementation to treat respiratory distress
- adrenaline or high doses of corticosteroids can be used to treat anaphylaxis
- CPR.

2.4.38 Emergencies occurring in obstetric situations and neonates

What you need to learn

- You need to be able to describe obstetric situations which require emergency intervention (dystocia).
- Outline potential neonatal emergencies:
  - apnoea
  - congenital abnormalities.
- Describe the first-aid management of a collapsed neonate:
  - resuscitation techniques
  - warmth
  - associated drug treatment
  - fluid therapy.

Dystocia

Dystocia is the term used to describe difficulty in parturition. It can be obstructive or non-obstructive.

Maternal dystocia

This is where the problem is caused by the mother (eg uterine inertia, small birth canal).

Foetal dystocia

This is where the problem is caused by the foetus (eg oversize).

Obstructive dystocia

- A puppy or kitten has become stuck in the birth canal (usually due to an oversized foetus or narrow birth canal).
- The dam will strain unproductively.
- If the pup or kitten can't be removed by careful traction a caesarian section will be necessary.

Non-obstructive dystocia

- The uterus is failing to contract strongly enough to expel the foetuses (known as primary uterine inertia).

- The symptoms can vary. Usually the owner will be concerned because the dam has entered the first stage of labour but has not progressed. There is sometimes a green discharge at the vulva indicating placental separation.
- Various treatments are used to encourage the uterus to contract.
- Caesarian section may be necessary if the foetuses become distressed.

Neonatal emergencies

- Lack of oxygen (hypoxia) is the main cause of death of neonates at birth.
- Apnoea (not breathing) occurs fairly commonly in neonates. Neonates therefore often require resuscitation, particularly after delivery by caesarian section.
- The neonates should be removed from the foetal membranes.
- Fluid from the nose and mouth should be cleared. Suction or gentle swinging with the head down can help.
- Respiration can be encouraged by gentle chest compressions.
- A respiratory stimulant such as doxapram may be administered (usually under the tongue).
- Artificial respiration can be performed by blowing gently into the mouth and nose of the neonate.
- External cardiac massage may be used if the heart is not beating.
- Once the neonates are breathing well they should be kept warm in a lined box until they are returned to the dam.
- The neonates should be examined carefully for congenital defects such as cleft palate, umbilical/inguinal hernias or obvious deformities.
- Fading puppy or kitten syndrome can result in high mortality rates. Signs of general weakness can appear within hours of birth. The animals are usually dehydrated and fail to suck. Treatment is unrewarding and the puppy or kitten usually dies. Possible causes are parvovirus infection, low birth weight, trauma during parturition, and congenital abnormalities.

First-aid treatment

First-aid treatment involves keeping the dam comfortable and quiet while the situation is assessed by a veterinary surgeon. Placing the animal in a dark kennel will reduce stress.

Older animals or those for which labour has been prolonged may require supportive treatment such as fluid therapy. If the foetuses have died there is a risk of infection and endotoxic shock, so the dam must be monitored carefully.

2.4.39 Poisons

What you need to learn

☙ You need to be able to explain what is meant by the term 'poison'.

☙ Describe principles of first-aid treatment for poisons that have been:
  ☙ ingested
  ☙ inhaled
  ☙ absorbed.

☙ Explain the service provided by the poison centre/bureau.

☙ Describe the general principles of collection and storage of samples if poisoning is suspected.

What is 'poison'?

A poison is a substance which when inhaled, ingested or absorbed into the body will cause adverse effects. Poisoning can happen with an accident, overdose (eg flea spray), allergic reactions, carelessness (leaving medication where a pet can find it) or ignorance (treating animals with human medication such as paracetamol). Malicious poisoning is extremely rare.

Poisons can be:

• **Medicines**: almost any medication taken at a high dose is toxic. Poisoning with ibuprofen and aspirin is commonly seen. Toxicity from illegal drugs such as marijuana (cannabis) is occasionally seen.
• **Pesticides**: weed killers, insecticides (including flea products), slug pellets and rodenticides (rat bait) are poisonous.
• **Foodstuffs**: raisins, chocolate, alcohol are toxic to some animals.
• **Household chemicals**: antifreeze, petrol and oil, cleaning fluids and wood treatments can be poisonous.
• **Plants**: poisonous plants include laburnum, foxglove, deadly nightshade and yew.
• **Bites**: bites from adders are occasionally seen.
• **Stings**: multiple wasp and bee stings can have toxic effects.

Obtaining an accurate history is vital in suspected cases of poisoning. Important questions are:

• What poison has been ingested?
• How much of the poison has been ingested?
• How long ago was the poison ingested?

Poisons can be inhaled (eg carbon monoxide), ingested (taken in through the mouth, the most common route), or absorbed across the skin and mucous membranes (stings, insecticides such as organophosphates).

First-aid treatment

First aid in poisoning aims to:

- **Remove the source of toxicity.** Poisons can be adherent to the coat. A collar which prevents licking should be applied, then the coat should be cleaned as soon as possible once the animal is stable.
- **Prevent further absorption of the ingested poison.** This often involves stimulating emesis (vomiting). Emetic substances (those used to induce emesis) include xylazine, apomorphine, washing soda crystals and ipecachuana syrup. Vomiting should not be induced if the poison is corrosive. Gastric contents remain in the stomach for approximately 4 hours so there is no point inducing emesis more than 4 hours after ingestion. Gastric lavage involves anaesthetising the patient and flushing the stomach with tepid water to remove all of the gastric contents. Adsorbents such as activated charcoal are used to bind to the toxin preventing absorption through the gut wall. Cathartics speed the elimination of unabsorbed poisons in the faeces. Examples are sorbitol and magnesium sulphate. These can cause dehydration and should be used with care.

Treat cases of poisoning with an antidote if one is available. Examples of antidotes are vitamin K (used to treat warfarin toxicity), naloxone (treats opiate toxicity), and antivenins (treats bites from poisonous snakes, spiders and fish).

Treatment of symptoms depends on the poison but usually involves supportive treatment such as fluid therapy. If convulsions occur these should be treated as described. Close monitoring is very important to assess deterioration or recovery.

The Veterinary Poisons Information Service (VPIS)

The Veterinary Poisons Information Service (VPIS) provides 24-hour information for veterinary surgeons. It can:

- supply data on the clinical effect of most poisons
- advise on antidotes
- advise on treatment methods.

Collection and storage of samples

When investigating the cause of a suspected poisoning, various samples can be collected and sent for laboratory analysis. Samples should always be collected aseptically to prevent contamination and erroneous results. Suspected poisons can be also toxic to the handler so precautions such as plastic gloves should be taken when obtaining samples.

Samples can be taken pre- or post-mortem:

• Whole blood should be sent in an EDTA or heparin tube (eg heavy metal toxicity).
• Plasma or serum should be sent in a clotting tube (eg chocolate toxicity).
• Brain, kidney and liver samples from a post-mortem should be frozen before transport to the lab.
• Stomach contents (or gastric lavage fluid) can be collected in a waterproof bag or vial. This can be frozen if necessary.
• Foodstuffs and water can be sent in a watertight container. These should be refrigerated or frozen.
• Environmental samples (bedding or soil samples) should also be collected if they are indicated in a poisoning case.

2.4.40   Organs of special sense

What you need to learn

☙ You need to be able to explain the principles of managing the common injuries which may occur to the organs of special sense:
  ☙ eye
  ☙ nose
  ☙ ear.

Emergencies involving the eye

Ophthalmic emergencies are rarely life threatening on their own. Emergency treatment is merited because they are often associated with severe pain, and vision can be lost unless prompt treatment is provided.

Ophthalmic emergencies include:

• glaucoma (raised intra-ocular pressure)
• proptosis (forward displacement of the globe)
• uveitis (inflammation of the uveal tract: iris, ciliary body and choroid)
• deep or melting corneal ulcers
• corneal lacerations, perforations and foreign bodies.

First-aid measures are limited and usually involve pain relief only until the veterinary surgeon attends. In cases of proptosis the globe should be regularly moistened with a lubricant to prevent desiccation while a treatment plan is formulated.

Emergencies involving the nose

First aid in cases where the nose has been injured involves maintenance of an airway and treatment of wounds. Inhalation of noxious fumes can damage the nasal cavity. Swelling of the lining can occlude the airways. Animals can usually breathe through the mouth but may require supplemental oxygen. Nasal foreign bodies should normally be removed by the veterinary surgeon.

Emergencies involving the ear

First aid in cases where the ear has been injured usually involves control of haemorrhage and treatment of wounds. Injuries to the pinna bleed profusely. Bleeding can be controlled by bandaging the ear to the head, taking care not to occlude the airways. Aural foreign bodies should normally be removed by the veterinary surgeon. Ruptured eardrums can be left to heal naturally providing there is no concurrent disease.

Vestibular syndrome

See page 353.

See page 353.

2.4.41   Seizures, fits and convulsions

What you need to learn

* You need to be able to describe the features of an epileptiform convulsion and outline the common causes of fits.
* Describe the first-aid management of a convulsing animal:
  * prevention of injury
  * quiet environment
  * sedation.
* Describe other causes of fits.

Seizures

Seizures result from disruption of the electrical activity in the brain. Epilepsy is the term used to describe recurrent seizures. Prolonged fitting known as status epilepticus is potentially life threatening.

Causes of seizures can be divided into:

• Seizures in the normal brain as a response to metabolic or toxic abnormalities: the disease is extracranial (outside the brain). Examples are hypoglycaemia, and circulating toxins due to liver or kidney failure.
• Seizures caused by disease of the structure of the brain: the disease is

intracranial (within the brain). Examples are brain tumours, trauma, inflammation of the brain (encephalitis) and hydrocephalus (build-up of CSF in the ventricles).
• Idiopathic epilepsy: in these cases the seizures result from a chemical imbalance in the brain. It is not associated with intra- or extracranial disease. Idiopathic epilepsy is not uncommon in dogs but very rare in the cat. The first seizure is usually seen when the animal is 1 to 4 years old. Seizures can be triggered by stress.

An epileptiform seizure can be divided into three phases:

• During the pre-ictal phase (a few minutes before the fit starts) the animal is often restless or excitable.
• During the vital phase of the seizure the animal usually loses consciousness for a variable period of time. There is often loss of continence. Paddling of the legs while recumbent and jerky movements usually occur.
• During the post-ictal phase (after the seizure) the animal is often disorientated and restless. The post-ictal phase usually lasts for a few hours but can be as long as a week.

Partial seizures can occur where the animal is unaware of its surroundings but does not lose consciousness. Twitching of part of the body may occur. Animals are completely normal in between seizures. Seizures often occur in clusters with an animal suffering a number of brief seizures of a period of a few hours.

• A thorough history should be obtained to identify possible causes of the seizure.
• First aid involves preventing injury to the animal and handlers during the fit.
• Medical treatment (anti-convulsants such as phenobarbitone and diazepam) will be given if the fit is prolonged (status epilepticus), or during a cluster of fits.
• The animal should be carefully moved away from objects which may cause injury.
• The room should be darkened and noise kept to a minimum.
• Make owners aware that an animal may bite during a seizure so it should be handled with great care.

2.4.42   Hypothermia and hyperthermia

What you need to learn

☘ You need to understand the different causes and possible conditions of hypo- and hyperthermia.
☘ State the first-aid treatment of hypo- and hyperthermia.

Hypothermia (abnormally low body temperature, usually following exposure to cold)

Causes of hypothermia include exposure to cold temperatures for prolonged periods; immersion in cold water; and in smaller animals, loss of heat because of a wet coat. Hypothermia can also result from prolonged anaesthesia. In advanced stages of disease the body temperature can start to fall.

First-aid treatment involves prevention of further heat loss and warming the animal slowly. Prevention of further heat loss can be achieved through:

- drying the coat thoroughly using towels or a warm (not hot) hair dryer
- wrapping the patient in bubble wrap or a heat-reflecting blanket.

Warming can be achieved using:

- heat pads and warmed wheat bags
- hot-water bottles
- warmed intravenous fluid.

The action of anaesthetic drugs should be reversed where possible (eg medetomidine can be reversed using atipamezole). The rectal temperature of the animal should be monitored until it returns to normal.

Hyperthermia (excessive rise in body temperature)

Animals lose heat in a variety of ways including sweating, panting and dilation of the skin blood vessels. Causes of hyperthermia include:

- overheating (eg in a car on a warm day)
- inability to dissipate heat (eg over-exercising on a warm day, or respiratory compromise).

Obese animals are more prone to hyperthermia as fat layers provide insulation – preventing heat loss. First-aid treatment involves removing the cause of hyperthermia (eg take the dog out of the car, cease exercise) and aiding heat loss.

Cooling can be achieved by:

- spraying or immersing the animal in cool water (not cold water as this causes constriction of skin blood vessels preventing heat loss)
- setting up an air flow using a fan or a draught to allow heat to dissipate through evaporation, this also eases respiration by providing plenty of fresh air

• cold intravenous fluids.

The temperature must be monitored until it is within one degree of normal.

With severe hyperthermia brain damage and even death can occur.

Multiple choice questions

1. An example of a disinfectant which is inactivated by organic material but will kill spores; will cause corrosion of instruments if undiluted and cannot be used as a skin antiseptic for dogs and cats would be:
   - ☐ A   isopropyl alcohol 70%
   - ☐ B   iodine
   - ☐ C   phenol
   - ☐ D   hypochlorite

2. Which of the following would be a normal parameter for an adult border collie bitch:
   - ☐ A   temperature 101.2°F
   - ☐ B   temperature 37.0°C
   - ☐ C   respiratory rate 35 breaths per minute
   - ☐ D   heart rate 200 beats per minute

3. Hypovolaemic shock may be indicated by:
   - ☐ A   an increased pulse rate
   - ☐ B   a pulse deficit
   - ☐ C   a weak 'thready' pulse
   - ☐ D   a strong, jerky pulse

4. Following reduction of a luxated hip, which of the following bandages could be applied?
   - ☐ A   Spica
   - ☐ B   Robert Jones
   - ☐ C   Ehmer sling
   - ☐ D   Velpeau sling

5. In relation to a cat's diet, which of the following is the least accurate?
   - ☐ A   the higher the biological value the more protein should be fed
   - ☐ B   taurine is an essential amino acid
   - ☐ C   arachidonic acid is derived from animal protein
   - ☐ D   taurine deficiency may lead to degeneration of the retina

6. When a particular drug potentiates the effect of another, this is known as:
   - ☐ A a reaction
   - ☐ B an interaction
   - ☐ C the half life
   - ☐ D the therapeutic effect

7. Opioid drugs are:
   - ☐ A anti inflammatory
   - ☐ B steroidal
   - ☐ C usually Schedule 2 controlled drugs
   - ☐ D cytotoxic

8. Drugs which selectively kill bacteria are known as:
   - ☐ A bacteriostatic
   - ☐ B fugicidal
   - ☐ C anaerobic
   - ☐ D bacteriocidal

9. A drug which is administered by the parenteral route:
   - ☐ A is painless and poorly absorbed
   - ☐ B is injectable and may have a direct effect
   - ☐ C has a poor systemic effect
   - ☐ D is topical with a direct action

10. An injection which is administered alongside the spinal cord is known as:
    - ☐ A intrathecal
    - ☐ B epidural
    - ☐ C sub-conjunctival
    - ☐ D intra-peritoneal

11. Which of the following emergencies could be the most life threatening, requiring immediate first aid and veterinary attention?
    - ☐ A hyperthermia
    - ☐ B prolapsed eye ball
    - ☐ C status epilepticus
    - ☐ D dystocia

12. According to the Veterinary Surgeons Act 1966, which of the following is the least accurate?
    - ☐ A an RTA involving a cat should be reported to the police
    - ☐ B a veterinary surgeon is obliged to give first aid to any injured animal
    - ☐ C anyone can perform first aid in the absence of a veterinary surgeon
    - ☐ D injured wild animals and stray dogs may have first aid administered by the RSPCA

13. Which of the following signs would indicate death?
    - ☐ A cyanotic mucous membranes, fast capillary refill time
    - ☐ B one pupil dilated, corneal reflex
    - ☐ C no cardiac output, pale mucous membranes
    - ☐ D apnoea, slow capillary refill time

14. Which type of shock may manifest itself if a patient had a severe inflammatory response to staphylococci infection?
    - ☐ A anaphylactic shock
    - ☐ B hypovolaemic shock
    - ☐ C cardiogenic shock
    - ☐ D endotoxic shock

15. If a dog was exhibiting signs of a distended fluid filled abdomen, cold extremities and pale mucous membranes you would be most likely to suspect:
    - ☐ A peritonitis
    - ☐ B ruptured liver or spleen
    - ☐ C herniation of gut contents
    - ☐ D gastric dilation volvulus

16. Immediate first aid treatment for a thermal burn would consist of:
    - ☐ A warming with a dry heat
    - ☐ B neutralising the substance
    - ☐ C application of a moist sterile dressing
    - ☐ D cooling with cold water

17. Vestibular syndrome:
    - ☐ A is a stroke common in older dogs
    - ☐ B is often idiopathic
    - ☐ C results in nystagmus and seizures
    - ☐ D occurs as a result of a cerebrovascular accident

18. The most suitable first aid treatment for a dog with haemorrhage to its right brachial artery would be to apply:
    - ☐ A pressure close to the jugular vein
    - ☐ B a tourniquet close to the base of the tail
    - ☐ C a pressure dressing to the hock and plantar region
    - ☐ D pressure medial to the elbow

19. A cathartic:
    - ☐ A may result in dehydration
    - ☐ B results in emesis
    - ☐ C may be used to treat rat poisoning
    - ☐ D will prevent absorption of a toxin from the intestines by binding the substance

20. The first priority when resuscitating a neonate should be:
  - ☐ A blowing gently close to the external nares
  - ☐ B swinging in an arc
  - ☐ C apply doxapram under the tongue
  - ☐ D remove the amniotic membrane

Level 2

Portfolio tips

Introduction

Your portfolio is a collection of evidence to demonstrate your practical competence and the standard that you have reached during your Veterinary Nursing (VN) NVQ training. It will provide an excellent training aid and may form the basis of your 'VN record of achievement'.

All NVQs require the completion of a portfolio that is appropriate to the level. There are actually five NVQ levels but veterinary nursing only involves Levels 2 and 3.

Even though VN students must also reach a successful outcome in the RCVS external examinations to achieve the NVQ certificate, they actually benefit more than most. The required format of the VN portfolio is authentically set out in the log sheets and most other important information and advice is given in the guidance notes for each portfolio module. This generally means that providing that the guidelines are rigidly adhered to and each log sheet block is completed as indicated, most of the important NVQ standards will be covered. The guidelines will give you all of the information that you need. If you are required to demonstrate three different species, then by obtaining three different cases you will have started to cover the scope as required by the standards.

It is important that when you start your training you begin to read and understand how to use the VN Objective Syllabus and the NVQ Occupational Standards. The syllabus will aid in how much you need to know about a particular subject and should be used in conjunction with your course provider (college) notes and as a study aid to prepare you for the RCVS external examinations.

Assessments and completion of log sheets can take place even if a particular subject has not been covered at college. Often most of the background knowledge required for a log will be familiar to you and relevant to normal work in veterinary practice. Subsequent logs and questions asked by your assessor at the completion of a module will then include your current academic knowledge.

All NVQ portfolios should show this natural progression. This means that it is not necessary for your early logs to be perfect.

Questions will be asked where some Performance Criteria (PC) or scope has not been met as satisfactory. Your assessor will include these on the actual log sheet. You are required to enter the answer in your own handwriting. An extra sheet of questions and your answers may also be included. Remember that this evidence should also state your name, enrolment number and be dated and signed by yourself and your assessor.

Occupational standards

What you need to know

- **The standards** are sectioned into Units (Level 2 has CU2, CU5 and VN 1 to 6 and Level 3 consists of VN 7 to 13).The 'CU' units are those that are common to all other NVQs, while the VN units relate directly to veterinary nursing.

  Each unit is then subdivided into elements that contain most of the detail.

- **The elements** relate to the modules of your portfolio and the introduction guidance notes at the beginning of each module list the units that are relevant. Each unit has an introduction explaining what it is all about.

- **Use the standards constantly** as a reference to help when deciding which case to choose, as a basis for ideas and as a checklist when writing a log. They must be used consistently by your assessor, especially when you will be observed and assessed for each case log. Write the case up within a week of your assessment stating on the log what you did and why. Use the PCs to help you do this.

- **The Performance Criteria** set out what you must do and how to perform a task. You will probably cover these in your day-to-day practical work without actually being aware of them. Each PC must be included in your evidence, but all of them will not necessarily appear in one log. A completed module must include them all and be relevant to the scope.

- **Knowledge and understanding** is the underpinning knowledge that is required to competently perform a particular task. This is also detailed in the syllabus.

  Be aware that including college timetables as evidence of subjects covered in college does not demonstrate your current knowledge. Your assessor, however, will need a copy of your timetable for planning your assessments.

- **The scope** gives the range (it used to be known as the range) of different circumstances necessary to display your competent practical skills. It should help you to decide on a particular case study.

All of the PCs in the element will apply to each individual scope. Including all of the PCs from only one scope will not be sufficient evidence. Each set must be included somewhere in the portfolio, not necessarily in one place or module.

For example, if you choose euthanasia as an assessment and log for Module 2c, you should study Unit VN5 to check on exactly what should be included. Element 5.1, the support of clients during provision of veterinary services, particularly applies to euthanasia, but only covers one part each of Part A and Part B of the scope. This means that the rest of the PCs for that scope must be covered elsewhere. The other elements (5.2, 5.3, 5.4) must also be covered. Element 5.2 states that you should advise clients on reproduction and neonatal care, and that this species should be different to the species you describe in relation to euthanasia.

All of this seems very daunting but it's not as complicated as it seems. Follow your assessor's advice and use the scope to check that everything listed has been included at some point in any log.

Your euthanasia Module 2c detailed client information log can include the possible situations and differences met when dealing with different species and different types of client.

Clients often ask for advice in relation to reproduction and the care of neonates. Your assessor can refer to your handling of these situations in Module 2a. This log is completed by your assessor and may be used to show a great many of the Unit 5 scopes.

- **The notes** show any special requirements for the assessment. They often relate to the suitability of submitting evidence produced from a simulation assessment.

Simulations are not ideal evidence but there are instances when they may be appropriate. Health and safety assessments are often suitable so that safety is not compromised and first-aid cases where a natural event may not arise can be used. Only a small number of simulations may be used at each level and both you and your assessor must indicate on the log sheet if a simulation was used.

RCVS annexes

What you must do

- **Photocopy** annexes when you first receive the portfolio, along with copies of the log sheets. Extra copies can be downloaded from the

RCVS website (www.rcvs.org.uk). Some of the actual master copies will continue for both Level 2 and 3 (annexes A, Ci and Ciii) but all of the others will need to be new sheets for Level 3.

• **Present** all of the annexes with any completed case logs at the time of any visit or interim submission.

• It is your responsibility to **keep all up-to-date.**

• **Annex A**
Complete this as soon as you receive the portfolio.

• **Annex B**
This is the **only** sheet that may be easier for you to complete as you finish Modules 1–5 or 6–11. It will, however, be necessary to submit a temporary contents page when your portfolio has an interim IV check.

• **Annex C**
Promptly record all absences from your Training Practice (TP) and ensure that the Practice Principal signs this record of your holidays or other absence, at the time. Academic training should be signed by your college course tutor following each term or residential block as appropriate. It is vital that the RCVS and your current and receiving Approved Centre (VNAC), are immediately informed of any change of circumstances.

• **Annex D**
Remember to ask all assessors and witnesses to sign the authentication sheet as you complete and they sign off each log. This is a safeguard just in case that particular person should leave the employment of the practice. Qualified and listed VNs and veterinary surgeons, other than your named assessor or mentor, can act as 'evidence gatherers' but they must then write, date and sign a 'witness statement'. This will be discussed with you at your weekly tutorial when that relevant log will be signed and dated by you and your assessor, and details of the witness observation are stated in the 'comments' boxes. Witness statements should be positioned in your portfolio following that particular case log.

• **Annex E**
Update weekly by yourself and your assessor at your tutorial planning session. This is really your assessor's responsibility and should be discussed with you. However you may need to 'chase them up' occasionally! Your portfolio is designed to be a working document and must be updated and reviewed regularly. The RCVS advises that your assessor plans and reviews your work on a weekly basis. Obviously in a busy practice there will be many missed opportunities and situations where planned evidence gathering and

assessments may need to be delayed; these can be indicated on the plan and action rescheduled for a later date.

With your assessor's approval institute a notice board in a prominent position in the practice that regularly informs other team members and your assessor of **what you need to do.**

Photocopy plenty of tracking sheets and use these for your own personal tracking as well as the smart 'official' version that will need to be checked and submitted. The Internal Verifier (IV) from your VNAC will tick off and date each module box when complete. You could tick off each box when a relevant log is complete or every time you work on a log. This will help you to track your progress and remind you of important little details such as vocabulary and phraseology to be included.

Case log format

What you need to do

- You may choose to **word process, type** or **handwrite** the case logs. Obviously if you are computer literate it is easier to amend or alter computer files before your assessor checks your work, and it is neater. Do not forget to back up and save!

 You may, however, still be required to handwrite any extra evidence and add this to your printed words. This is excellent valid proof of authenticity.

 Also expect the 'neatness' to be adulterated, by your assessor's 'scribbling' all over the log! This is standard practice to show the IV how well the assessor is judging your work.

- **Handwriting must be legible** and in blue or black pen. Pencil is unacceptable.

 Black ink photocopies better. Remember to photocopy all of your work, to guard against loss, before submitting the original for verification.

- Never use **correction fluid,** except to obliterate client details (for confidentiality). You can cross out with just a pen line through a word or phrase; it does not need signing at this point but your assessor may use the opportunity to state why a correction was made or the mistake could be mentioned by you in your comments box. It shows that you understand the error and the reasoning behind the correction. It also gives you something 'meaningful' to enter in the comments box! It is often a problem when trying to compose a relevant comment that has significance to the case yet has already been referred to.

- **The comments box** should include your reflection of the case. This could indicate other methods or ideas which may not have been used in that particular case but which you have read about or studied elsewhere. For example, there are a number of ways to bandage a tail tip. Provided that each method is functional, comfortable for the patient and looks professional, all would be acceptable.

For another entry it may be useful to include important details which did not seem suitable to enter in any of the other boxes. The details are, however, important to include to actually demonstrate some of the PCs not already covered.

Example: Log sheet 5b – Basic First Aid

Element VN 3.3 Administer emergency first aid to animals
PCs covered, just by comments: 4, 5, 8, 10

---

8   **Student's comments to include confirmation of your role and any additional detail not given previously:**

The owner was very worried about the apparent blood loss. This appeared to be worse than it actually was because the dog was continually shaking its head and blood was splattered in the owner's car and the waiting room. I am pleased that I was able to pacify and calm the owner by immediately assessing the situation and applying a bandage to control the haemorrhage. I checked that the client understood the possibility of a general anaesthetic to suture the wound and helped them to complete the consent form in readiness for the arrival of the vet. This also helped to reduce their anxiety.

- Use **bullet points,** provided that major points are clarified and descriptions are included. Bullets are much clearer and 'pointed' than long sentences and are easier for you to construct and the assessor and verifier to read.

- **Extend the blocks** on the log sheets as required or even use the back of the log sheet if further space is needed. An extra sheet may be used but make sure that it is set out with the appropriate headings and is signed and dated by yourself and your assessor and included on your contents sheet.

Generally the original size of the block is a good indication for the amount of detail required. Appendices can be used where detail is required.

- **Enter ALL case log boxes,** even Yes ☐ and No ☐. In some instances this may seem repetitive but will be relevant to that particular case and to ensuring that all of the standards have been covered.

The patient's weight and age must always be included. It is vital that you enter your name, RCVS enrolment number and signature on every single log.

Remember also that your portfolio is a working document so each log sheet will need to be presented to your assessor and signed by them shortly after completion (ideally within 1 week).

Your assessor must also complete all of their relevant boxes, including their comments box. Many assessors are often reluctant to do this!

- **Abbreviations** are acceptable but they must be accompanied by the full word with a brief explanation when each is used for the first time.

Example
'The VS (Veterinary Surgeon) advised that Billy was dispensed clindamycin which is a POM (Prescription Only Medicine) which can only be dispensed by a VS to animals under their care.'

You may find it easier to use an appendix for abbreviations but then the first time you use the abbreviation you would need to refer to the appendix.

- Similarly an appendix could be used for **clinical parameters** so that you don't need to keep stating what the norm is. These can include normal TPR for all common species. However in some instances where the clinical measurement is vastly different and relevant to the case then the normal should still be stated.

Example
'The dog's CRT > 2 s. The capillary refill time was greater than normal which should be less than 2 seconds. This may have been due to the haemorrhage and it was important that I monitored this about every 10–15 minutes in order to assess when his blood pressure was beginning to return to normal. To do this I pressed on the dog's gums with my index finger, released and then observed how long it took for the colour to return to the blanched area. Because the dog was unconscious this was the most suitable mucous membrane to observe'.

So on subsequent logs only the CRT needs to be mentioned

because you will already have met the standard required in the first instance.

Be aware that anything you mention **should be explained,** but may not need to be in great detail especially in Level 2. If you state that a patient was *'given a drip which was warmed up'*, then you must state what the drip was and how it was heated. Also include a brief explanation of the purpose of administering the drip. It is not important for great detail in this instance as Fluid Therapy is included in Level 3 work. At Level 3 you would be expected to explain the choice of the drip, calculate the rate of administration and explain the monitoring. This also applies particularly to anaesthetics.

In Level 3 detailed explanation is expected. For example Module 6a requires three tests to demonstrate knowledge of blood biochemistry. You must comment on the results and reasons for high and low results for every test included in the profile.

Always state the **dilution of disinfectants** and antiseptic solutions.

• Use **correct terminology**; although this not essential for the first logs progression must be seen. Initially you may want to include the basic meaning to show your knowledge.

Example
'emesis (vomiting)'

• **Correct spelling** is vitally important, particularly for veterinary terminology.

Use of **English language** should be correct. Poor use will be noted and commented on by your assessor/verifier. It is not always necessary that you rewrite logs correctly initially but you will be required to demonstrate considerable improvement by the last dated logs of Level 3. This demonstrates natural progression.

Inform your assessor initially if you do have a particular problem such as dyslexia, or you just find it difficult to express yourself in sentence form. They will make allowances for this. It may need to be reported on IV reports but this will be to your advantage and confidentiality will always be respected. Bullet points may be particularly useful here.

• Dose rate **calculations** must include 'mg per kg body weight'. Otherwise the calculation will be meaningless. Equations and all reckoning should be shown. In the case of topical medicines, a calculation may not be appropriate. In Modules 2b and 5c, note the strength/concentration of the drug and therefore a mention of the dose as appropriate, e.g. 'each application will contain approximately (**? number**) mg.

- Use **generic drug names** throughout. There are just a few exceptions to this rule, especially Module 2c when discussing information relayed to clients. Here the trade name will be required to be listed first, however even in this instance both names should be stated.

- Only include **extra evidence** if it can be directly attributable to you and is relevant to the case. Module guidelines state where extra evidence is required such as hospitalisation observation records (5a) and patient-monitoring records (9c). Again always remember the importance of confidentiality and obliterate all client details.

  Commercially produced leaflets, data sheets and other relevant notes such as the practice pre- and post-operative sheets will not enhance your evidence unless you clearly state the purpose of the inclusion and highlight the parts relevant to your assessment.

  Include any extra evidence following the particular log and remember to add a page number and adjust your contents sheet accordingly.

- **Appendices** can be the most useful way to show extra evidence and at the same time demonstrate the depth of your knowledge. They can be used to avoid the duplication of information, but should only be used for details that remain the same throughout, such as kennel accommodation, bedding and cleaning protocols (Module 5a) or basic preparation of an animal for surgery (Module 9c).

  Detailed descriptions of the type of kennels, size, materials, benefits and problems can be described and photos can even be included.

- The appendix must be signed and dated by yourself and the assessor and don't forget to include your RCVS enrolment number, which should be included in virtually every sheet of your portfolio.

- Appendices should be clearly cross referenced between case logs and additional information is included in that log box. It is not sufficient to just state '*ref Appendix 2*' without referring to which section of the Appendix applies and any other special details relevant to the case. For instance this information would be vital for Module 9c.

- **Cross-reference** wherever practical. For example, for Module 5a details of the medication and its method of administration can be cross referenced to Module 5c which deals solely with administration. This means that the same patient and all the relevant details can be used for both, saving you time and effort.

A Module 7a medical nursing case could be cross referenced to a 7b Fluid therapy case. Expanded details about the fluid can then be discussed in 7b and only needs to be referred to in Module 7a box 7.

The module guidelines indicate where cross referencing would be suitable, but your assessor will also help you to plan and decide on suitable cases at your tutorial sessions.

• Ensure that all **dates** are consistent, including those on the planning sheet (Annex F) and authentication sheet (Annex D) which should tally with a planned assessment/log sheet. Double check each date.

Whenever an IV visits your practice they will actually spot check individual clinical records to ensure authenticity and currency of case logs.

What to do if your assessor leaves the training practice

• **Don't panic.** There is usually another member of the practice team who is keen to begin assessor training.

• **Contact your IV** who can offer help and advice on any portfolio aspect. They may even be able to arrange for a qualified assessor to countersign some of your case log assessments witnessed by unqualified evidence gatherers.

Finally you should:

• Be guided by your assessor. It is often tempting to choose really exciting cases, but although they may be interesting and thought provoking, they may not include all of the evidence needed for the standards, and may not be suitable to cross reference.

• Be immensely proud of your portfolio! It is the perfect way to demonstrate your practical veterinary nursing skills and show your huge commitment to NVQ VN training achievement.

Margaret E Blezard
VN CertEd D Units 32,33,34,35

Calculations

The use of calculators is **not** permitted in the written RCVS examinations.

Try not to think of these calculations as mathematical problems but what you routinely perform on a daily basis when dispensing medicines and diluting solutions in practice.

What you need to learn

- Standard units of weight and volume.
- Calculating percentage solutions.
- Calculating drug dosages for injectable and oral administration.
- Dilution of concentrated stock solutions.
- Making up solutions.

Standard units of weight

The most common units of weight are:

milligram (mg) = 1000 µg (microgram)
gram (g) = 1000 mg
kilogram (kg) = 1000 g.

It is important that the dosage rate and weight of the patient are in the same units. If the weight of the patient is given in pounds (lb) but the dosage rate is given in mg/kg the weight of the patient must be converted to kilograms by dividing the weight of the patient in pounds by 2.2 (1 kg = 2.2 lb).

Standard units of volume

The most common units of volume are:

millilitres (ml)
litre (L) = 1000 ml
decilitre (dl) = 100 ml.

Percentage solutions

- A solution is a solid (solute) dissolved in a liquid (solvent).
- A percentage solution expresses the weight of solute relative to the volume of liquid. ie weight to volume (w/v).
- A 1% solution contains 1 g of solute dissolved in 100 ml of water.
- As 1 g is equivalent to 1000 mg a 1% solution contains 1000 mg of solute dissolved in 100 ml of water.

To make subsequent calculations quicker you can use this information in the following way.

In 100 ml of a 1% solution are 1000 mg of solute.

Therefore in 1 ml there are $\dfrac{1000}{100} \times 1 = 10$ mg

In other words a 1% solution contains 10 mg/ml.

To convert the concentration of a solution expressed in % into mg/ml simply multiply the % figure by 10.

Utilising this method a:

- 2% solution contains 20 mg/ml
- 5% solution contains 50 mg/ml
- 10 % solution contains 100 mg/ml.

Calculating drug dosages

It is vital that student veterinary nurses are aware of the importance of calculating the correct dosage of a drug to be administered to a patient.

Remember it can mean the difference between life and death!

Calculation protocol

- Work out the correct weight of the patient.
- Calculate the total dose using the weight of the patient and the correct dosage rate.
- Calculate the amount of the drug to be given to the patient. This would be the volume of an injectable drug or the number of tablets if the drug was to be administered orally.

Injectable drug calculations

You must remember the following:

Total dose required = dosage rate × weight of patient
Ensure the units are the same.

$$\text{Volume required} = \frac{\text{total dose required}}{\text{concentration of the drug (amount of drug/ml)}}$$

Example

A 10 kg dog requires 10 mg/kg of a drug. What volume of a 2% solution should be administered?

Substitute the values into the equations.

Dose required = dosage rate × weight of patient
$$= 10 \times 10 = 100 \text{ mg}$$

$$\text{Volume required} = \frac{\text{total dose required}}{\text{Concentration of the drug}}$$

Total dose is 100 mg. The concentration of the drug is 20 mg/ml as a 2% solution is being used. (See previous notes.)

Therefore the volume required is $\frac{100}{20} = 5$ ml

If the weight of the dog was given in pounds ie, 22 lb it would be necessary to first convert the weight into kilograms to enable the calculation to be completed: 22 ÷ 2.2 = 10 kg.

Oral drug calculations

You must remember as with injectable drug calculations:

Total dose required = dosage rate × weight of patient

Then number of tablets required $= \frac{\text{total dosage}}{\text{strength of the tablets}}$

Example

A 5 kg cat requires 10 mg/kg of a drug daily. How many 50 mg tablets should be dispensed for a 5-day course of treatment?

Total dose required = 10 × 5 = 50 mg

Tablets required $= \frac{50}{50} = 1$ tablet /day

For a 5-day course five tablets should be dispensed.

How much have you learnt?

1 How many milligrams equal a gram?

2 The number of millilitres in a litre is?

3 What is the conversion factor to change pounds to kilograms?

4 A 2.5% solution expressed in mg/ml is?

5 An 8% solution expressed in mg/ml is?

6 The number of millilitres in a decilitre is?

7 A solution containing 50 mg/ml expressed as a % is?

8 Calculate the volume of 1% Rapinovet (propofol) needed to induce a premedicated 4 kg cat if the dosage rate is 6 mg/kg.

9 Calculate the volume of a 5% antibiotic solution needed to treat a 20 kg dog if the dosage rate is 10 mg/kg.

10 Calculate the number of amoxycare 40 mg tablets required for a 4 kg cat if the dosage rate is 10 mg/kg administered for 7 days.

The answers can be found in this chapter.

Dilution of concentrated stock solutions

This is an important concept as solutions often have to be diluted in veterinary practice for various purposes including dilution of disinfectants according to the manufacturers instructions.

You must remember:

Amount of stock solution required = $\dfrac{\text{strength required}}{\text{stock strength}} \times$ total volume required

Example

Calculate the volume of pure Milton required to prepare 1 litre of a 5% solution.

A pure solution is a 100% solution.

Simply substitute the values in the equation.

Amount of Milton required = $\dfrac{5}{100} \times 1000 = 50$ ml

50 ml of Milton in 950 ml of water will give 1 litre of a 5% solution of Milton.

Making up solutions

Veterinary nursing students often have to make up solutions in practice.

Using previous knowledge 1 ml of a 1% solution contains 10 mg of solute.

Therefore 100 ml of a 1% solution will contain 100 mg of a solute. A litre (1000 ml) of a 1% solution will contain 1000 mg of solute.

Example

How many grams of solute are required to make up 500 ml of a 1% solution?

Each ml should contain 10 mg

Therefore 500 ml should contain 10 × 500 = 5000 mg

1000 mg = 1 g

Therefore 5000 mg = 50 g

Lorraine Allan
BVSc MRCVS PGCE

Multiple choice questions

1. The weight of a 44 lb dog in kilograms is:
   - ☐ A 20 kg
   - ☐ B 22 kg
   - ☐ C 40 kg
   - ☐ D 44 kg

2. A 2.5% solution contains:
   - ☐ A 0.25 mg/ml
   - ☐ B 2.5 mg/ml
   - ☐ C 25 mg/ml
   - ☐ D 250 mg/ml

3. The volume of 2.5% thiopentone needed to anaesthetise a 10 kg dog if the dosage rate is 25 mg/kg is:
   - ☐ A 2.5 ml
   - ☐ B 10 ml
   - ☐ C 12.5 ml
   - ☐ D 25 ml

4. The volume of 2% Rompun® needed to sedate a 5 kg cat if the dosage rate is 3 mg/kg is:
   - ☐ A 0.2 ml
   - ☐ B 0.25 ml
   - ☐ C 0.5 ml
   - ☐ D 0.75 ml

5. How much 10% amoxycillin injection should be administered to a 25 kg dog if the dosage rate is 5 mg/kg?
   - ☐ A 0.25 ml
   - ☐ B 1.25 ml
   - ☐ C 2.5 ml
   - ☐ D 12.5 ml

6. A 22 kg dog requires an antibiotic injection. The drug is contained in a 10% solution and the dosage rate is 5 mg/kg. The volume required is:
   - ☐ A 0.5 ml
   - ☐ B 2.5 ml
   - ☐ C 5 ml
   - ☐ D 10 ml

7. What volume of pure Savlon is needed to prepare 500 ml of a 5% solution?
   - ☐ A 1.25 ml
   - ☐ B 5 ml
   - ☐ C 10 ml
   - ☐ D 12.5 ml

8. How many prednisolone tablets (2.5 mg) should be dispensed for a 5 kg cat if the dosage rate is 0.25 mg/kg twice a day and the course of treatment is 5 days?
   - ☐ A 1 tablet
   - ☐ B 2.5 tablets
   - ☐ C 5 tablets
   - ☐ D 10 tablets

9. How many grams of sodium nitrate are needed to make 500 ml of a 5% solution?
   - ☐ A 15 g
   - ☐ B 20 g
   - ☐ C 25 g
   - ☐ D 50 g

10. How many Drontal Plus tablets should be dispensed for a 30 kg Labrador if the dosage rate is 1 tablet/22 lb body weight?
    - ☐ A 2
    - ☐ B 3
    - ☐ C 4
    - ☐ D 5

Level 2

Multiple choice answers

Unit 1: Health and safety

1. Answer: B
   Controlled drugs should be returned to the manufacturer or disposed of in 'special' clinical waste.

2. Answer: D
   The incident must be recorded but this is not the first priority.

3. Answer: C
   The Health and Safety at Work Act controls all aspects of providing a safe working environment.

4. Answer: C
   Rabies is a notifiable disease and suspect cases must be reported immediately to DEFRA.

5. Answer: B
   Thyroid shields are a type of protection from X-rays.

6. Answer: B
   Vectors are live carriers of infective agents.

7. Answer: C
   For electrical burns the first priority should always be to switch off the current.

8. Answer: C
   Personal safety is the first priority of any first-aid situation.

9. Answer: A
   Allowing fresh air into the room is essential but not until the cat has been confined.

10. Answer: A

Unit 2: Communication, record keeping and practice organisation

1. Answer: D.
   Non-verbal communication such as eye contact and posture may help but it is important to stay calm then call for extra help as necessary.

2. Answer: D
   After listening you should remain calm and try to deal with the problem promtly. No member of the team should ever be blamed.

3. Answer: B
   Reactions to grief and loss may occur at different stages but usually follow a particular sequence.

4. Answer: D
   Personal reflection with assessor support is essential.

5. Answer: B
   An organised system divided into specific areas.

6. Answer: B

7. Answer: C
   The neighbour can only be informed of client details if the owner has authorised permission in the presence of a witness.

8. Answer: B
   Clients have a right to request a second opinion.

9. Answer: C
   Libel is defamation by the written word, while objectivity and discretion refer to the discussion only of what is relevant to the case, whilst taking confidentiality into account.

10. Answer: C
    All employee details and client details are confidential under the Data Protection Act 1998. Specific insurance companies can be informed of their client's pet's booster records.

Unit 3: Anatomy and physiology

1. Answer: B
   Mitochondria are the 'power houses' of the cell. Enzymes located on the cristae of the mitochondria are involved in the production of adenosine triphosphate which acts as an energy store
   (A) Lysosomes contain hydrolytic enzymes which when released can lyse, destroy old or dying cells.
   (C) Ribosomes manufacture protein.
   (D) The golgi apparatus receives lipids and proteins from the endoplasmic reticulum packages then dispatches them to different sites both within and outside the cell.

2. Answer: C

It is important in wafting the ova along the oviduct towards the uterus. Peristalis of the smooth muscle in the wall of the oviduct also plays an important role. This type of epithelium is also found lining the epididymis which facilitates the movement of spermatozoa towards the vas deferens.

(A) The oesophagus is lined by non-keratinised stratified squamous epithelia which is protective in function.

(B) The trachea is lined with simple ciliated pseudostratified epithelia which is an important component of the mucocilary carpet which protects the lower respiratory tract.

(D) The bladder is lined with transitional epithelia which is capable of stretching as the bladder expands.

3. Answer: A

Neurones are the basic cells of the nervous system. There are different types unipolar, bipolar and multipolar.

(B) Nephrons are the functional units of the kidney.

(C) Neuroglia are the supportive and protective cells of the central nervous system.

(D) Neutrophils are granular white blood cells which are phagocytic.

4. Answer: B

The haploid number is half the normal chromosome complement of the cell (the diploid number). It occurs during meiotic division of the reproductive cells, ie the ova and sperms.

5. Answer: D

(A) lines the pleural cavity

(B) covers the abdominal organs

(C) covers the thoracic organs.

6. Answer: B

Examples of irregular bones are vertebrae, long bones are the femur and humerus and short bones are the carpals and tarsals.

7. Answer: A

(B) mesocephalic

(C) and (D) brachycephalic.

8. Answer: B

(A) os calcis: the Achilles/calcanean tendon inserts here

(C) scapular tuberosity is the origin of the biceps brachii

(D) tibial crest: the quadriceps femoris inserts here via the patellar ligament.

9. Answer: C

The gastrocnemius muscle has a reciprocal action on the stifle and hock.

10. Answer: C

The correct sequence outermost to innermost is dura, arachnoid then pia mater which is closely adherent to the brain and spinal cord. There is no such structure as the epidural mater. There is however the epidural space.

11. Answer: D

(A) the limbus is the region where the cornea and sclera meet
(B) the sclera is the outermost layer of the eye
(C) the choroid is the middle layer which is richly supplied with blood vessels.

12. Answer: B

(A) lymphocytes are responsible for antibody production
(C) platelets and clotting factors cause clotting
(D) neutrophils and monocytes are phagocytic.

13. Answer: D

Commonest types of leucocytes are neutrophils then lymphocytes, monocytes and eosinophils. Basophils are very rare in the dog and cat.

14. Answer: D

The right atrioventricular valve and the tricuspid valve are the same valve.
The left semilunar valve is the aortic valve.

15. Answer: A

(B) trypsinogen is involved in protein digestion but is produced by the pancreas before being released into the small intestine
(C) amylase is involved in carbohydrate digestion and is also produced by the pancreas
(D) lipase is involved in the digestion of fats.

16. Answer: C

Oxytocin is produced by the posterior pituitary and causes uterine contractions and the 'let down' of milk.

17. Answer: C

(A) the prescapular is found at the point of the shoulder.
(B) the axillary in the axilla of the foreleg
(C) the inguinal is found in the groin.

18. Answer: B

(A) tidal volume
(C) functional residual capacity
(D) residual volume.

19. Answer: C
    (A) the innermost layer of the uterus
    (B) the middle layer of the heart composed of cardiac muscle
    (D) part of the broad ligaments of the uterus, it suspends the uterus from the dorsal abdominal wall.

20. Answer: B
    Urea is produced by the liver and excreted by the kidney.

Unit 4: Principles of animal management and nursing

1. Answer: D
   Hypochlorite is a bleach.

2. Answer: A
   (B) subnormal
   (C) bradypnoea
   (D) tachycardia.

3. Answer: C

4. Answer: C
   Would support a hip joint following reduction or surgery.

5. Answer: A
   Less protein is required because more can be utilised by the body.

6. Answer: B
   Reaction relates to a patient's adverse reaction and the therapeutic effect is the intended effect of the drug.

7. Answer: C.
   Opioids include morphine and pethidine which are controlled by special Schedule 2 regulations.

8. Answer: D.
   -cidal refers to killing. A static will slow or prevent growth. Anaerobic affects bacteria which do not require oxygen for growth.

9. Answer: B.
   Parenteral describes an injected medication with a good systemic effect.

10. Answer: A.
    The intrathecal route is into subdural space (cerebrospinal fluid). Typically used for myelogram contrast media studies.

11. Answer: C
    Severe persistent fitting

12. Answer: A
    Cats are classed as wild animals and there is no legal obligation.

13. Answer: C
    (D) would indicate impending death

14. Answer: D
    A response to severe infection by bacteria

15. Answer: B
    All are signs of severe closed abdominal injury, resulting in internal haemorrhage.

16. Answer: D
    A thermal burn occurs due to the application of dry or moist heat

17. Answer: B
    Unknown cause which may result in nystagmus but not usually convulsions

18. Answer: D.

19. Answer: A
    Used occasionally when an animal has consumed a poisonous substance, to speed up elimination by the faeces. May result in other side effects.

20. Answer: D
    Then progress to clear the airway

Calculations

1. Answer: A
   1 kg = 2.2 lb
   $$\frac{44}{2.2} = 20 \text{ kg}$$

2. Answer: C
   A 1% solution contains 10 mg/ml
   Therefore a 2.5% solution contains $2.5 \times 10 = 25$ mg/ml

3. Answer: B
   Dose required = $25 \times 10 = 250$ mg
   2.5% thiopentone contains 25 mg/ml
   $$\text{Volume required} = \frac{250}{25} = 10 \text{ ml}$$

4. Answer: D
   Dose required = $3 \times 5 = 15$ mg
   2% Rompun contains 20 mg/ml
   $$\text{Volume required} = \frac{15}{20} = 0.75 \text{ ml}$$

5. Answer: B
   Dose required = 5 × 25 = 125 mg
   10% amoxycillin contains 100 mg/ml
   Volume required = $\dfrac{125}{100}$ = 1.25 ml

6. Answer: C
   First convert the weight of the dog to kg
   $\dfrac{22}{2.2}$ = 10 kg
   Dose required = 5 × 10 = 50 mg
   A 10 % solution contains 100 mg/ml
   Volume required = $\dfrac{50}{100}$ = 0.5 ml

7. Answer: D
   Amount of stock = $\dfrac{\text{strength required}}{\text{stock strength}}$ × total volume
   $\quad = \dfrac{2.5}{100}$ × 500
   $\quad = 12.5$ ml

8. Answer: C
   Dose required = 0.25 × 5 = 1.25 mg/dose
   $\qquad\qquad\qquad = 0.5$ a tablet
   Give twice a day for 5 days.
   0.5 × 2 × 5 = 5 tablets

9. Answer: C
   A 5% solution contains 50 mg/ml
   500 ml contains 50 × 500 = 25 000 mg 1000 mg = 1g
   25 000 mg = 25 gm

10. Answer: B
    Convert no of tablets/lb to no/kg.
    Weight of dog in kg = $\dfrac{22}{2.2}$ = 10 kg
    Dose required = 1 tablet/10 kg.
    Dog weighs 30 kg therefore needs 3 tablets.

Terms associated with digestion

Digestion

This is the breakdown of food into its component units so that it can be absorbed by the cells of the body.

Digestion starts in the stomach in dogs and cats and continues into the small intestine.

Deglutition

This is the process by which food/fluid is moved from the mouth into the lower oesophagus and stomach.

Deglutition is commonly known as swallowing.

Peristalsis

This is the rhythmical contraction of the smooth muscle layers in the gut wall which serves to push ingesta along the digestive tract.

Peristalsis moves ingesta distally from the mouth towards the anus.

Absorption

This is the uptake of the products of digestion into the cells of the body.

Catabolic reaction

A catabolic reaction is one in which a substance is broken down into smaller units.

Anabolic reaction

In an anabolic reaction smaller units are joined together to make larger molecules.

Basal Metabolic Rate (BMR)

This is the rate at which energy must be used to maintain the vital functions such as respiration, heartbeat, peristalsis and biosynthesis (construction of proteins and other molecules).

The BMR is high in young animals to allow for growth. BMR levels off in mature animals and then declines with old age.

Polymerisation

Polymerisation is the joining together of single molecular units (monomers) to create strings of units (polymers).

For example: The creation of polypeptides from amino acids is a polymerisation reaction with amino acids being the monomers and the polymer being the polypeptide.

Amino acid

Amino acids are the building blocks which make up proteins.

They are molecules which contain mainly carbon, hydrogen, oxygen and nitrogen.

There are 20 common amino acids. They join together in various combinations.

Amino acids are joined together by peptide bonds.

A short string of amino acids is called a polypeptide.

A protein is a longer string of amino acids joined with peptide bonds.

Peptide

Peptide bonds join amino acids together in polypeptides and proteins.

Polypeptide

A polypeptide is a short chain of amino acids joined by peptide bonds.

Protein

Proteins are long chains of amino acids. They perform many activities in the body.

Numerous substances and structures such as enzymes, antibodies, body tissues, haemoglobin to name just a few consist of proteins.

The three dimensional shape of a protein (ie how the chain of amino acids is folded) is important in determining its function.

Enzyme

An enzyme is a protein which acts as a biological catalyst. This means that it can speed up or slow down reactions within the body.

Enzymes are very specific so that one enzyme will only catalyse one specific reaction. For this reason many thousands of different enzymes are found within each cell.

Carbohydrate
A carbohydrate is a compound containing carbon (C), hydrogen (H) and oxygen (O), usually in the proportion 1:2:1.

Sugars and starches are carbohydrates.

An example of a carbohydrate is glucose which contains $C_6H_{12}O_6$.

Monosaccharide
A monosaccharide is an individual sugar molecule.

Glucose, galactose and fructose are examples of monosaccharides.

Disaccharide
A disaccharide is a pair of joined monosaccharides.

Examples of disaccharides are sucrose (made from one glucose molecule + one fructose molecule) and lactose (made from one glucose molecule + one galactose molecule).

Polysaccharide
A polysaccharide is a polymer consisting of a number of joined monosaccharide molecules.

Glycogen, cellulose and starches are examples of polysaccharides.

Glycogen is a polymer of glucose molecules. It is insoluble in water and so is useful for storing glucose within cells. Large stores of glycogen are found in the liver and muscles.

Fatty acid
Fats, or lipids consist of two components: fatty acids and glycerol. There are a number of different types of fatty acids.

Fats are insoluble in water and are used as storage molecules for energy.

Level 2

Index

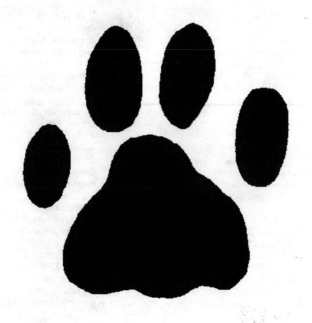

Good luck with your exams